Internal Medicine: Advanced Principles and Practice

Internal Medicine: Advanced Principles and Practice

Editor: Harriet Jacobs

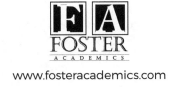

www.fosteracademics.com

www.fosteracademics.com

Cataloging-in-Publication Data

Internal medicine : advanced principles and practice / edited by Harriet Jacobs.
   p. cm.
Includes bibliographical references and index.
ISBN 978-1-63242-704-5
1. Internal medicine. 2. Medicine. I. Jacobs, Harriet.
RC46 .I58 2019
616--dc23

© Foster Academics, 2019

Foster Academics,
118-35 Queens Blvd., Suite 400,
Forest Hills, NY 11375, USA

ISBN 978-1-63242-704-5 (Hardback)

This book contains information obtained from authentic and highly regarded sources. Copyright for all individual chapters remain with the respective authors as indicated. All chapters are published with permission under the Creative Commons Attribution License or equivalent. A wide variety of references are listed. Permission and sources are indicated; for detailed attributions, please refer to the permissions page and list of contributors. Reasonable efforts have been made to publish reliable data and information, but the authors, editors and publisher cannot assume any responsibility for the validity of all materials or the consequences of their use.

Trademark Notice: Registered trademark of products or corporate names are used only for explanation and identification without intent to infringe.

Contents

Preface IX

Chapter 1 **Differences in the health transition patterns of migrants and non-migrants aged 50 and older** 1
Matias Reus-Pons, Clara H. Mulder, Eva U. B. Kibele and Fanny Janssen

Chapter 2 **A model of access combining triage with initial management reduced waiting time for community outpatient services: a stepped wedge cluster randomised controlled trial** 16
Katherine E. Harding, Sandra G. Leggat, Jennifer J. Watts, Bridie Kent, Luke Prendergast, Michelle Kotis, Mary O'Reilly, Leila Karimi, Annie K. Lewis, David A. Snowdon and Nicholas F. Taylor

Chapter 3 **Medications that reduce emergency hospital admissions** 26
Niklas Bobrovitz, Carl Heneghan, Igho Onakpoya, Benjamin Fletcher, Dylan Collins, Alice Tompson, Joseph Lee, David Nunan, Rebecca Fisher, Brittney Scott, Jack O'Sullivan, Oliver Van Hecke, Brian D. Nicholson, Sarah Stevens, Nia Roberts and Kamal R. Mahtani

Chapter 4 **Epidemiological and genomic determinants of tuberculosis outbreaks in First Nations communities** 40
Alexander Doroshenko, Caitlin S. Pepperell, Courtney Heffernan, Mary Lou Egedahl, Tatum D. Mortimer, Tracy M. Smith, Hailey E. Bussan, Gregory J. Tyrrell and Richard Long

Chapter 5 **Specific microRNA signatures in exosomes of triple-negative and HER2-positive breast cancer patients undergoing neoadjuvant therapy within the GeparSixto trial** 52
Ines Stevic, Volkmar Müller, Karsten Weber, Peter A. Fasching, Thomas Karn, Frederic Marmé, Christian Schem, Elmar Stickeler, Carsten Denkert, Marion van Mackelenbergh, Christoph Salat, Andreas Schneeweiss, Klaus Pantel, Sibylle Loibl, Michael Untch and Heidi Schwarzenbach

Chapter 6 **Healthcare costs and utilization associated with high-risk prescription opioid use** 68
Hsien-Yen Chang, Hadi Kharrazi, Dave Bodycombe, Jonathan P. Weiner and G. Caleb Alexander

Chapter 7 **Malaria elimination in remote communities requires integration of malaria control activities into general health care: an observational study and interrupted time series analysis** 79
Alistair R. D. McLean, Hla Phyo Wai, Aung Myat Thu, Zay Soe Khant, Chanida Indrasuta, Elizabeth A. Ashley, Thar Tun Kyaw, Nicholas P. J. Day, Arjen Dondorp, Nicholas J. White and Frank M. Smithuis

Chapter 8	**Quantifying the impact of social groups and vaccination on inequalities in infectious diseases using a mathematical Model**	89

James D. Munday, Albert Jan van Hoek, W. John Edmunds and Katherine E. Atkins

Chapter 9	**Vaccination with chemically attenuated *Plasmodium falciparum* asexual blood-stage parasites induces parasite-specific cellular immune responses in malaria-naïve Volunteers**	101

Danielle I. Stanisic, James Fink, Johanna Mayer, Sarah Coghill, Letitia Gore, Xue Q. Liu, Ibrahim El-Deeb, Ingrid B. Rodriguez, Jessica Powell, Nicole M. Willemsen, Sai Lata De, Mei-Fong Ho, Stephen L. Hoffman, John Gerrard and Michael F. Good

Chapter 10	**Breaking bread: examining the impact of policy changes in access to state-funded provisions of gluten-free foods**	117

Myles-Jay Linton, Tim Jones, Amanda Owen-Smith, Rupert A. Payne, Joanna Coast, Joel Glynn and William Hollingworth

Chapter 11	**Pretreatment chest x-ray severity and its relation to bacterial burden in smear positive pulmonary tuberculosis**	125

S. E. Murthy, F. Chatterjee, A. Crook, R. Dawson, C. Mendel, M. E. Murphy, S. R. Murray, A. J. Nunn, P. P. J. Phillips, Kasha P. Singh, T. D. McHugh and S. H. Gillespie

Chapter 12	**Complex interactions between malaria and malnutrition**	136

D Das, R F Grais, E A Okiro, K Stepniewska, R Mansoor, S van der Kam, D J Terlouw, J Tarning, K I Barnes and P J Guerin

Chapter 13	**How are health-related behaviours influenced by a diagnosis of pre-diabetes?**	150

Eleanor Barry, Trisha Greenhalgh and Nicholas Fahy

Chapter 14	**Trends in, and factors associated with, HIV infection amongst tuberculosis patients in the era of anti-retroviral therapy**	167

Joanne R. Winter, Helen R. Stagg, Colette J. Smith, Maeve K. Lalor, Jennifer A. Davidson, Alison E. Brown, James Brown, Dominik Zenner, Marc Lipman, Anton Pozniak, Ibrahim Abubakar and Valerie Delpech

Chapter 15	**Participatory design of an improvement intervention for the primary care management of possible sepsis using the Functional Resonance Analysis Method**	179

Duncan McNab, John Freestone, Chris Black, Andrew Carson-Stevens and Paul Bowie

Chapter 16	**Avoidable waste of research related to outcome planning and reporting in clinical trials**	198

Youri Yordanov, Agnes Dechartres, Ignacio Atal, Viet-Thi Tran, Isabelle Boutron, Perrine Crequit and Philippe Ravaud

Chapter 17	**Thresholds of socio-economic and environmental conditions necessary to escape from childhood malnutrition: a natural experiment in rural Gambia**	209

Mayya Husseini, Momodou K Darboe, Sophie E Moore, Helen M Nabwera and Andrew M Prentice

Chapter 18 **Determinants of the urinary and serum metabolome in children from
six European Populations** 218
Chung-Ho E. Lau, Alexandros P. Siskos, Léa Maitre, Oliver Robinson,
Toby J. Athersuch, Elizabeth J. Want, Jose Urquiza, Maribel Casas, Marina Vafeiadi,
Theano Roumeliotaki, Rosemary R. C. McEachan, Rafaq Azad, Line S. Haug,
Helle M. Meltzer, Sandra Andrusaityte, Inga Petraviciene, Regina Grazuleviciene,
Cathrine Thomsen, John Wright, Remy Slama, Leda Chatzi, Martine Vrijheid,
Hector C. Keun and Muireann Coen

Chapter 19 **Quantifying the risk of local Zika virus transmission in the contiguous US
during the 2015–2016 ZIKV epidemic** 236
Kaiyuan Sun, Qian Zhang, Ana Pastore-Piontti, Matteo Chinazzi, Dina Mistry,
Natalie E Dean, Diana Patricia Rojas, Stefano Merler, Piero Poletti, Luca Rossi,
M Elizabeth Halloran, Ira M Longini Jr and Alessandro Vespignani

Permissions

List of Contributors

Index

Preface

This book aims to highlight the current researches and provides a platform to further the scope of innovations in this area. This book is a product of the combined efforts of many researchers and scientists, after going through thorough studies and analysis from different parts of the world. The objective of this book is to provide the readers with the latest information of the field.

Internal medicine is a medical specialty, which deals with the diagnosis, prevention and treatment of diseases in adults. Specialists in this field are involved in the management of complex multisystem disease conditions, such as weight loss, chest pain, dyspnoea, fatigue, etc. as well as multiple chronic diseases or comorbidities. Some of the subspecialties in this field are allergy, asthma and immunology, endocrinology, hematology, gastroenterology, rheumatology, etc. This book is compiled in such a manner, that it will provide in-depth knowledge about the current practices and procedures of internal medicine. The aim of this book is to present the new researches that have transformed this discipline and aided its advancement. It is a vital tool for all researching or studying internal medicine as it gives incredible insights into emerging trends and concepts.

I would like to express my sincere thanks to the authors for their dedicated efforts in the completion of this book. I acknowledge the efforts of the publisher for providing constant support. Lastly, I would like to thank my family for their support in all academic endeavors.

Editor

Differences in the health transition patterns of migrants and non-migrants aged 50 and older in southern and western Europe (2004–2015)

Matias Reus-Pons[1,2], Clara H. Mulder[1*], Eva U. B. Kibele[3] and Fanny Janssen[1,4]

Abstract

Background: Most previous research on migrant health in Europe has taken a cross-sectional perspective, without a specific focus on the older population. Having knowledge about inequalities in health transitions over the life course between migrants and non-migrants, including at older ages, is crucial for the tailoring of policies to the demands of an ageing and culturally diverse society. We analyse differences in health transitions between migrants and non-migrants, specifically focusing on the older population in Europe.

Methods: We used longitudinal data on migrants and non-migrants aged 50 and older in 10 southern and western European countries from the Survey of Health, Ageing and Retirement in Europe (2004–2015). We applied multinomial logistic regression models of experiencing health deterioration among individuals in good health at baseline, and of experiencing health improvement among individuals in poor health at baseline, separately by sex, in which migrant status (non-migrant, western migrant, non-western migrant) was the main explanatory variable. We considered three dimensions of health, namely self-rated health, depression and diabetes.

Results: At older ages, migrants in Europe were at higher risk than non-migrants of experiencing a deterioration in health relative to remaining in a given state of self-rated health. Western migrants had a higher risk than non-migrants of becoming depressed, while non-western migrants had a higher risk of acquiring diabetes. Among females only, migrants also tended to be at lower risk than non-migrants of experiencing an improvement in both overall and mental health. Differences in the health transition patterns of older migrants and non-migrants remained robust to the inclusion of several covariates, including education, job status and health-related behaviours.

Conclusions: Our findings indicate that, in addition to having a health disadvantage at baseline, older migrants in Europe were more likely than older non-migrants to have experienced a deterioration in health over the study period. These results raise concerns about whether migrants in Europe are as likely as non-migrants to age in good health. We recommend that policies aiming to promote healthy ageing specifically address the health needs of the migrant population, thereby distinguishing migrants from different backgrounds.

Keywords: Health transitions, Migration, Ageing, Europe

---

* Correspondence: c.h.mulder@rug.nl
[1]Population Research Centre, Faculty of Spatial Sciences, University of Groningen, Groningen, The Netherlands
Full list of author information is available at the end of the article

Background

As European societies become older and more diverse [1], the study of the health of older migrants in Europe is becoming increasingly relevant. Having detailed knowledge on how health transitions differ between migrants and non-migrants over the life course is crucial in assessing the future healthcare demands of a society that is becoming older and more culturally diverse [2]. Having such knowledge is also helpful for policymakers who are attempting to adapt their interventions to achieve health equity, which is one of the main pillars of European healthcare systems and policies [3].

Most of the previous research on older migrants' health in Europe has taken a cross-sectional perspective. These studies showed that, regardless of a generally lower socioeconomic status, migrants tend to live longer than non-migrants; this so-called 'migrant mortality paradox' has been observed across the life course, including at older ages [4, 5]. However, previous research has also acknowledged that, compared to non-migrants, older migrants in Europe can expect to live a smaller number of years and a smaller share of their remaining life expectancy in good health [6]. Indeed, compared to older non-migrants, older migrants in Europe tend to have poorer self-rated health, more chronic conditions, worse functioning and higher rates of depression [4, 6–9]. Longitudinal studies can provide a more complete picture than cross-sectional studies of how health and health inequalities evolve over the life course of individuals, and can provide valuable information about the causes of such inequalities.

Several studies have investigated the health differences between migrants and non-migrants in a longitudinal manner [10–16]. These studies have found that migrants, who often have a health advantage relative to non-migrants at arrival, tend to experience steeper rates of health decline with age and length of stay; thus, the health status of migrants tends to converge with that of non-migrants. However, only two of these previous studies specifically focused on the older population [14, 16]. A specific focus on the older population is essential for gaining a better understanding of healthy ageing in a multicultural context, the implications of which vary from maintaining the ability to work at older working ages, which is in itself a protective health factor, to increased quality of life and the possibility to live independently at advanced ages [17].

Furthermore, all of the abovementioned studies examining how the health transitions of migrants and non-migrants differ have been focused on the United States of America (USA) or Canada; yet, whether their findings are also valid in a European context remains unclear. A majority of the older migrants who currently live in western Europe arrived before the early 1970s as labour migrants, or from neighbouring countries or former colonies [1]. We know that many years after migration, older migrants in Europe tend to be disadvantaged relative to non-migrants in terms of self-rated health, chronic conditions, functioning, limitations and depression [4, 6–9]. This is an important difference with respect to the USA and Canada, where older migrants have been shown to have an overall health advantage relative to non-migrants at baseline [14, 16]. On the one hand, this implies that, in Europe, the migrant health advantage at the time of arrival disappears by the time migrants have reached age 50. On the other hand, if migrants in Europe were to maintain steeper rates of health decline than non-migrants at older ages, this would inevitably lead to an increase of migrant health inequalities.

To our knowledge, only a single study so far has described how the health transition patterns of older migrants and non-migrants in Europe differ [18], focusing on the extent to which these two groups maintained good health and experienced health recovery. The authors found that, as compared to non-migrants, older migrants had a lower probability to remain in good health, and a lower probability to experience an improvement in health. However, their paper did not consider other health variables besides self-rated health, and they did not attempt to explain the differences in health transitions between older migrants and non-migrants based on their demographic, socioeconomic or lifestyle-related characteristics.

Moreover, previous studies on the differences in the health transition patterns of older migrants and non-migrants either did not distinguish migrants according to their place of origin [16], or focused on very specific origin groups, such as Hispanic [14] or eastern European [18]. The specific origin of migrants is likely to play an important role in determining differences in health transitions relative to non-migrants. For example, the health status of migrants at the time of arrival is determined to a large extent by the physical, socioeconomic and political environment of their country or area of origin [19]. In addition, the context of origin may affect migrant health transition patterns at older ages, since specific diseases that tend to develop later in life, such as stomach cancer, may be associated with deprivation during childhood [19].

The aim of the present longitudinal study is to analyse the differences in the health transition patterns of migrants and non-migrants, specifically focusing on the older population in Europe, and to illustrate how a range of individual health determinants contribute to explaining these differences in health transition patterns. In our analysis, we incorporate three dimensions of health, namely a subjective measure of overall health (self-rated health), a measure of mental health (depression) and a measure of physical health (diabetes). As in previous migrant health research [6, 20–23], we also distinguish between western and non-western migrants.

Methods
Setting
Our study population consisted of individuals aged 50 and older who participated in the Survey of Health, Ageing and Retirement in Europe (SHARE). Research on individuals aged 50 and older is common in the literature on health at older ages [4–9, 14], and starting from this relatively young age enabled us to study not only health deterioration but also health improvement (which is less common at more advanced ages).

Since 2004, SHARE has been collecting panel data on the health status, the socioeconomic status and the social networks of older individuals in European countries and Israel [24]. For our analysis, we selected data from countries in western and southern Europe only, namely Austria, Belgium, Denmark, France, Germany, Italy, the Netherlands, Spain, Sweden and Switzerland. We excluded eastern European countries because they have very different migration histories than western European countries, with most remaining mainly emigration countries [25]. We used data from waves 1 (2004–2005), 2 (2006–2007), 4 (2011–2012), 5 (2013) and 6 (2015) [26–30]. At each wave, refreshment samples were drawn to increase the sample size and to compensate for panel attrition [24]. We included respondents in wave 1 and in the successive refreshment samples for whom health data were available for at least two waves. Data from wave 6 were not available for the Netherlands, leading to a greater proportion of transitions ending in attrition for this country. Results from a sensitivity analysis excluding the Netherlands from the data remained in the same direction, although occasionally an effect lost statistical significance.

Dependent variable
We defined health transitions (see analysis below), our dependent variable, based on health status at baseline and follow-up. Although self-rated health is often dichotomised into good or more and less-than-good (e.g. [10]), this might conceal certain transition patterns to and from fair health. A recent study showed that the variations in self-rated health response patterns are not strongly related to migrant origin, but rather to the survey language [31]. SHARE questionnaires are provided in the national languages only, which helps reduce the potential variability in the response patterns of migrants versus non-migrants within each country. However, the likelihood of assessing one's health in a certain way might differ between countries, especially because the term 'fair' has distinct connotations in different languages [31]. Moreover, although the validity of self-rated health is well documented in cross-sectional research, reported changes in self-rated health over time might be caused by changes in expectations or in the awareness of health problems [32]. We therefore considered an additional measure of mental health (depression), and an additional measure of physical health (diabetes).

Answers to the question: "Would you say your health is…?" (originally in five categories) were recoded into three categories, i.e. as indicating good (excellent, very good or good), fair or poor self-rated health. Depression was measured using the EURO-D scale [33], which consists of 12 items, namely depression, pessimism, death wish, guilt, sleep, interest, irritability, appetite, fatigue, concentration, enjoyment and tearfulness. Individuals with a EURO-D scale score of more than three were classified as suffering from depression [34]. Respondents who answered "yes" to the question: "Has a doctor ever told you that you had any diabetes or high blood sugar?" were considered to have diabetes.

We converted the data into a person-wave format, allowing as many person-wave observations (health status at baseline combined with health status at follow-up) as possible per respondent. In order to minimise the number of observations ending in loss to follow-up, we also included observations from non-consecutive waves when health information was missing in intermediate waves. Observations from non-consecutive waves represented 3–5% of all observations among non-migrants, western migrants and non-western migrants, and occurred more often among younger, less educated and non-retired respondents. We took into account the differential time of exposure in different transitions by including the pairs of waves as a control variable (see below).

The analytical sample for the analysis of self-rated health consisted of 66,660 respondents who contributed 127,136 person-wave observations. Of these, 116,537 corresponded to non-migrants, 7854 to western migrants and 2745 to non-western migrants. Because a given respondent may provide an answer to one health question but not to another, the samples for analysing depression ($n = 124{,}167$) and diabetes ($n = 127{,}042$) were slightly different.

Independent variables
We defined migrants, our main independent variable, as those respondents who were not born in their current country of residence. As in previous migrant health research [6, 20–23], we distinguished between migrants with a western or non-western origin. We defined western migrants as those born in Europe (except Turkey), North America, Oceania or Japan [6, 23]. Data restrictions did not allow us to distinguish more specific categories of migrant origins, nor motives for migration. The distinction between western and non-western

migrants allowed us to account for the role of the context of origin. The environmental, socioeconomic and political context in the country of origin of migrants has an important role in determining their baseline health status and this is especially relevant when the countries involved can be positioned in different stages of the epidemiologic transition [19]. Moreover, the culture and behaviours of non-European migrants are more distant from those of the host society [35]. The vast majority of western migrants in our data (98%) were of European origin. The majority of non-western migrants had been born in one of the following five countries, namely Morocco, Algeria, Turkey, Indonesia and Congo.

We included age to adjust for different age structures in the migrant and non-migrant populations, and country of residence and wave to adjust for contextual differences across space and time. We additionally adjusted for other factors known to be related to health. Being married or partnered is associated with better health outcomes [36]. Poor socioeconomic status is strongly associated with both poor physical and poor mental health outcomes [32, 37, 38]. While job status captures an individual's current socioeconomic status, level of education also partially reflects socioeconomic position during childhood and youth [39]. Health-related behaviours, and particularly body mass index (BMI), exercise habits and smoking history, are all strongly associated with health outcomes [40].

All covariates, except for an indicator for the pair of waves to which the observation pertained, were measured at the initial wave of each observation (baseline), namely age, country of residence and length of residence in that country, marital status, socioeconomic status (education, job status) and health-related behaviours (BMI, smoking, physical activity). Age was recoded into 5-year age groups up to 85+. Length of residence (up to 10 years and 10 years or longer) was derived from the year of migration and the year when the interview took place; this distinction was also used in a previous study [23] to demonstrate that the initial healthy migrant effect wears off with increasing length of stay, effectively finding differences in the health status of migrants relative to non-migrants according to the length of residence in the country. Distinguishing shorter periods was not feasible because 94% of older migrants in our data had been living in the countries of destination for more than 10 years. We coded marital status into four categories as married[1] (consisting of the categories "married and living together with spouse" and "registered partnership"), separated (consisting of the categories "married and living separated from spouse" and "divorced"), single ("never married") and widowed. International Standard Classification of Education 1997 codes of highest level of education were recoded into four categories as primary education or lower (codes 0 and 1),

secondary education (codes 2 and 3), higher education (codes 4, 5 and 6), and other (consisting of the categories "still in education" and "other"). Current job status was recoded into four categories as retired, economically active ("employed" or "self-employed"), unemployed or economically inactive ("unemployed", "permanently sick or disabled" or "homemaker") and other. We used the original BMI coding of underweight (< 18.5), normal weight (18.5–24.9), overweight (25–29.9) and obese (> 30). We also maintained the dichotomous coding for ever having smoked (yes/no), and the four categories indicating how frequently the respondent engaged in either vigorous or moderate activities as more than once a week, once a week, one to three times a month, and hardly ever or never. In SHARE, vigorous activities are defined as sports, heavy housework and physically demanding jobs, while moderate activities include less demanding forms of exercise such as gardening, cleaning the car or going for a walk.

Statistical analysis

We performed two-sided tests to assess whether the differences in the background characteristics and the health status at baseline between older migrants (western and non-western) and non-migrants were statistically significant.

We applied multinomial logistic regression models separately by sex. While other methods, such as ordered logistic regression models, would have allowed to retain the original five-category self-rated health variable, such methods would not allow distinguishing health deterioration from health improvement. More importantly, we would have to exclude observations ending in attrition, which would potentially bias our findings.

We ran separate models for transitions starting in good, fair and poor self-rated health, since the possible health transitions were restricted by the health status at baseline. Compared to the reference category (remaining in the same health status), those initially in good health could experience transitions leading to health deterioration (to fair health or to poor health) or to attrition (either to death or to loss to follow-up). Those initially in fair health could experience health improvement (to good health), health deterioration (to poor health) or be lost to attrition. Those initially in poor health could experience health improvement (to fair health or to good health) or be lost to attrition (Fig. 1).

Similarly, we ran separate models for those transitions starting in a non-depressed state, and for those transitions starting in a depressed state. Compared to remaining non-depressed, the possible transitions were experiencing health deterioration (becoming depressed), and being lost to attrition. Likewise, compared to remaining depressed, the possible transitions were experiencing health improvement (recovering from depression) and being lost to attrition.

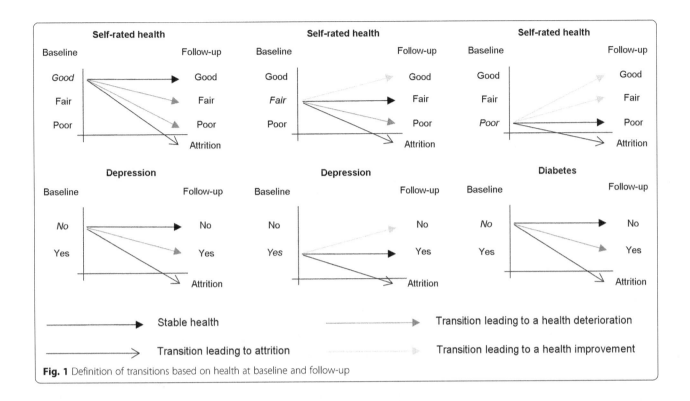

Fig. 1 Definition of transitions based on health at baseline and follow-up

For diabetes, we only considered transitions starting in a healthy state (non-diabetic), because recovery is unlikely, although healthier lifestyles have been shown to mitigate its negative effects on health (e.g. [41]). Compared to remaining in a healthy state (non-diabetic), the possible transitions were experiencing health deterioration (becoming diabetic) and being lost to attrition.

Unfortunately, the data did not allow us to differentiate transitions leading to death from those leading to loss to follow-up. However, we modelled transitions leading to attrition (either death or loss to follow-up) as a competing risk in each of the analyses. This is important because, unfortunately, attrition cannot be seen as random since death is obviously a health outcome and loss to follow-up may also be related to health problems.

We estimated robust standard errors [42, 43] to take into account the fact that the same respondent may be observed several times (transition or no transition). Models were run in three steps. In step 1, we included migrant origin (non-migrant, western migrant or non-western migrant) and controlled for age, country of residence and wave. In step 2, we additionally controlled for each respondent's length of residence in the country, marital status, highest level of education attained and current job status. Finally, in step 3, we additionally controlled for BMI, having ever smoked and frequency of engaging in vigorous and moderate activities.

Results

Descriptive findings

Table 1 shows the absolute and the relative distributions of the person-wave observations according to individual characteristics at baseline by migrant origin, for the sample used in the analysis of self-rated health deriving from data on older respondents (aged 50 and older) in 10 southern and western European countries in SHARE (2004–2015). Compared to non-migrants, the proportion of males was lower among western migrants, but higher among non-western migrants. While western migrants had a similar age profile to that of non-migrants, non-western migrants tended to be younger. The vast majority of migrants had been living in the current country of residence for more than 10 years. Compared to non-migrants, all migrants were more likely to be separated and less likely to be married, non-western migrants were less likely to be widowed and western migrants were less likely to be single. While larger shares of both western and non-western migrants than of non-migrants were highly educated, the share of non-western migrants with primary education or lower was also larger. In line with their younger age structure, non-western migrants were less likely than non-migrants to be retired, and more likely to be economically active, unemployed or economically inactive, whereas the job status profile of western migrants was very similar to that of non-migrants. Non-western migrants were less likely than both non-migrants and western migrants to report

Table 1 Person-wave observations[a] according to individual characteristics at baseline by migrant origin (2004–2015)

	Non-migrants		Western migrants		Non-western migrants	
	N	%	N	%	N	%
Sex						
Male	53,353	45.8	3267*	42.8*	1482*	50.0*
Female	63,184	54.2	4370*	57.2*	1480*	50.0*
Age, years						
50–54	24,258	20.8	1590	20.8	1052*	35.5*
55–59	22,012	18.9	1336*	17.5*	635*	21.4*
60–64	20,125	17.3	1344	17.6	465	15.7
65–69	16,994	14.6	1202*	15.7*	345*	11.6*
70–74	13,860	11.9	911	11.9	223*	7.5*
75–79	10,070	8.6	655	8.6	137*	4.6*
80–84	5875	5.0	409	5.4	75*	2.5*
85+	3343	2.9	190	2.5	30*	1.0*
Length of residence (years)						
0–9	0	0.0	450	5.9	191	6.5
10+	116,537	100.0	7172	94.1	2763	93.5
Marital status						
Married	85,089	73.1	5353*	70.1*	2095*	70.8*
Separated	10,092	8.7	898*	11.8*	406*	13.7*
Single	7010	6.0	396*	5.2*	173	5.8
Widowed	14,285	12.3	989	13.0	287*	9.7*
Education						
Primary or lower	32,385	27.8	1385*	18.2*	894*	30.3*
Secondary	55,767	47.9	3467*	45.4*	1100*	37.3*
Higher	27,773	23.8	2614*	34.3*	879*	29.8*
Other	536	0.5	163*	2.1*	74*	2.5*
Job status						
Retired	54,888	47.4	3664	48.3	874*	29.7*
Active	37,019	31.9	2412	31.8	1124*	38.3*
Unemployed or inactive	22,472	19.4	1418	18.7	872*	29.7*
Other	1537	1.3	89	1.2	68*	2.3*
BMI						
Underweight	1365	1.2	123*	1.6*	37	1.3
Normal weight	45,393	39.8	2897	38.6	1213	42.0
Overweight	47,382	41.6	3198	42.6	1107*	38.3*
Obese	19,807	17.4	1281	17.1	530	18.4
Ever smoked						
No	60,766	52.3	3929	51.7	1656*	56.1*
Yes	55,433	47.7	3671	48.3	1294*	43.9*

Table 1 Person-wave observations[a] according to individual characteristics at baseline by migrant origin (2004–2015) *(Continued)*

	Non-migrants		Western migrants		Non-western migrants	
	N	%	N	%	N	%
Vigorous activities						
More than once a week	43,078	37.1	2851	37.5	936*	31.8*
Once a week	15,866	13.7	1022	13.5	345*	11.7*
One to three times a month	9538	8.2	540*	7.1*	200*	6.8*
Hardly ever or never	47,700	41.1	3185	41.9	1466*	49.7*
Moderate activities						
More than once a week	83,372	71.8	5578*	73.4*	1909*	64.7*
Once a week	14,959	12.9	925	12.2	466*	15.8*
One to three times a month	5806	5.0	356	4.7	153	5.2
Hardly ever or never	12,053	10.4	739	9.7	423*	14.3*
TOTAL	116,537		7637		2962	

Source: Own calculations based on data from respondents aged 50 and older in 10 southern and western European countries in SHARE (2004–2015)
*Proportion statistically significantly different from that of non-migrants ($p < 0.05$), except for length of residence (difference between western and non-western migrants)
[a]These observations pertain to the sample used in the analysis of self-rated health transitions (see methods section for information on the various samples). The comparison of the background characteristics of the person-wave observations of migrants and non-migrants in the samples used in the analyses of depression and diabetes followed the same pattern

frequently engaging in vigorous and moderate activities. However, in terms of smoking and BMI, non-western migrants had a slightly healthier profile, as the shares of non-western migrants who had ever smoked or were overweight were smaller than those of both non-migrants and western migrants.

Table 2 shows the counts and the proportions of the different categories of the person-wave observations according to health by sex and migrant origin. At baseline, older western migrants had worse self-rated health outcomes than older non-migrants. Although the self-rated health of non-western migrants at baseline did not seem to differ from that of non-migrants, non-western migrants were more likely to report diabetes or depression. Migrants, especially those of non-western origin, were more likely to have made transitions leading to death or loss to follow-up, and less likely to have experienced no transition (stable good health, stable poor health) than non-migrants. These patterns were present among both males and females. Among females only, compared to non-migrants, western migrants were less likely to experience an improvement in self-rated health and non-western migrants were less likely to recover from depression.

Health deterioration

The differences between older migrants and older non-migrants in the likelihood of experiencing health deterioration were robust to the inclusion of a wide variety of covariates that are strongly associated with health outcomes and transitions (socioeconomic status, health-related behaviours, marital status). We therefore show only the coefficients for the fully adjusted model. The complete results, including all steps and the effects of all covariates, as well as the models showing the risk of experiencing transitions leading to attrition (death or loss to follow-up) are shown in the appendix (Additional file 1).

Table 3 shows the risk of experiencing a transition relative to remaining in a given state of self-rated health on the logit scale, by sex. We found that, among those initially in good self-rated health, both older western and older non-western migrants faced a higher risk than older non-migrants of deteriorating health as compared to maintaining good health. The effect of being a migrant on health deterioration tended to be stronger for transitions leading to poorer states of health. That is, the difference in the risk of experiencing a transition between migrants and non-migrants was higher for transitions leading from good to poor health than for transitions leading from good to fair health. These patterns were found for both sexes, although the differences in the risk of health deterioration between non-western female migrants and female non-migrants were not statistically significant. Among females only, migrants had a higher risk of experiencing health deterioration as compared to remaining in fair health, while the risk of transitioning from fair to poor health did not seem to differ much between male migrants and male non-migrants.

Table 4 shows the risk of experiencing a transition in mental health (depression) as compared to remaining in a given state of health. For both sexes, older western migrants had a higher risk than older non-migrants of

Table 2 Person-wave observations according to health at baseline and follow-up by sex and migrant origin (2004–2015)

Males	Non-migrants		Western migrants		Non-western migrants	
	N	%	N	%	N	%
TOTAL: good health[a] (baseline)	37,241	69.8	2183*	66.8*	1013	68.4
Stable good health	23,541	63.2	1287*	59.0*	553*	54.6*
Health deterioration	4933	13.2	299	13.7	129	12.7
Good health to death/loss to follow-up	8767	23.5	597*	27.3*	331*	32.7*
TOTAL: poor health (baseline)	16,112	30.2	1084*	33.2*	469	31.6
Stable poor health	7573	47.0	466*	43.0*	167*	35.6*
Health improvement	3288	20.4	190	17.5	92	19.6
Poor health to death/loss to follow-up	5251	32.6	428*	39.5*	210*	44.8*
TOTAL: non-depressed (baseline)	43,159	82.8	2599	81.3	1050*	75.3*
Stable non-depressed	28,302	65.6	1582*	60.9*	583*	55.5*
Health deterioration	3576	8.3	221	8.5	83	7.9
Non-depressed to death/loss to follow-up	11,281	26.1	796*	30.6*	384*	36.6*
TOTAL: depressed (baseline)	8941	17.2	598	18.7	344*	24.7*
Stable depressed	2946	32.9	164*	27.4*	101	29.4
Health improvement	3014	33.7	203	33.9	99	28.8
Depressed to death/loss to follow-up	2981	33.3	231*	38.6*	144*	41.9*
TOTAL: non-diabetic (baseline)	46,858	87.9	2850	87.3	1230*	83.2*
Stable non-diabetic	33,123	70.7	1869*	65.6*	739*	60.1*
Health deterioration	1545	3.3	83	2.9	51	4.1
Non-diabetic to death/loss to follow-up	12,190	26.0	898*	31.5*	440*	35.8*
TOTAL: diabetic (baseline)	6461	12.1	413	12.7	248*	16.8*
Females	Non-migrants		Western migrants		Non-western migrants	
	N	%	N	%	N	%
TOTAL: good health[a] (baseline)	41,424	65.6	2682*	61.4*	928	62.7
Stable good health	25,887	62.5	1600*	59.7*	514*	55.4*
Health deterioration	6016	14.5	383	14.3	123	13.3
Good health to death/loss to follow-up	9521	23.0	699*	26.1*	291*	31.4*
TOTAL: poor health (baseline)	21,760	34.4	1688*	38.6*	552	37.3
Stable poor health	11,338	52.1	863	51.1	242*	43.8*
Health improvement	4293	19.7	264*	15.6*	90	16.3
Poor health to death/loss to follow-up	6129	28.2	561*	33.2*	220*	39.9*
TOTAL: non-depressed (baseline)	42,621	68.9	2794*	65.6*	830*	59.1*
Stable non-depressed	25,932	60.8	1589*	56.9*	441*	53.1*
Health deterioration	6057	14.2	389	13.9	111	13.4
Non-depressed to death/loss to follow-up	10,632	24.9	816*	29.2*	278*	33.5*
TOTAL: depressed (baseline)	19,194	31.1	1463*	34.4*	574*	40.9*
Stable depressed	8129	42.4	609	41.6	236	41.1
Health improvement	5712	29.8	401	27.4	119*	20.7*
Depressed to death/loss to follow-up	5353	27.9	453*	31.0*	219*	38.2*

Table 2 Person-wave observations according to health at baseline and follow-up by sex and migrant origin (2004–2015) *(Continued)*

TOTAL: non-diabetic (baseline)	56,917	90.2	3923	89.8	1294*	87.5*
Stable non-diabetic	41,465	72.9	2717*	69.3*	820*	63.4*
Health deterioration	1460	2.6	100	2.5	40	3.1
Non-diabetic to death/loss to follow-up	13,992	24.6	1106*	28.2*	434*	33.5*
TOTAL: diabetic (baseline)	6218	9.8	445	10.2	185*	12.5*

Source: Own calculations based on data from respondents aged 50 and older in 10 southern and western European countries in SHARE (2004–2015)
*Proportion statistically significantly different from that of non-migrants ($p < 0.05$)
aThe category "good" self-rated health consists of the original categories "excellent", "very good" and "good". Additional analyses revealed that the proportions of transitions within these three original states did not differ between older migrants and non-migrants

becoming depressed as compared to remaining non-depressed. The risk of becoming depressed did not seem to differ between non-western migrants and non-migrants.

Table 5 shows the risk of becoming diabetic as compared to remaining non-diabetic. The risk of acquiring diabetes was substantially higher for older non-western migrants than for older non-migrants. Western female migrants were also at a higher risk of becoming diabetic than female non-migrants.

The effects of all covariates on the risk of health deterioration were rather similar regardless of the specific dimension of health considered (self-rated health, depression or diabetes) (Additional file 1). The risk of health deterioration increased with age. Lower socioeconomic status and risky health-related behaviours were associated with a greater likelihood of experiencing transitions leading to poorer health outcomes. The risk of health deterioration decreased with increasing levels of education. Respondents who were economically active were less likely than those who were retired to have experienced health deterioration. Being unemployed or economically inactive was associated with a higher risk of health deterioration than being retired, especially among males. The effect of the socioeconomic covariates on the risk of health deterioration remained similar after adjusting for health behaviours. Being underweight, overweight or obese, having ever smoked, and exercising less frequently were all factors that substantially increased the risk of transitioning to a poorer health status.

Health improvement

In general, the risk of experiencing an improvement in health as compared to remaining in a given state of self-rated health for older migrants did not seem to differ from that of older non-migrants (Table 3). Western female migrants were less likely than female non-migrants to have experienced an improvement from poor to fair, and from fair to good self-rated health as compared to maintaining poor or fair health, respectively. Non-western male migrants tended to be more likely than male non-migrants to have experienced an improvement from poor to good health as compared to maintaining poor health.

Older female migrants, and especially those of non-western origin, were less likely than older female non-migrants of experiencing a recovery from depression as compared to remaining depressed (Table 4). Among males, the risk of recovering from depression as compared to remaining depressed did not seem to differ between migrants and non-migrants.

The effects on the risk of experiencing an improvement in health among older migrants and non-migrants remained very similar in size and in the same direction after all of the covariates had been included in the analysis (Additional file 1). The likelihood of health improvement decreased with age. Single and separated respondents were less likely to have experienced an improvement in health than married respondents. The risk of health improvement was lower among those with primary education or lower than among those with secondary education. Respondents who were economically active were more likely than those who were retired to have experienced an improvement in health, while the opposite was the case among respondents who were unemployed or economically inactive. Being underweight, overweight or obese, having ever smoked, and exercising less frequently were associated with a reduced likelihood of recovery. These effects were similar regardless of the dimension of health considered (self-rated health, depression or diabetes). The effect of socioeconomic status on the risk of health improvement remained similar in terms of direction and size after additionally controlling for health behaviours.

Discussion

Summary of the results

We applied multinomial regression models to longitudinal data on self-rated health, depression and diabetes derived from the Survey of Health, Ageing and Retirement in Europe (2004–2015) to examine differences in the health transition patterns of migrants and non-migrants aged 50 and older in 10 southern and western European countries. We found that, at older ages, western migrants had poorer self-rated health at baseline than non-migrants, while non-western migrants were more likely than non-migrants to have diabetes or

Table 3 Effects[a] (logit) of experiencing a transition in self-rated health, by sex (2004–2015)

Effects (logit) of transitioning as compared to remaining in good (or more) self-rated health

	Males (N = 39,807)				Females (N = 43,839)			
Log pseudo-likelihood	−35,304				−38,987			
Pseudo R^2	0.0735				0.0820			
	to fair health		to poor health		to fair health		to poor health	
	b	SE	b	SE	b	SE	b	SE
Origin: non-migrants (ref)								
Western migrants	0.19**	0.08	0.37**	0.16	0.21***	0.07	0.29*	0.16
Non-western migrants	0.20*	0.12	0.45*	0.25	0.19	0.12	0.21	0.26

Effects (logit) of transitioning as compared to remaining in fair self-rated health

	Males (N = 12,763)				Females (N = 16,944)			
Log pseudo-likelihood	−15,648				−20,737			
Pseudo R^2	0.0606				0.0583			
	to good health		to poor health		to good health		to poor health	
	b	SE	b	SE	b	SE	b	SE
Origin: non-migrants (ref)								
Western migrants	0.03	0.12	0.02	0.15	−0.20**	0.09	0.26**	0.12
Non-western migrants	0.14	0.18	−0.24	0.25	0.19	0.16	0.41**	0.20

Effects (logit) of transitioning as compared to remaining in poor self-rated health

	Males (N = 4430)				Females (N = 5850)			
Log pseudo-likelihood	−5187				−6892			
Pseudo R^2	0.0676				0.0746			
	to good health		to fair health		to good health		to fair health	
	b	SE	b	SE	b	SE	b	SE
Origin: non-migrants (ref)								
Western migrants	0.23	0.25	−0.10	0.19	−0.31	0.24	−0.35**	0.16
Non-western migrants	0.91**	0.40	0.16	0.35	−0.07	0.40	−0.09	0.27

Source: Own calculations based on data from respondents aged 50 and older in 10 southern and western European countries in SHARE (2004–2015)
[a]The effects shown pertain to the fully adjusted model. Results for the intermediate steps are shown in the appendix
* $p < 0.1$, ** $p < 0.05$, *** $p < 0.01$

depression. We also found that older migrants in Europe were at higher risk than older non-migrants of experiencing health deterioration as compared to remaining in a given state of self-rated health. Western migrants had a higher risk than non-migrants of becoming depressed, while non-western migrants had a higher risk of acquiring diabetes. Among females only, migrants also tended to be at lower risk than non-migrants of experiencing an improvement in both overall and mental health. Even after the inclusion of several covariates that are strongly associated with health, differences in the health transition patterns of older migrants and non-migrants remained largely unexplained.

Interpretation of the results

We found that, over the study period, older migrants in Europe were more likely than older non-migrants to have experienced health deterioration and, among females only, less likely to have experienced health improvement. This finding seems to be in line with the steeper rates of health decline among migrants with age and the passage of time, previously observed both at younger adult ages and at older ages [13, 14, 16, 44]. Our results may be explained by the cumulative disadvantage theory [45, 46], which postulates that migrants suffer from the negative effects of having a relatively low socioeconomic position throughout their life course, including detrimental effects on their health. Indeed, migrants often experience material deprivation, poor working conditions, social isolation and limited access to services [47]. Furthermore, failure to meet socioeconomic aspirations, and in particular perceived downward social mobility as compared to the expectations had the person not migrated, can result in an even greater health burden for migrants [48].

Table 4 Effects[a] (logit) of experiencing a transition in mental health, by sex (2004–2015)

Effects (logit) of becoming depressed as compared to remaining non-depressed				
	Males (N = 46,137)		Females (N = 45,076)	
Log pseudo-likelihood	−36,011		−38,987	
Pseudo R^2	0.0673		0.0666	
	b	SE	b	SE
Origin: non-migrants (ref)				
Western migrants	0.17**	0.08	0.15**	0.07
Non-western migrants	0.02	0.13	0.00	0.12
Effects (logit) of recovering from depression as compared to remaining depressed				
	Males (N = 9612)		Females (N = 20,249)	
Log pseudo-likelihood	− 9788		−20,395	
Pseudo R^2	0.0730		0.0676	
	b	SE	b	SE
Origin: non-migrants (ref)				
Western migrants	0.15	0.12	−0.24***	0.08
Non-western migrants	0.01	0.16	−0.37***	0.13

Source: Own calculations based on data from respondents aged 50 and older in 10 southern and western European countries in SHARE (2004–2015)
[a]The effects shown pertain to the fully adjusted model. Results for the intermediate steps are shown in the appendix
** $p < 0.05$, *** $p < 0.01$

Among males only, the risk of experiencing a health improvement did not seem to differ between migrants and non-migrants. Previous research showed that (non-western) migrants tend to suffer more often from infectious diseases and occupational injuries, which, compared to most non-communicable diseases, are more likely to lead to recovery in case of survival [47, 49–51]. It might be possible that recovery from these causes mitigates the negative effects migrants bear due to a general social and economic disadvantage over their life courses. We may speculate that, because of the particularly pronounced gendered social and labour-market position among migrants of mainly non-western origin (e.g. [52]), female migrants might be less prone to occupational injuries and therefore also less likely to recover.

Table 5 Effects[a] (logit) of becoming diabetic as compared to remaining non-diabetic, by sex (2004–2015)

	Males (N = 50,001)		Females (N = 60,094)	
Log pseudo-likelihood	−32,819		−36,874	
Pseudo R^2	0.0766		0.0834	
	b	SE	b	SE
Origin: non-migrants (ref)				
Western migrants	0.10	0.12	0.25**	0.12
Non-western migrants	0.56***	0.17	0.43**	0.19

Source: Own calculations based on data from respondents aged 50 and older in 10 southern and western European countries in SHARE (2004–2015)
[a]The effects shown pertain to the fully adjusted model. Results for the intermediate steps are shown in the appendix
** $p < 0.05$, *** $p < 0.01$

We also found that, at older ages, migrants had poorer health at baseline than non-migrants. This finding is in line with results from previous studies in Europe [4, 6–9]. Although migrants tend to have a health advantage relative to non-migrants at the time of arrival (e.g. [53]), their health tends to decline at a faster pace starting just a few years after arrival [13, 44, 54]. This might explain why, many years after migration, older migrants in Europe tend to be in poorer general health than non-migrants. However, the initial health advantage of migrants does not seem to have reversed by the time they reach old age in the USA or Canada, where steeper rates of health decline among migrants at older ages lead to a decrease in migrant health inequalities and thus to convergence in health between older migrants and non-migrants [14, 16]. In contrast, higher risks of health deterioration and lower risks of health improvement among older migrants in Europe will lead to an increase in migrant health inequalities and thus to divergence in health between older migrants and non-migrants.

Our findings also show that migrant origin plays a role in explaining differences in the health transition patterns of older migrants and non-migrants. The risk of experiencing a deterioration in self-rated health and the risk of acquiring diabetes tended to be higher among older non-western migrants than among older western migrants. In particular, the higher risk of developing diabetes among non-western migrants is likely due to a combination of genetic and physiological factors, conditions during early life such as malnutrition, and potential changes in health-related behaviours after migration [55, 56]. Although the risk of becoming depressed did not differ between non-western migrants and non-migrants, non-western migrants were more likely to have depression than both non-migrants and western migrants at baseline.

However, it was unexpected that non-western male migrants were more likely to experience transitions leading from poor to good self-rated health as compared to remaining in poor health. Given the small sample size of non-western male migrants initially in poor self-rated health ($N = 120$), the effect of outliers in this group might be large. Indeed, 13 non-western male migrants transitioned from poor to good health. These respondents were much younger than non-migrants in this group (below 65), and were more often unemployed or economically inactive. These characteristics did not correspond with the general characteristics of non-western male migrants initially in poor health (results not shown), thereby suggesting that these 13 respondents correspond to cases of acute illness and subsequent recovery.

Evaluation of data and methods
This study provided new insights into the health transition patterns of older migrants and non-migrants in 10 countries in southern and western Europe by considering measures of overall, mental and physical health. However, some limitations in the data and methods need to be considered.

First, SHARE is not designed to adequately subsample the migrant subpopulation. However, underrepresentation of migrants in our data proved to be only moderate. According to Eurostat data for 2011 [57], migrants represented 9.1% of the population aged 50 and older in the 10 countries studied, whereas in our data based on SHARE, migrants only contributed 8.3% of the person-wave observations. Nevertheless, migrants in the sample are very likely to be selective because SHARE questionnaires are provided in the national languages only. Thus, only migrants who have a good command of the country's language are eligible. Although the observed pattern of stronger health deterioration among migrants follows the pattern of previous studies outside Europe [10–16], further studies may want to investigate whether our findings can indeed be generalised to the population level. In addition, small migrant sample sizes hampered the classification of migrants beyond a broad western versus non-western typology. Furthermore, the data for all of the countries were pooled together. Although we controlled for the effect of country of residence to broadly consider the spatial, social and institutional context, the impact of this context could well be dissimilar for migrants and non-migrants. For instance, integration policies or public attitudes towards migrants are aspects of the policy and societal context that may affect migrants and their health in particular (e.g. [58]).

Second, due to data restrictions, we were unable to distinguish transitions leading to death from those leading to loss to follow-up. The respondents in SHARE are traced and followed if they relocate within the country, and their mortality is recorded via end-of-life interviews with a proxy respondent, who could be a family or household member, a neighbour or another person socially related to the deceased [24]. A recent study compared the mortality rates in SHARE with those from the Human Mortality Database, and concluded that SHARE underestimates mortality [59]. Although transitions leading to attrition (either death or loss to follow-up) were modelled as a competing risk, the results of this part of the analysis are difficult to interpret. Given that older migrants may have a mortality advantage over older non-migrants in Europe, or at least in certain European countries [4, 5], our results suggest that migrants are more likely to be lost to follow-up than non-migrants. Considering the (rather debated) possibility that older non-migrants in poor health might return to their country of origin, as suggested by the "salmon bias" hypothesis [60], our results may underestimate the relative disadvantage of migrants in transitioning to poorer states of health. Additionally, given that we could not distinguish mortality from losses to follow-up, the relevance of our findings could be challenged by arguing that mortality is the ultimate health outcome. Nevertheless, we argue that general health also matters, and has a clear impact on people's quality of life [61]. Thus, we believe our findings have implications relevant to health-related policies and healthcare provision.

Third, we could observe a maximum of four person-wave observations per respondent. Respondents first entered the survey in different waves, and not all of the respondents made it to the final wave due to death or loss to follow-up. Because the number of transitions observed per individual was relatively small, we were unable to analyse longer health trajectories. Considerably more effort should be devoted to gathering comparative longitudinal migrant health data across Europe.

Finally, the coefficients for being a migrant might be influenced by an unmeasured residual effect of socioeconomic status on the risk of experiencing a given health transition. Migrants tend to be in a disadvantaged position with respect to non-migrants in a similar socioeconomic position [62]. Yet, the role of socioeconomic status in the health of migrants is complex and not yet well understood; moreover, the various dimensions of socioeconomic status may affect the health of migrants and non-migrants differently [63]. By controlling for the highest level of education and job status only, we may not be able to accurately capture socioeconomic differences between older migrants and non-migrants. Had we been able to include additional control variables indicating socioeconomic status (e.g. income), these might have further explained the inequalities in health transitions between migrants and non-migrants.

Conclusion

Our study is the first to analyse and explain the differences in the overall, physical and mental health transition patterns of older migrants and non-migrants in a European context. Our results show that older migrants in Europe were more likely than older non-migrants to have experienced health deterioration and, among females only, less likely to have experienced an improvement in health. These patterns were visible for self-rated health, depression and diabetes, and seem to be in line with the social and economic disadvantage migrants tend to experience over their life courses. The transition patterns in terms of depression or diabetes can be thought as examples of how transition patterns in mental and physical health, respectively, shaped transition patterns in overall health. Our results also show that the differences in the health transition patterns of older migrants and non-migrants remained largely unexplained even after a range of socioeconomic indicators and health-related behaviours were taken into account.

Our results raise concerns about whether migrants in Europe are as likely as non-migrants to age in good health, and suggest that general policies aimed at improving health among the older population, such as policies that promote healthier lifestyles or broader socioeconomic policies that seek to tackle socioeconomic inequalities, might not suffice to effectively reduce health inequalities between migrants and non-migrants. We recommend that policies aiming to promote healthy ageing specifically address the health needs of the migrant population, thereby distinguishing migrants from different backgrounds.

Future research should investigate the role of specific diseases and conditions, and the extent to which the context in the country or area of origin and in the country of residence explain the differences in health and health transitions between older migrants and non-migrants. The findings of these studies may, for example, be used to help formulate healthy ageing policies that target specific diseases and conditions that affect migrants in particular, to design more inclusive integration policies and to create campaigns to promote more favourable public attitudes towards migrants.

Endnotes

[1]Although this is not completely accurate, we use the term "married" to denote both respondents that were married and living with their spouse, and respondents who were in a registered partnership. Registered partnership is a rare category in the data, which was found mainly in Sweden, the Netherlands, and Belgium (5–10% of cases). No information was available on whether those in a registered partnership were actually living with their partner. Neither was information available on informal cohabitation.

Abbreviations
BMI: body mass index; SHARE: Survey of Health, Ageing and Retirement in Europe; USA: United States of America

Acknowledgements
This paper uses data from SHARE Waves 1, 2, 3 (SHARELIFE), 4, 5, and 6 (DOIs: https://doi.org/10.6103/SHARE.w1.600, https://doi.org/10.6103/SHARE.w2.600, https://doi.org/10.6103/SHARE.w3.600, https://doi.org/10.6103/SHARE.w4.600, https://doi.org/10.6103/SHARE.w5.600, https://doi.org/10.6103/SHARE.w6.600), see Börsch-Supan et al. [24] for methodological details. The SHARE data collection has been primarily funded by the European Commission through FP5 (QLK6-CT-2001-00360), FP6 (SHARE-I3: RII-CT-2006-062193, COMPARE: CIT5-CT-2005-028857, SHARELIFE: CIT4-CT-2006-028812) and FP7 (SHARE-PREP: N°211909, SHARE-LEAP: N°227822, SHARE M4: N° 261982). Additional funding from the German Ministry of Education and Research, the Max Planck Society for the Advancement of Science, the U.S. National Institute on Aging (U01_AG09740-13S2, P01_AG005842, P01_AG08291, P30_AG12815, R21_AG025169, Y1-AG-4553-01, IAG_BSR06-11, OGHA_04-064, HHSN271201300071C) and from various national funding sources is gratefully acknowledged (see www.share-project.org).

Funding
University of Groningen and Vrije Universiteit Brussel.

Authors' contributions
MR-P performed the statistical analyses, drafted and finalised the manuscript. All authors contributed to the design of the study and interpretation of results, and approved the final version of the manuscript. CM participated in the data analysis and critically reviewed the manuscript. EK critically reviewed the manuscript. FJ contributed to drafting and provided detailed review of the manuscript.

Competing interests
The authors declare that they have no competing interests.

Author details
Population Research Centre, Faculty of Spatial Sciences, University of Groningen, Groningen, The Netherlands. [2]Interface Demography, Department of Sociology, Vrije Universiteit Brussel, Brussels, Belgium. Statistical Office Bremen, Bremen, Germany. [4]Netherlands Interdisciplinary Demographic Institute, The Hague, The Netherlands.

References

1. Lanzieri G. Fewer, older and multicultural?: projections of the EU populations by foreign/national background. Luxemburg: Eurostat; 2011.
2. International Organization for Migration. Migrant health: better health for all in Europe. Geneva: International Organisation for Migration; 2009.
3. Nørredam M, Krasnik A. Migrants' access to health services. In: Rechel B, Mladovsky P, Devillé W, Rijks B, Petrova-Benedict R, McKee M, editors. Migration and health in the European Union. Berkshire: Open University Press; 2011. p. 67–80.
4. Carnein M, Milewski N, Doblhammer G, Nusselder WJ. Health inequalities of immigrants: patterns and determinants of health expectancies of Turkish migrants living in Germany. In: Doblhammer G, editor. Health among the elderly in Germany: new evidence on disease, disability and care need. Leverkusen: Barbara Budrich; 2014. p. 157–90.
5. Reus-Pons M, Vandenheede H, Janssen F, Kibele EUB. Differences in mortality between groups of older migrants and older non-migrants in Belgium, 2001-09. Eur J Pub Health. 2016;26:992–1000.
6. Reus-Pons M, Kibele EUB, Janssen F. Differences in healthy life expectancy between older migrants and non-migrants in three European countries over time. Int J Public Health. 2017;62:531–40.
7. Solé-Auró A, Crimmins EM. Health of immigrants in European countries. Int Migr Rev. 2008;42:861–76.
8. Aichberger MC, Schouler-Ocak M, Mundt A, Busch MA, Nickels E, Heimann HM, Ströhle A, Reischies FM, Heinz A, Rapp MA. Depression in middle-aged and older first generation migrants in Europe: results from the Survey of Health, Ageing and Retirement in Europe (SHARE). Eur Psychiat. 2010;25:468–75.
9. Lanari D, Bussini O. International migration and health inequalities in later life. Ageing Soc. 2012;32:935–62.
10. Newbold KB. Self-rated health within the Canadian immigrant population: risk and the healthy immigrant effect. Soc Sci Med. 2005;60:1359–70.
11. De Maio FG, Kemp E. The deterioration of health status among immigrants to Canada. Glob Public Health. 2010;5:462–78.
12. So L, Quan H. Coming to Canada: the difference in health trajectories between immigrants and native-born residents. Int J Public Health. 2012;57:893–904.
13. Kim I-H, Carrasco C, Muntaner C, McKenzie K, Noh S. Ethnicity and postmigration health trajectory in new immigrants to Canada. Am J Public Health. 2013;103:96–104.
14. Gubernskaya Z. Age at migration and self-rated health trajectories after age 50: understanding the older immigrant health paradox. J Gerontol Ser B-Psychol Sci Soc Sci. 2015;70:279–90.
15. Reynolds MM, Chernenko A, Read JG. Region of origin diversity in immigrant health: moving beyond the Mexican case. Soc Sci Med. 2016;166:102–9.
16. Garcia MA, Reyes AM. Physical functioning and disability trajectories by age of migration among Mexican elders in the United States. J Gerontol Ser B-Psychol Sci Soc Sci. 2017; https://doi.org/10.1093/geronb/gbw167.
17. Kristiansen M, Razum O, Tezcan-Güntekin H, Krasnik A. Aging and health among migrants in a European perspective. Public Health Rev. 2016;37:20.
18. Lanari D, Bussini O, Minelli L. Self-perceived health among eastern European immigrants over 50 living in western Europe. Int J Public Health. 2015;60:21–31.
19. Razum O, Twardella D. Time travel with Oliver Twist-towards an explanation for a paradoxically low mortality among recent immigrants. Tropical Med Int Health. 2002;7:4–10.
20. Lindström M, Sundquist J, Östergren PO. Ethnic differences in self reported health in Malmö in southern Sweden. J Epidemiol Community Health. 2001;55:97–103.
21. Hosper K, Nierkens V, Nicolaou M, Stronks K. Behavioural risk factors in two generations of non-western migrants: do trends converge towards the host population? Eur J Epidemiol. 2007;22:163–72.
22. Arnold M, Razum O, Coebergh JW. Cancer risk diversity in non-western migrants to Europe: an overview of the literature. Eur J Cancer. 2010;46:2647–59.
23. Vandenheede H, Willaert D, de Grande H, Simoens S, Vanroelen C. Mortality in adult immigrants in the 2000s in Belgium: a test of the 'healthy-migrant' and the 'migration-as-rapid-health-transition' hypotheses. Tropical Med Int Health. 2015;20:1832–45.
24. Börsch-Supan A, Brandt M, Hunkler C, Kneip T, Korbmacher J, Malter F, Schaan B, Stuck S, Zuber S, on behalf of the SHARE Central Coordination Team. Data resource profile: the Survey of Health, Ageing and Retirement in Europe (SHARE). Int J Epidemiol. 2013;42:992–1001.
25. Castles S, Miller MJ. The age of migration. 5th ed. Basingstoke: Palgrave Macmillan; 2014.
26. Börsch-Supan A. Survey of Health, Ageing and Retirement in Europe (SHARE) wave 1. Release version: 6.0.0. SHARE-ERIC. 2017. http://dx.doi.org/10.6103/SHARE.w1.600.
27. Börsch-Supan A. Survey of Health, Ageing and Retirement in Europe (SHARE) wave 2. Release version: 6.0.0. SHARE-ERIC. 2017. http://dx.doi.org/10.6103/SHARE.w2.600.
28. Börsch-Supan A. Survey of Health, Ageing and Retirement in Europe (SHARE) wave 4. Release version: 6.0.0. SHARE-ERIC. 2017. http://dx.doi.org/10.6103/SHARE.w4.600.
29. Börsch-Supan A. Survey of Health, Ageing and Retirement in Europe (SHARE) wave 5. Release version: 6.0.0. SHARE-ERIC. 2017. http://dx.doi.org/10.6103/SHARE.w5.600.
30. Börsch-Supan A. Survey of Health, Ageing and Retirement in Europe (SHARE) wave 6. Release version: 6.0.0. SHARE-ERIC. 2017. http://dx.doi.org/10.6103/SHARE.w6.600.
31. Seo S, Chung S, Shumway M. How good is "very good"? Translation effect in the racial/ethnic variation in self-rated health status. Qual Life Res. 2014;23:593–600.
32. Kunst AE, Bos V, Lahelma E, Bartley M, Lissau I, Regidor E, Mielck A, Cardano M, Dalstra JA, Geurts JJ, Helmert U, Lennartsson C, Ramm J, Spadea T, Stronegger WJ, Mackenbach JP. Trends in socioeconomic inequalities in self-assessed health in 10 European countries. Int J Epidemiol. 2005;34:295–305.
33. Prince MJ, Reischies F, Beekman AT, Fuhrer R, Jonker C, Kivela SL, Lawlor BA, Lobo A, Magnusson H, Fichter M, van Oyen H, Roelands M, Skoog I, Turrina C, Copeland JR. Development of the EURO-D scale - a European Union initiative to compare symptoms of depression in 14 European centres. Bri J Psychiat. 1999;174:330–8.
34. Dewey ME, Prince MJ. Mental health. In: Börsch-Supan A, Brugiavini A, Jürges H, Mackenbach J, Siegrist J, Weber G, editors. Health, ageing and retirement in Europe - first results from the Survey of Health, Ageing and Retirement in Europe. Mannheim: Mannheim Research Institute for the Economics of Ageing (MEA); 2005. p. 108–17.
35. Gorodzeisky A, Semyonov M. Terms of exclusion: public views towards admission and allocation of rights to immigrants in European countries. Ethnic Racial Stud. 2009;32:401–23.
36. Carr D, Springer KW. Advances in families and health research in the 21st century. J Marriage Fam. 2010;72:743–61.
37. Nazroo JY. The structuring of ethnic inequalities in health: economic position, racial discrimination, and racism. Am J Public Health. 2003;93:277–84.
38. Mackenbach JP, Stirbu I, Roskam AR, Schaap MM, Menvielle G, Leinsalu M, Kunst AE. Socioeconomic inequalities in health in 22 European countries. N Engl J Med. 2008;358:2468–81.
39. Bhopal R, Hayes L, White M, Unwin N, Harland J, Ayis S, Alberti G. Ethnic and socio-economic inequalities in coronary heart disease, diabetes and risk factors in Europeans and south Asians. J Public Health Med. 2002;24:95–105.
40. World Health Organization. Joint WHO/FAO expert consultation on diet, nutrition and the prevention of chronic diseases. WHO technical report series 916. Geneva: WHO; 2003.
41. Chen L, Pei JH, Kuang J, Chen HM, Chen Z, Li ZW, Yang H. Effect of lifestyle intervention in patients with type 2 diabetes: a meta-analysis. Metabolism. 2015;64:338–47.
42. Huber PJ. The behavior of maximum likelihood estimates under nonstandard conditions. Proceedings of the Fifth Berkeley Symposium on Mathematical Statistics and Probability. 1967;1:221–33.
43. White H. A heteroskedasticity-consistent covariance matrix estimator and a direct test for heteroskedasticity. Econometrica. 1980;48:817–38.
44. Goldman N, Pebley AR, Creighton MJ, Teruel GM, Rubalcava LN, Chung C. The consequences of migration to the United States for short-term changes in the health of Mexican immigrants. Demography. 2014;51:1159–73.
45. Angel JL, Buckley CJ, Sakamoto A. Duration or disadvantage? Exploring nativity, ethnicity, and health in midlife. J Gerontol Ser B-Psychol Sci Soc Sci. 2001;56:S275–84.
46. Dannefer D. Cumulative advantage/disadvantage and the life course: cross-fertilizing age and social science theory. J Gerontol Ser B-Psychol Sci Soc Sci. 2003;58:S327–37.

47. Gushulak B, Pace P, Weekers J. Migration and health of migrants. In: Koller T, editor. Poverty and social exclusion in the WHO European region: health systems respond. Copenhagen: WHO Regional Office for Europe; 2010. p. 257–81.
48. Alcántara C, Chen C, Alegría M. Do post-migration perceptions of social mobility matter for Latino immigrant health? Soc Sci Med. 2014;101:94–106.
49. Rechel B, Mladovsky P, Ingleby D, Mackenbach JP, McKee M. Migration and health in an increasingly diverse Europe. Lancet. 2013;381:1235–45.
50. Deboosere P, Gadeyne S. Adult migrant mortality advantage in Belgium: evidence using census and register data. Population. 2005;60:655–98.
51. Anthamatten P, Hazen H. An introduction to the geography of health. Abingdon (Oxford): Routledge; 2011.
52. Huschek D, de Valk HAG, Liefbroer AC. Gender-role behavior of second-generation Turks: the role of partner choice, gender ideology and societal context. Adv Life Course Res. 2011;16:164–77.
53. De Maio FG. Immigration as pathogenic: a systematic review of the health of immigrants to Canada. Int J Equity Health. 2010;9:27.
54. Norredam M, Agyemang C, Hoejbjerg-Hansen OK, Petersen JH, Byberg S, Krasnik A, Kunst AE. Duration of residence and disease occurrence among refugees and family reunited immigrants: test of the 'healthy migrant effect' hypothesis. Tropical Med Int Health. 2014;19:958–67.
55. Hales CN, Barker DJP. Type 2 (non-insulin-dependent) diabetes mellitus: the thrifty phenotype hypothesis. Diabetologia. 1992;35:595–601.
56. Sniderman AD, Bhopal R, Prabhakaran D, Sarrafzadegan N, Tchernof A. Why might South Asians be so susceptible to central obesity and its atherogenic consequences? The adipose tissue overflow hypothesis. Int J Epidemiol. 2007;36:220–5.
57. Eurostat. http://ec.europa.eu/eurostat. Accessed 3 Feb 2018.
58. Malmusi D. Immigrants' health and health inequality by type of integration policies in European countries. Eur J Pub Health. 2015;25:293–9.
59. Solé-Auró A, Michaud P-C, Hurd M, Crimmins E. Disease incidence and mortality among older Americans and Europeans. Demography. 2015;52:593–611.
60. Abraído-Lanza AF, Dohrenwend BP, Ng-Mak DS, Turner JB. The Latino mortality paradox: a test of the "salmon bias" and healthy migrant hypotheses. Am J Public Health. 1999;89:1543–8.
61. Uitenbroek DG, Verhoeff AP. Life expectancy and mortality differences between migrant groups living in Amsterdam, the Netherlands. Soc Sci Med. 2002;54:1379–88.
62. Nazroo JY. Genetic, cultural or socio-economic vulnerability? Explaining ethnic inequalities in health. Sociol Health Ill. 1998;20:710–30.
63. Nielsen SS, Hempler NF, Krasnik A. Issues to consider when measuring and applying socioeconomic position quantitatively in immigrant health research. Int J Environ Res Public Health. 2013;10:6354–65.

A model of access combining triage with initial management reduced waiting time for community outpatient services: a stepped wedge cluster randomised controlled trial

Katherine E. Harding[1,2]*, Sandra G. Leggat[2], Jennifer J. Watts[3], Bridie Kent[4], Luke Prendergast[2], Michelle Kotis[5], Mary O'Reilly[1], Leila Karimi[2], Annie K. Lewis[1,2], David A. Snowdon[1,2] and Nicholas F. Taylor[1,2]

Abstract

Background: Long waiting times are associated with public community outpatient health services. This trial aimed to determine if a new model of care based on evidence-based strategies that improved patient flow in two small pilot trials could be used to reduce waiting time across a variety of services. The key principle of the Specific Timely Appointments for Triage (STAT) model is that patients are booked directly into protected assessment appointments and triage is combined with initial management as an alternative to a waiting list and triage system.

Methods: A stepped wedge cluster randomised controlled trial was conducted between October 2015 and March 2017, involving 3116 patients at eight sites across a major Australian metropolitan health network.

Results: The intervention reduced waiting time to first appointment by 33.8% (IRR = 0.663, 95% CI 0.516 to 0.852, $P = 0.001$). Median waiting time decreased from a median of 42 days (IQR 19 to 86) in the control period to a median of 24 days (IQR 13 to 48) in the intervention period. A substantial reduction in variability was also noted. The model did not impact on most secondary outcomes, including time to second appointment, likelihood of discharge by 12 weeks and number of appointments provided, but was associated with a small increase in the rate of missed appointments.

Conclusions: Broad-scale implementation of a model of access and triage that combined triage with initial management and actively managed the relationship between supply and demand achieved substantial reductions in waiting time without adversely impacting on other aspects of care. The reductions in waiting time are likely to have been driven, primarily, by substantial reductions for those patients previously considered low priority.

Keywords: Waiting lists, Access, Appointments and schedules, Outpatients, Community health

---

* Correspondence: katherine.harding@easternhealth.org.au
[1]Eastern Health, Level 2/5 Arnold Street, Box Hill, VIC 3128, Australia
[2]La Trobe University, Kingsbury Drive, Bundoora, VIC 3086, Australia
Full list of author information is available at the end of the article

Background

Excessive waiting times for care can be a problem for both patients and health services [1]. Access issues are often associated with emergency departments [2, 3] and surgical procedures [4, 5]. However, sub-acute and community-based services also suffer from the constant pressure of lengthy waiting lists [6–9]. Delays in access to care for these services have been associated with poorer patient outcomes [10, 11], anxiety [12], and reduced engagement with services [13, 14].

Delays in care can result in waiting lists or queues. Delays, and hence waiting lists, are the result of a disparity between demand for a service and the capacity available to meet this demand [15]. Queueing theory is the equation that defines the relationship between demand, capacity and wait time [16]. Queues or waiting lists are formed when demand is higher than capacity [16]. Shortages in markets are often corrected through a "price signal", but this mechanism is ineffective in public health services where consumers face subsidised prices and costs to consumers do not change in response to rise in demand. On the supply side, individual providers may not be responsive to price signals due to wages paid as salary or other government regulation. Hence, alternative strategies are needed to mitigate the adverse effects of long waiting times.

One strategy is to use short-term strategies such as immediate and temporary increases in supply to "clear" a waiting list; however, this does not resolve the underlying problem and waiting lists are likely to simply recur [17]. Another common strategy is to focus attention on managing the waiting list, for example, by dedicating staff to monitoring patients on the list, setting up data systems to record waiting list data or creating complex sorting or triage systems to prioritise patients according to need. These systems can help the most urgent patients to access timely care, but often do not assist in reducing overall waiting time; conversely, they may contribute to the problem by diverting resources from clinical care to administrative processes associated with managing the waiting list [17, 18].

In contrast, promising results have been reported from strategies that address patient flow by reducing complexity in booking systems, combining triage with initial management and/or actively managing the relationship between supply and demand [18, 19]. Trials in this area have focussed primarily on emergency departments (for example by placing a senior physician at triage to commence treatment and quickly manage simple cases) [20] and primary care settings (the Advanced Access approach, for example, reduces time for pre-booked appointments, opening sufficient space for patients needing same-day or next-day consultations with their local doctor) [21]. Preliminary evidence is also available from isolated studies in single services to suggest that patient flow interventions that utilise one or more of these elements may be effective in other types of community outpatient services [22–25].

Long waits for services are a problem for community outpatient services with negative consequences for patients and service providers. Of the various strategies that have been tried to reduce waiting time, there are several elements that show promise of effectiveness but evidence is limited to small, single-site studies or from extrapolation of evidence from emergency departments and primary care settings. It is not known whether a model of care that brings these key elements together can be successful in reducing waiting time across a variety of community-based outpatient health services. This trial aimed to determine whether a model of access that combines triage with initial management and allows supply to be responsive to demand fluctuations can be used to reduce waiting time across multiple community outpatient services.

Methods

Design

A stepped wedge cluster randomised controlled trial was conducted [26] in accordance with the published trial protocol [27]. Trial data collection was completed from October 2015 to March 2017. Data were collected from all sites for a 12-week pre-intervention control period. A new site then implemented the intervention every 4 weeks, commencing February 2016. Following the implementation period of 12 weeks at each site, intervention data were collected for a minimum of 12 weeks at all sites (Fig. 1).

The trial was registered with the Australian and New Zealand Clinical Trial Registry (ACTRN12615001016527) [27] and ethical approval was provided by the Human Research Ethics Committee of the health network. Funding was provided by the Australian National Health and Medical Research Council (APP1076777) and the Victorian Department of Health and Human Services.

Setting

The health network in which the trial took place provides care to a population of more than 700,000 people in eastern metropolitan Melbourne, Australia, and adjacent rural communities. The eight sites within this network that took part in the study met the criteria of providing community outpatient services. For the purposes of the trial, "community outpatient services" were considered to include community health services and sub-acute ambulatory care services (SACS). In Australia, public community health services provide allied health, community nursing services and medical services (within multi-disciplinary teams) to improve health and well-being. They may assist in recovery after an illness or injury, provide support in the management of chronic

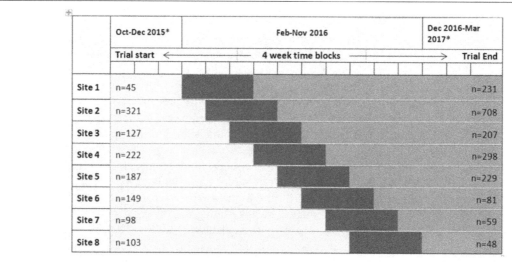

Fig. 1 Stepped Wedge trial design. *Excludes period from December 25 to end of January in each year of the trial. Light shade denotes control period, the dark shade the implementation period, and medium shade the intervention period

health conditions, support children with development disabilities or participate in health promotion activities. SACS also offer community-based care, but are usually co-located with other services provided within public health networks [28]. Services are often associated with a hospital admission prevention strategy or follow-up after a hospital stay. For example, they may include specialist, multi-disciplinary teams for assessment and management of conditions such as dementia, incontinence, falls or outpatient multi-disciplinary rehabilitation programs. Sites were selected for inclusion in the trial from 28 community outpatient services within the network that participated in a preliminary study exploring managers' perceptions of factors that affect waiting lists [9]. Selection for the current trial was based on suitability for the intervention and approval from service managers. Community outpatient services in the network were eligible to participate if they typically provided care over series of appointments, used waiting lists to manage demand and reported the length of their waiting lists to be reasonably stable over the previous 2 years.

Intervention

All sites used a waiting list to manage demand in the pre-intervention period, with new patients offered appointments as they could be accommodated in clinician schedules. Specific Timely Appointments for Triage (STAT) has been described in detail previously [27]. The fundamental principle of the intervention is that the rate of demand is calculated, and the number of new appointments required each week to keep up with demand is protected in clinician schedules. Patients are allocated an initial appointment immediately after referral (minimising processes associated with access and triage), and prioritisation decisions shift from priority of access to the service to a focus on priority of need for ongoing services after initial assessment. Clinicians make these decisions based on clinical judgement, with access to both a complete picture of client needs and the context of demand for the service.

In line with similar interventions in other settings [21], the intervention began with short-term, targeted interventions involving a small injection of resources that aimed to reduce or clear the backlog of waiting patients. Participating sites were free to use these resources in whatever way they deemed most effective; possibilities included, but were not limited to, employing additional short-term staff, increasing hours of part-time staff or contracting work to private providers. No additional ongoing resources were provided. Team leaders and mangers at each site led the implementation, with project officers from the research team providing education about the intervention and informal support and consultation as required during the implementation period [27].

Participants

Routinely collected data were analysed from all patients who had their first appointment with the site within the control and intervention periods at each site. New patients were not recruited during the 12-week implementation period, and data collection was also suspended at all sites during the Christmas holiday period because several participating sites either closed or markedly reduced services during this period. Service use of all participating patients was followed for 12 weeks from the date of first appointment.

Randomisation

The order of intervention for the eight sites was determined through generation of a random sequence using an online randomisation generator (http://www.randomization.com). This was performed in a concealed manner using a single block by a researcher not involved in recruitment or data collection. Service providers were not informed of the order of implementation until eight sites had been recruited and consented to the project.

Outcome measures

The primary outcome was time in days from referral to first appointment at the level of the patient. Secondary outcome data were collected to determine impacts of the change in model of access on other aspects of service provision at the level of the patient. These were as follows: the rate of missed appointments, the total number of appointments received, the proportion of patients discharged at the end of 12 weeks, the time between the first and second appointment, and the number of unplanned admissions and resulting number of unplanned days spent in hospital in the 6 months following the first appointment with the included site as a marker of adverse events.

Additional variables were collected at both patient and site levels to evaluate the impact of other factors that may have influenced outcomes. These included age, sex, date of referral (reflecting season) and size of the site. The ratio of referrals from the same 12-week time periods over 2 years was also collected for each site as an indicator of any changes in service demand over the course of the project.

Patients attending for the first time during the study period and therefore meeting eligibility for inclusion in the sample were identified prospectively from clinician schedules. Primary and secondary outcome data were then collected from the health network database for each of these patients. Information from databases was supplemented with manual checking of clinician schedules and written referrals to verify accuracy of data or follow up missing information as required.

Other outcome measures

Health utilisation, cost data, quality of life and service satisfaction data were collected from a sample of 557 patients across the eight sites that contributed to a health economics analysis. In-depth interviews were also conducted with 20 staff members who experienced the change to evaluate the process of implementing the STAT model. Findings of these additional analyses will be reported separately.

Sample size

A sample of 2496 participants was estimated as the minimum required to detect a mean difference with small to medium effect size in waiting time at 5% level of significance, power of 80% and an intraclass correlation coefficient (ICC) of $\rho = 0.01$ [29, 30]. The calculation estimated approximately 26 admissions per site per 4-week block of data collection. The sample size calculation was based on conservative estimates of the effect size detected in the pilot trial ($\delta = .65$) [22] consistent with similar effect sizes observed in studies of Advance Access in general practice settings [31], as well as the number of steps, the number of baseline measurements and the number of measurements between steps in the stepped wedge design.

Statistical analysis

Waiting time (a count variable) from referral to first scheduled appointment was modelled using generalised mixed effects models assuming a negative binomial dependent variable to allow for over-dispersion. The model was used to assess the effectiveness of the intervention while adjusting for potential confounders such as patient age, patient gender, referral season (summer, autumn, winter and spring), size of the site and demand ratio. A random effect was included for clustering within the site to allow for within-site correlation. Since the intervention effect was likely to vary across clusters, we followed the advice of Davey et al. [32] and ensured that this was adequately modelled. To do so, we introduced a slope random effect for treatment. As a sensitivity analysis, a Gaussian linear mixed effects model was used, allowing for different variances within clusters and both a random intercept and slope were fitted to the log of waiting time plus one. Analyses were completed using the statistical package R version 3.3.3 [33].

Results

Data were collected from 3113 participants, 1252 in the pre-intervention period and 1861 in the post-intervention period. Characteristics of the sample are included in Table 1. Patient characteristics appeared well matched between control and intervention periods, although differing lengths of time in the control and intervention period for each site due to the trial design contributed to some observed differences. For example, the greater number of patients referred for physiotherapy services and musculoskeletal disorders in the post intervention group was accounted for by site 2 (the largest site) having a short pre and long post intervention period.

The eight sites varied both in the nature of the client group (age range, conditions) and service characteristics (size, rural or metropolitan catchment area and staffing mix). Service demand was stable through the period of the trial for five sites; three sites had substantial increases in number of referrals received. Characteristics of included sites are shown in Table 2.

Table 1 Participant characteristics

Patient characteristics	Control period n = 1252	Intervention period n = 1861
Gender [n (%)]		
Female	743 (59%)	1172 (63%)
Male	509 (41%)	689 (37%)
Age [years, mean(SD)]	43 (30)	41 (29)
Referral reason [n (%)]		
Musculoskeletal	408 (33%)	862 (46%)
Neurological	113 (9%)	51 (3%)
Developmental assessment	304 (24%)	340 (18%)
Incontinence	350 (28%)	511 (27%)
General function (e.g. falls, mobility, home assessment)	77 (6%)	97 (5%)
Referral source [n (%)]*		
Hospital	243 (19%)	279 (15%)
Medical practitioner	412 (33%)	673 (36%)
Self/relative/carer	146 (12%)	151 (8%)
Community service provider	450 (36%)	757 (41%)
First discipline appointment n (%)		
Physiotherapist	695 (56%)	1333 (72%)
Occupational therapist	64 (5%)	70 (4%)
Speech pathologist	179 (14%)	96 (5%)
Nurse	238 (19%)	241 (13%)
Medical specialist	62 (5%)	106 (6%)
Social worker	9 (1%)	6 (< 1%)
Dietician	5 (< 1%)	9 (< 1%)

*One patient with missing data in each group

Table 2 Characteristics of participating sites

Site characteristics	Number of sites n = 8
Classification (n)	
Community health service	4
Multidisciplinary SAC clinic	3
Allied Health Outpatient service	1
Service size (clinical EFT) (median, IQR)	2.7 (1.5–3.3)
Primary catchment area	
Rural	2
Metropolitan	4
Mixed	2
Disciplines represented (n)	
Single-discipline service	3
2–3 disciplines	4
> 3 disciplines	1
Target age group (n)	
Paediatric	3
Adult	4
Mixed	1
Primary condition (n)	
Continence	2
Neurological	1
Developmental disorders	3
Mixed (ortho/neuro/general frailty)	2
Stability of demand	
No substantial change (< 10% difference, year 1 to year 2)	5
25–50% increase	1
50–75% increase	2

Stability of demand was calculated by comparing the number of referrals received from Sept. to Nov. in 2015 (all sites pre intervention) and the same period in 2016 (with each site in either the implementation or post implementation period)

Implementation of the intervention

The intervention was implemented as planned at each of the eight sites. The mean waiting time of the last 20 patients to be seen at the end of the implementation phase for each site was 33% lower than the mean waiting time for the first 20 patients referred at the start of the implementation phase. This suggests that short-term waitlist reduction strategies (the first component of the intervention) had some effect. A variety of methods, alone or in combination, were used to reduce the numbers of waiting patients during the implementation phase, including extra hours for existing staff (5 sites), additional administrative hours to manage bookings and audit the waitlist (4 sites), employment of additional temporary clinical and/or administrative staff (4 sites) and contracting private service providers (1 site). On average, the investment in waitlist reduction strategies at each site was equivalent to 5% of the annual salary budget (mean AUD$9000) at each site over the 12-week implementation period (range 0.5 to 10%).

Effect of the intervention: waiting time

The intervention resulted in a 33.7% mean reduction in waiting time until first appointment (IRR = 0.663, 95% CI 0.516 to 0.852, $P = 0.001$) (Table 3). Waiting time decreased from a median of 42 days (IQR 19 to 86) in the control period to a median of 24 days (IQR 13 to 48) in the intervention period. The reduction in waiting time during the intervention period was observed to be accompanied by a reduction in variability in waiting time; there appeared to be fewer patients waiting long periods in the intervention period compared with the control period (Fig. 2). Age and gender were significant covariates (age: IRR = 0.997, 95% CI 0.995 to 0.998, $P < 0.001$; gender: IRR = 0.931, 95% CI 0.883 to 0.982, $P = 0.008$), with the mean waiting time estimated to decrease 0.3%

Table 3 The effect of STAT on time from referral to first appointment (primary outcome)

	Intervention N = 1861	Control N = 1252	Adj ratio (95% CI)	ICC
Waiting time, *days*				
Mean (SD)	35.6 (33.6)	60.0 (55.2)	IRR 0.663 (0.516 to 0.852)	0.058
Median (IQR)	24 (13–48)	42 (19–86)		

IRR incident rate ratio, *ICC* intra-cluster correlation coefficient, *Adj ratio* adjusted ratio indicates that other factors, such as potential confounders, have been included in the model

per year of increasing age (i.e. older patients were more likely to have shorter waiting times) and, on average, males had an estimated 6.9% lower waiting times than females. Both of these covariates were further tested for interactions with the intervention. Neither interactions were significant suggesting that intervention effects did not significantly differ with respect to gender or age. The findings from the sensitivity analysis were similar in regard to statistical significance and hence not reported further.

Effect of intervention: secondary outcomes

There were no differences in the total number of appointments in the first 12 weeks and the number of days from the first to the second appointment between the intervention and control periods (Table 4). There was little difference in the observed proportion of patients discharged in the first 12 weeks (approximately 50%). However, taking account of clustering, there were reduced odds that patients during the intervention period would be discharged in the first 12 weeks.

Patients in the intervention period were more likely to miss a scheduled appointment compared to patients in the control period (OR 1.557, 95% CI 1.019 to 2.222). This finding was consistent with observations that the rate of missed appointments increased from 11% in the control period to 16% in the intervention period.

Regarding patient outcomes, there was no difference between the intervention and control periods for the likelihood of having an unplanned hospital admission within 6 months after the first outpatient appointment.

Discussion

The STAT model (Specific Timely Appointments for Triage) is designed to reduce waiting times for community outpatient services by booking patients directly into protected assessment appointments and combining triage with initial management as an alternative to a waiting list and triage system. A constant rate of patient flow is maintained and calculated to match the rate of referral, and service providers are encouraged to make priority decisions about ongoing treatment in the context of demand. This is the first time that this model has been trialled on a broad scale with multiple services. Findings suggest that the STAT model accounted for a 34% reduction in waiting time after controlling for clustering by site, similar to results of pilot trials conducted in community rehabilitation (42% reduction in waiting time) [22] and physiotherapy outpatients (22% reduction in waiting time) [25]. Thus, this is a feasible way to reduce waiting time across a broad range of community outpatient services, resulting in improved access to care and increased patient flow.

Reductions in waiting time achieved with STAT also appear to be comparable with other patient flow initiatives reported in community outpatient settings, although direct comparison is difficult due to heterogeneity in the ways in which wait times are measured. For example, there was a 23% reduction in median waiting time for a prosthetics clinic through changing scheduling to a modified walk-in system, rather than scheduled appointments [24]; Lynch et al. achieved a 70% reduction in the number of people on a waiting list for mental health services with an intervention that addressed the residual waitlist in combination with new approaches to treatment and triage [23]; and Maddison et al. described a reduction in waiting time for musculoskeletal services despite an increase in referrals through creation of a back pain pathway [34]. In contrast to these studies that all described interventions developed specifically for the services in which they were conducted, the current trial provides evidence of a structured approach that can be used to reduce waiting time across a broad range of settings.

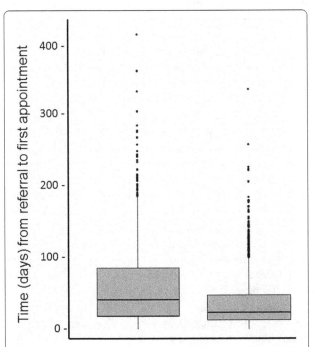

Fig. 2 Waiting time for control (left) and intervention (right) periods. Median represented by bar, 25th and 75th percentiles represented by box and upper and lower quartiles represented by whiskers

Table 4 The effect of STAT on secondary outcomes

	Intervention $n = 1861$	Control $n = 1252$	Adj ratio (95% CI)	ICC
Appointments missed per patient, n				
Mean (SD)	0.5 (0.7)	0.4 (0.9)	IRR 1.18 (1.04 to 1.35)	0.01
Median (IQR)	0 (0–1)	0 (0–1)		
Time from the 1st to 2nd appointment, *days*, n				
Mean (SD)	28.5 (18.5)	28.8 (18.5)	IRR 1.03 (0.98 to 1.09)	0.03
Median (IQR)	23 (13–42)	21 (14–39)		
Appointments in first 12 weeks, n				
Mean (SD)	2.4 (2.1)	2.1 (1.7)	IRR 0.99 (0.93 to 1.05)	0.01
Median (IQR)	2 (1–3)	2 (1–3)		
Patients discharged at 12 weeks, %	50.7	48.5	OR: 0.77 (0.60 to 0.99)	0.08
Unplanned admission days, n				
Mean (SD)	0.4 (4.0)	0.3 (3.5)	IRR 1.33 (0.49 to 3.59)	0.00
Median (IQR)	0 (0–0)	0 (0–0)		
Proportion of patients with unplanned hospital admissions within 6 months, %	2.3	2.7	OR 1.039 (0.51 to 2.13)	0.24

IRR incident rate ratio, *OR* odds ratio, *ICC* intra-cluster correlation coefficient, *Adj ratio* adjusted ratio indicates that other factors, such as potential confounders, have been included in the model

Stability of demand is an important element in the effectiveness and sustainability of the STAT model. Similar to the Advanced Access developed for use in primary care [21], STAT is based partly on the observation that many services have a relatively stable demand, indicated by a waitlist that shows little variation in length over time. Patients are therefore entering the service at a similar rate, but always several weeks or months behind. If the backlog can be cleared and patients brought into a service at a rate that is consistent with the rate of demand, it follows that the service should be able to maintain patient flow without a waiting list developing. However, a sustained increase in demand is one notable risk to the model's success. This was observed in the current trial as, despite all sites recruited to the trial having reported reasonably stable waiting lists over the previous 2 years, data from two of the sites showed an increase in referrals of more than 50% over the equivalent period in the first compared with the second year of the project, and another site experienced an increase of 25–50%. Despite this, substantial reductions in waiting times were still observed across the eight sites in the trial. This implies that efficiencies driven by STAT may be able to compensate for some increase in demand, but it is likely that a point is reached where additional strategies (such as tightening eligibility criteria or increasing supply) are needed to address the imbalance between supply and demand to achieve ongoing reductions in waiting time. It is also possible that in some services reduced waiting time may stimulate demand, leading to an increase in people seeking the service [1].

In addition to reductions in waiting time, another important outcome was the observed reduction in variability of wait time (Fig. 2). Consistent with a previous pilot study evaluating the STAT model in physiotherapy outpatients [25], the greatest benefits of this intervention appear to have come to those who were previously waiting the longest. This reduction in variability may provide an explanation for how STAT was effective in reducing waiting time overall. This finding is important, as one of the criticisms of traditional waiting lists and triage systems is the risk that low priority patients are continually pushed down the list by those with higher priority ratings, sometimes to the point where they never get seen [8].

The intra-cluster correlation of 0.05 observed for the primary outcome of waiting time was substantially higher than the estimate of 0.01 that was used to determine the sample size in the protocol [27]. This suggests that there was a higher degree of variability between the clusters than originally anticipated and that the impact of the intervention varied to some degree across sites. Given the diversity of sites included in the trial, it is not surprising that there may be site-specific factors that influence the success of the model. The STAT model requires a significant shift in the way that clinicians prioritise their workload, and response to change is likely to have differed to some degree across sites. It is possible also that the STAT model may be more applicable to some settings than others. The planned exploration of the perceptions of key stakeholders at sites where STAT was implemented using qualitative methods will provide insights on the human and service factors that influenced success.

One component of the STAT model is a one-off strategy to reduce the existing backlog prior to implementing the model. A small investment of resources was allocated to each site to facilitate this, and it could be argued that the observed reductions in waiting time were simply a reflection of short-term changes directly related to those additional resources. However, previous literature has shown that single injections of resources, without changes to service delivery, are unlikely to make a sustainable difference to waiting times [35, 36]. STAT is also consistent with other waiting time initiatives that have advocated approaches combining one-off backlog reduction strategies followed by the implementation of patient flow interventions [21, 24]. In the current trial, a comparison of mean waiting times for a small sample of consecutive patients entering the service immediately before and after the waitlist reduction strategies provides some indication of their impact. The 33% reduction in waiting time observed at the conclusion of implementation of targeted waitlist reduction strategies was consistent with the 34% reduction measured across the entire trial. This would suggest that the initial gains made during the backlog reduction strategies were maintained by the STAT model, regardless of the timing of the intervention and relative length of the follow-up period within the stepped wedge design, which continued for up to 10 months.

One perceived risk of an intervention that allows patient flow into a service at a steady rate is the possibility that a "hidden" waitlist is created, where patients receive a first appointment promptly but then wait for a second appointment. The current trial showed no difference in the time from first to second appointment when considering the data across all sites. This finding suggests that concerns about secondary delays were unfounded and that clinicians were prioritising second appointments equally.

There was an increase in the proportion of patients who failed to attend at least one appointment in the intervention period, which was surprising given that failure to attend rates have previously been negatively associated with waiting time [13]. A possible explanation is that patients in the intervention group were given information about their appointment time soon after referral rather than being placed on a waiting list for an interim period. Although overall waiting time reduced during the intervention period, the time between being given an appointment and the appointment itself increased. For example, where previously a patient might wait 6 weeks to receive notification of an appointment 1 week later, with STAT this same patient receives notification after 1 week for an appointment 3 weeks later. Forgotten appointments become more likely and could be mitigated by strategies such as SMS reminders [37].

This trial was conducted in eight community outpatient sites that differed from each other in a number of ways. They provided a range of services to patients ranging from infants to the frail elderly, some treated chronic conditions and others provided short-term follow-up to acute injuries. All sites, however, shared the common features of providing non-emergency services to patients over a series of outpatient appointments. These observations suggest that the STAT model is likely to be generalisable to a wide range of outpatient services provided that they have these features. STAT encourages clinicians to change the focus of decisions about patient priority; rather than triage decisions influencing access to the service, prioritisation is instead directed at the rationing of resources for ongoing treatment. In order for this to work, there needs to be some flexibility in the way that services are delivered. For example, clinicians working in these types of services can choose to see patients less frequently, for shorter appointments, or move patients from individual to group sessions during times of high demand. Results of this trial suggest that STAT is likely to be applicable to any non-emergency outpatient service with stable demand and flexibility in service delivery decisions, regardless of the type of service provided.

A major strength of this trial is the use of a stepped wedge cluster randomised controlled trial design, an emerging trial design in health service delivery evaluations that offers several benefits over other parallel cluster designs [26, 38]. The rigour of this method and the involvement of multiple sites offers clear advantages over other commonly used methods for evaluation of patient flow or waiting list interventions, such as single-site studies [23, 39], quality improvement methods [40, 41] or retrospective analyses of health service datasets [42, 43]. The ICC for the primary outcome of waiting time was larger than hypothesised in our sample size estimation ($\rho = 0.058$ versus $\rho = 0.01$) [27], possibly due to greater variability than expected between sites. There were many possible sources of variation, including differences between clinicians, management of each of the sites, socioeconomic characteristics of the patient population and complexity of patient needs that were not measured in the trial. Despite this, all sites provided services for patients living in the community and the analysis took account of clustering. Further adequately powered studies could investigate the effect of variation, in particular the effect of STAT on subgroups of patients, such as those from lower socioeconomic backgrounds and those with more complex health needs [44, 45].

The stepped wedge design of this trial meant that the lengths of control and intervention data collection varied between sites. As a result, there were some differences in the characteristics of patients in the pre and post intervention data driven by differences between the services, but this was accounted for by clustering in the analysis. This aspect of the design also meant that the last site to receive the intervention had a follow-up period of only 3 months. It is possible that this was not long enough to measure the true effect of the intervention. Conversely, over a longer follow-up period, sustainability of the intervention may come into question, as the effect of the initial injection of resources wears off and support from the research team is withdrawn. The relatively short follow-up time (particularly for the last site to receive the intervention) is a limitation of the current trial, and further research is required to look at longer-term outcomes. A further challenge of the trial design was that it provided for little flexibility in the timing of implementation of the intervention, reducing backlogs and embedding new processes into practice. It is therefore likely that greater benefits may be achieved when implementing STAT without these limitations.

There were some minor deviations from the protocol due to the characteristics of the services selected for inclusion and availability of the required data. We intended to collect data on the number of patients on the waiting list at key time points for each service to assess the fidelity of the implementation strategies to reduce backlog at each site. It was not possible to collect these data across all sites due to differences in the way that waiting list data were recorded. Instead, we analysed waiting time for a sample of 20 consecutive patients at each time point rather than counting the number of patients on the waiting list. We also intended to analyse the number of group and individual appointments across sites and time periods to see whether the new model of care led to increased use of group appointments, as observed in a previous trial [22]; however, this was not necessary as the majority of the sites selected for inclusion in the trial did not offer group appointments as a treatment option.

Conclusion

A model of access and triage based on evidence-based strategies known to improve patient flow was successfully implemented on a broad scale, involving eight community outpatient services. Waiting time was reduced by 34%, and waiting time variability also decreased substantially, suggesting those people previously waiting the longest were likely to benefit most. This trial also demonstrated that evaluation of patient flow initiatives previously limited to single-site studies, quality improvement projects or retrospective analysis of health service data can be conducted using rigorous research methods to produce high-quality evidence for health care service providers.

Abbreviations

SACS: Sub-acute ambulatory care services; STAT: Specific Timely Appointments for Triage

Funding

This trial was funded by the National Health and Medical Research Council of Australia with a *Partnerships for Better Health Grant* (APP 1076777), with contributions from industry partners Eastern Health (in-kind) and the Victorian Department of Health and Human Services (direct and in-kind).

Acknowledgements

Nil

Authors' contributions

KH and NT led the inception of the project and development of the proposal, provided oversight for implementation of the intervention and collection of data and drafted the manuscript. SL, JW, BK, LK, MO and MK also contributed to the project design, interpretation of findings and editing of the manuscript. LP led the analysis of data and interpretation of findings. DS and AL implemented the intervention, collected data and contributed to the manuscript. All authors read and approved the final manuscript.

Competing interests

The authors declare that they have no competing interests.

Author details

Eastern Health, Level 2/5 Arnold Street, Box Hill, VIC 3128, Australia. [2]La Trobe University, Kingsbury Drive, Bundoora, VIC 3086, Australia. [3]Deakin University, 221 Burwood Highway, Burwood, VIC 3125, Australia. [4]University of Plymouth, Drake Circus, Plymouth, Devon PL4 8AA, UK. [5]Victorian Department of Health and Human Services, 50 Lonsdale Street, Melbourne, VIC 3000, Australia.

References

1. Rotstein GC, Alter D. Where does the waiting list begin? A short review of the dynamics and organization of modern waiting lists. Soc Sci Med. 2006; 62:3157–60.
2. Lambe S, Washington DL, Fink A, Laouri M, Liu H, Scura Fosse J, et al. Waiting times in California's emergency departments. Ann Emerg Med. 2003;41:35–44.
3. Kennedy J, Rhodes K, Walls CA, Asplin BR. Access to emergency care: restricted by long waiting times and cost and coverage concerns. Ann Emerg Med. 2004;43:567–73.
4. Oudhoff JP, Timmermans DR, Rietberg M, Knol DL, van der Wal G. The acceptability of waiting times for elective general surgery and the appropriateness of prioritising patients. BMC Health Serv Res. 2007;7:32.
5. Walters JL, Mackintosh S, Sheppard L. The journey to total hip or knee replacement. Aust Health Rev. 2012;36:130–5.
6. Lynch ME, Campbell FA, Clark AJ, Dunbar MJ, Goldstein D, Peng P, et al. Waiting for treatment for chronic pain - a survey of existing benchmarks: toward establishing evidence-based benchmarks for medically acceptable waiting times. Pain Res Manag. 2007;12:245–8.
7. Rastall M, Fashanu B. Hospital physiotherapy outpatient department waiting lists: a survey. Physiother. 2001;87:563–72.
8. Raymond MH, Demers L, Feldman DE. Waiting list management practices for home-care occupational therapy in the province of Quebec, Canada. Health Soc Care Community. 2015;24:154–64.
9. Harding KE, Robertson N, Snowdon DA, Watts JJ, Karimi L, O'Reilly M, et al. Are wait lists inevitable in subacute ambulatory and community health services? A qualitative analysis. Aust Health Rev. 2017;42:93–9.
10. Johnson DA, Sacrinty MT, Gomadam PS, Mehta HJ, Brady MM, Douglas CJ, et al. Effect of early enrollment on outcomes in cardiac rehabilitation. Am J Cardiol. 2014;114:1908–11.
11. Zigenfus GC, Yin J, Giang GM, Fogarty WT. Effectiveness of early physical therapy in the treatment of acute low back musculoskeletal disorders. J Occup Environ Med. 2000;42:35–9.
12. Harding KE, Leggat S, Bowers B, Stafford M, Taylor NF. Perspectives of clinicians and patients following introduction of a new model of triage that reduced waiting time: a qualitative analysis. Aust Health Rev. 2013;33:324–30.
13. Russell KL, Holloway TM, Brum M, Caruso V, Chessex C, Grace SL. Cardiac rehabilitation wait times: effect on enrolment. J Card Rehab Prev. 2011;31:373–7.
14. Westin AM, Barksdale CL, Stephan SH. The effect of waiting time on youth engagement to evidence based treatments. Com Ment Health J. 2014;50: 221–8.

15. Green L. Queueing analysis in health care. In: Hall R, editor. Patient flow: reducing delay in healthcare delivery. 2nd ed. Boston: Springer; 2013. p. 361–84.
16. Palvannan RK, Teow KL. Queueing for healthcare. J Med Syst. 2012;36:541–7.
17. Kreindler SA. Watching your wait: evidence-informed strategies for reducing health care wait times. Qual Manag Health Care. 2008;17:128–35.
18. Harding KE, Taylor NF, Leggat S. Do triage systems in healthcare improve patient flow? A systematic review of the literature. Aust Health Rev. 2011;35: 371–83.
19. Kreindler SA. Policy strategies to reduce waits for elective care: a synthesis of international evidence. Br Med Bull. 2010;95:7–32.
20. Terris J, Leman P, O'connor N, Wood R. Making an IMPACT on emergency department flow: improving patient processing assisted by consultant at triage. Emerg Med J. 2004;21:537–41.
21. Murray M, Berwick DM. Advanced access: reducing waiting and delays in primary care. JAMA. 2003;289:1035–40.
22. Harding KE, Leggat S, Bowers B, Stafford M, Taylor NF. Reducing waiting time for community rehabilitation services: a controlled before and after trial. Arch Phys Med Rehab. 2013;94:23–31.
23. Lynch G, Hedderman E. Tackling a long waiting list in a child and adolescent mental health service. Irish J Psych Med. 2006;23:103–6.
24. Jarl G, Hermansson L. A modified walk-in system versus scheduled appointments in a secondary-care prosthetic and orthotic clinic. Prosthetics Orthot Int. 2017:309364617728120. https://doi.org/10.1177/0309364617728120. [Epub ahead of print]
25. Harding K, Bottrell J. Specific Timely Appointments for Triage (STAT) reduced waiting lists in an outpatient physiotherapy service. Physiother. 2015;102:345–50.
26. Hemming K, Haines TP, Chilton PJ, Girling AJ, Lilford RJ. The stepped wedge cluster randomised trial: rationale, design, analysis, and reporting. BMJ. 2015; 350:h391.
27. Harding KE, Watts JJ, Karimi L, O'Reilly M, Kent B, Kotis M, et al. Improving access for community health and sub-acute outpatient services: protocol for a stepped wedge cluster randomised controlled trial. BMC Health Serv Res. 2016;16:364.
28. Victorian Department of Health. Health independence programs guidelines. (2008) https://www2.health.vic.gov.au/hospitals-and-health-services/patient-care/rehabilitation-complex-care/health-independence-program/hip-guidelines. Accessed 15 Jan 2018.
29. Woertman W, de Hoop E, Moerbeek M, Zuidema S, Gerritsen D, Teerenstra S. Stepped wedge designs could reduce the required sample size in cluster randomized trials. J Clin Epid. 2013;66:752–8.
30. Goldstein H. Multilevel statistical models. London: 3rd ed: Arnold; 2003.
31. Murray M, Bodenheimer T, Rittenhouse D, Grumbach K. Improving timely access to primary care: case studies of the advanced access model. JAMA. 2003;289:1042–6.
32. Davey C, Hargreaves J, Thompson JA, Copas AJ, Beard E, Lewis JJ, et al. Analysis and reporting of stepped wedge randomised controlled trials: synthesis and critical appraisal of published studies, 2010 to 2014. Trials. 2015;16:358.
33. R Core Team R. A language and environment for statistical computing. Vienna: R Foundation for Statistical Computing; 2017.
34. Maddison P, Jones J, Breslin A, Barton C, Fleur J, Lewis R, et al. Improved access and targeting of musculoskeletal services in northwest Wales: targeted early access to musculoskeletal services (TEAMS) programme. BMJ. 2004;329:1325–7.
35. Kenis P. Waiting lists in Dutch healthcare: an analysis from an organization theoretical perspective. J Health Org Manag. 2006;20:294–308.
36. Hanning M. Maximum waiting-time guarantee - an attempt to reduce waiting lists in Sweden. Health Policy. 1996;36:17–35.
37. Taylor N, Bottrell J, Lawler K, Benjamin D. Mobile phone short message service (SMS) reminders can reduce non-attendance in physical therapy outpatient clinics: a randomized controlled trial. Arch Phys Med Rehab. 2012;93:21–6.
38. Lamb SE. The case for stepped-wedge studies: a trial of falls prevention. Lancet. 2015;385:2556–7.
39. Titus D, Morris N. Reducing wait times to access outpatient physiotherapy. Physiother. 2011;97:eS1556.
40. Ho ET. Improving waiting time and operational clinic flow in a tertiary diabetes center. BMJ Qual Improv Rep. 2014;2(2). https://doi.org/10.1136/bmjquality.u201918.w1006. eCollection 2014.
41. Vose C, Reichard C, Pool S, Snyder M, Burmeister D. Using LEAN to improve a segment of emergency department flow. J Nurs Adm. 2014;44:558–63.
42. Sobolev B, Brown P, Zelt D, Kuramoto L. Waiting time in relation to wait-list size at registration: statistical analysis of a waiting-list registry. Clin Invest Med. 2004;27:298–305.
43. Vermeulen MJ, Stukel TA, Guttmann A, Rowe BH, Zwarenstein M, Golden B, et al. Evaluation of an emergency department lean process improvement program to reduce length of stay. Ann Emerg Med. 2014;64:427–38.
44. Fitzpatrick R, Norquist JM, Reeves BC, Morris RW, Murray DW, Gregg PJ. Equity and need when waiting for total hip replacement surgery. J Eval Clin Pract. 2004;10:3–9.
45. Johar M, Jones G, Keane MP, Savage E, Stavrunova O. Discrimination in a universal health system: explaining socioeconomic waiting time gaps. J Health Econ. 2013;32:181–94.

Medications that reduce emergency hospital admissions: an overview of systematic reviews and prioritisation of treatments

Niklas Bobrovitz[1,2*], Carl Heneghan[1,2], Igho Onakpoya[1,2], Benjamin Fletcher[1], Dylan Collins[1,3], Alice Tompson[1,4], Joseph Lee[1], David Nunan[1,2], Rebecca Fisher[1,5], Brittney Scott[6,7], Jack O'Sullivan[1,2], Oliver Van Hecke[1], Brian D. Nicholson[1], Sarah Stevens[1], Nia Roberts[8] and Kamal R. Mahtani[1,2]

Abstract

Background: Rates of emergency hospitalisations are increasing in many countries, leading to disruption in the quality of care and increases in cost. Therefore, identifying strategies to reduce emergency admission rates is a key priority. There have been large-scale evidence reviews to address this issue; however, there have been no reviews of medication therapies, which have the potential to reduce the use of emergency health-care services. The objectives of this study were to review systematically the evidence to identify medications that affect emergency hospital admissions and prioritise therapies for quality measurement and improvement.

Methods: This was a systematic review of systematic reviews. We searched MEDLINE, PubMed, the Cochrane Database of Systematic Reviews & Database of Abstracts of Reviews of Effects, Google Scholar and the websites of ten major funding agencies and health charities, using broad search criteria. We included systematic reviews of randomised controlled trials that examined the effect of any medication on emergency hospital admissions among adults. We assessed the quality of reviews using AMSTAR. To prioritise therapies, we assessed the quality of trial evidence underpinning meta-analysed effect estimates and cross-referenced the evidence with clinical guidelines.

Results: We identified 140 systematic reviews, which included 1968 unique randomised controlled trials and 925,364 patients. Reviews contained 100 medications tested in 47 populations. We identified high-to moderate-quality evidence for 28 medications that reduced admissions. Of these medications, 11 were supported by clinical guidelines in the United States, the United Kingdom and Europe. These 11 therapies were for patients with heart failure (angiotensin-converting-enzyme inhibitors, angiotensin II receptor blockers, aldosterone receptor antagonists and digoxin), stable coronary artery disease (intensive statin therapy), asthma exacerbations (early inhaled corticosteroids in the emergency department and anticholinergics), chronic obstructive pulmonary disease (long-acting muscarinic antagonists and long-acting beta-2 adrenoceptor agonists) and schizophrenia (second-generation antipsychotics and depot/maintenance antipsychotics).

(Continued on next page)

---

* Correspondence: niklas.bobrovitz@phc.ox.ac.uk
[1]Nuffield Department of Primary Care Health Sciences, University of Oxford, Radcliffe Observatory Quarter, Woodstock Road, Oxford OX2 6GG, United Kingdom
[2]Centre for Evidence-Based Medicine, University of Oxford, Oxford, United Kingdom
Full list of author information is available at the end of the article

> (Continued from previous page)
>
> **Conclusions:** We identified 11 medications supported by strong evidence and clinical guidelines that could be considered in quality monitoring and improvement strategies to help reduce emergency hospital admission rates. The findings are relevant to health systems with a large burden of chronic disease and those managing increasing pressures on acute health-care services.
>
> **Keywords:** Hospital admissions, Unplanned admissions, Emergency admissions, Unscheduled admissions, Pharmacology, Medication, Drug, Systematic review, Overview, Clinical guidelines

Background

Emergency hospital admissions place a major burden on patients and health-care systems. Large increases in emergency admissions can cause delays and cancellations of elective procedures, prolong emergency department waiting times and increase the risk of hospital-acquired infections [1–5]. Emergency admissions, which comprise 10% of the total health-care budget in some countries, also have significant financial effects [6, 7]. Rates of emergency hospital admissions are rising in many countries, creating emergency-care crises [6, 8, 9].

Identifying interventions that reduce emergency hospital admissions is, therefore, a priority for health services globally, and there have been large-scale evidence reviews to address this [10, 11]. However, a major gap in these systematic assessments has been the omission of medication therapy, which has the potential to reduce use of emergency health-care services. For example, a systematic review of randomised controlled trials (RCTs) has shown that aldosterone receptor antagonists reduce emergency admissions for heart failure by 21% over 20 months [12]. Despite these robust data, there have been no comprehensive reviews to identify and compare medications that effectively and safely prevent hospital admissions in different patient populations. Systematically identifying these beneficial medications is the first step towards monitoring and improving their use in practice. Given that there are existing mechanisms for quality measurement and improvement of clinical practices in many health systems, monitoring and improving medication use may be a feasible and efficient strategy to alleviate some of the burden of emergency admissions compared with the lengthy and expensive process of developing, testing and implementing new complex interventions.

The objectives of this study were to review systematically the evidence to identify medications that affect hospital admissions and prioritise therapies for quality improvement by assessing the quality of evidence and cross-referencing the findings with clinical guidelines.

Methods

Protocol and registration

We developed the methods using guidance on systematic reviews and overviews described in the *Cochrane Handbook of Systematic Reviews of Interventions* [13]. The protocol was registered (PROSPERO: CRD42014014779) [14] and published [15]. In our protocol, we specified that we would search for any type of intervention. This overview focuses on medications. Our subsequent overviews will describe the evidence for other types of interventions.

Types of reviews

We included systematic reviews of RCTs published in English that examined the effect of any medication on emergency hospital admissions in adults (16 years or older). We included reviews that searched two or more electronic databases and assessed and reported the quality of included studies. We defined a medication as any administered chemical or biological product. We included only reviews that reported at least one meta-analysed effect estimate for emergency hospital admissions that was not part of a composite measure. We defined an emergency hospital admission as an unanticipated admission or readmission to hospital that occurred at short notice because of a perceived need for immediate health care [16]. We did not consider admission to an emergency department or an observational unit to be a hospital admission. We excluded studies reporting only scheduled or elective hospital admissions. We excluded superseded Cochrane reviews. We excluded non-Cochrane reviews if all the RCT data on hospital admissions were included in a more recent review of the same intervention and patients. When two reviews reported identical clinical trial data, we selected the review that reported more detailed information, as judged by two of the authors through discussion and consensus (NB and IO).

Search strategy and study selection

We searched MEDLINE (OvidSP), PubMed, the Cochrane Database of Systematic Reviews & Database of Abstracts of Reviews of Effects, Google Scholar and the websites of ten national funding agencies and health charities, using broad search criteria from inception to February 2016. The search strategy was developed by a library and information scientist (NR). The websites of national funding agencies and health charities were identified using Google searches and by our academic-clinician co-authors. We also contacted experts in emergency admissions and reviewed the reference lists of included reviews to identify additional studies. Details of the search can be found in Additional file 1: Table S1 in the online supplement. Three authors (NB, IO and BF) independently screened titles, abstracts and full-text articles for inclusion. Discrepancies in article inclusion were resolved by discussion. Inter-rater reliability for agreement between authors for title/abstract screening and full-text screening was quantified using Cohen's kappa statistic .

Data extraction and quality assessment of reviews

In pairs, we independently extracted information in duplicate on the characteristics of the reviews and assessed their quality using the Assessing the Methodological Quality of Systematic Reviews (AMSTAR) tool [17]. We have provided summary AMSTAR scores when describing review characteristics to give a broad indication of quality; however, full results are also provided as summary scores may obscure important strengths or weaknesses [17]. One minor revision to the AMSTAR tool was made: for item 2 (was there duplicate study selection and data extraction?) reviews did not score 'yes' if data selection or extraction was done by one reviewer and checked by another. Information on specific treatment comparisons in the reviews was extracted by one author (NB) and verified by a second (IO, BF, DC, AT, JL, RF, DN, BS, JO, OH, BN or SS). Discrepancies in extracted information or quality assessment scores were resolved by discussion. All reviews and each extracted treatment comparison were assigned a unique identifying number (e.g. review 100 or comparisons 100a and 100b).

Prioritising therapies through quality assessment of meta-analysed effect estimates and cross-referencing treatments with clinical guidelines

We assessed the quality of meta-analysed effect estimates showing statistically significant effects on admissions. We used criteria from the Grading of Recommendations Assessment, Development and Evaluation (GRADE) Working Group [18]. Using these ratings, we prioritised therapies based on the strength of their evidence base. Quality assessments were completed by one reviewer (NB) and verified by a second (DN). Two generalist clinicians (JL and IO) provided judgements for the indirectness domain, which included assessments of the comparability of populations, interventions, comparators and outcomes between studies and of the applicability of the body of studies to the aims of this overview.

A minimal important threshold in effect had to be defined to utilise the GRADE method, specifically, the imprecision domain [18]. To our knowledge, there is no consensus on what defines a minimal important threshold for hospital admissions. The goal of this research is to manage rising rates of emergency hospital admissions; therefore, we picked a threshold that would achieve this: a 3% relative risk reduction. This threshold is equivalent to the population-adjusted average year-on-year increase in admissions in the UK over the past five years (2011–2016) [9, 19]. The UK is facing the worst emergency-care crisis of any high- or middle-income country that we are aware of. If we were able to identify and implement interventions for every patient group that reduced admission rates by 3%, then the overall admissions rate would cease to rise in the UK. In countries where annual increases are less than 3%, which includes most other high- and middle-income countries facing emergency-care pressures, these interventions would operate to reduce the annual rate of admissions.

We assessed the quality of subgroup effect estimates only if the subgroup analyses were pre-specified and met one or more of the following criteria:

- The subgroup estimate was calculated to explain the presence of substantial heterogeneity in the summary estimate ($I^2 \geq 50\%$ or chi-squared $P < 0.1$) [20].
- The subgroup estimate was calculated from a subset of trials at low risk of bias (as assessed by the original review authors).
- The subgroup estimate showed a significant reduction or increase in hospital admissions, while the summary estimate found no effect.

We considered high and moderate GRADE ratings to represent strong evidence, since the effect estimates are unlikely to change if additional studies are conducted [18, 21].

To prioritise the therapies further, we cross-referenced the list of medications supported by high- or moderate-quality evidence with clinical guidelines. We conducted this analysis to ensure that the overall balance of benefit to harm for the therapies had been judged acceptable by key health-care stakeholders. We first cross-referenced the list with National Institute for Health and Care Excellence (NICE) clinical guidelines [22]. NICE is the largest UK-based organisation providing guidance on clinical care across all disciplines. It was selected based on a consensus among our academic-clinician co-authors. NICE recommends therapies based on their clinical appropriateness, safety, cost-effectiveness and feasibility as judged by clinical experts, health economists, administrators, regulators and patients [23]. We then cross-referenced the short list of NICE-recommended treatments with guidelines in Europe and America. We identified the most recent guidelines by searching the National Guideline Clearinghouse maintained by the Agency for Healthcare Research and Quality. If we could not find a relevant guideline, we then searched for national medical associations and professional societies providing guidance on the treatment for the patient population of interest. The following guidelines were selected from search results by consensus among our clinical-academic co-authors: European Society of Cardiology [24, 25], European Atherosclerosis Society [26], American Heart Association/American College of Cardiology [27–29], European Respiratory Society [30], American Thoracic Society [31], European Psychiatric Association [32] and the American Psychiatric Association [33]. To be considered guideline-based, the treatment must have been recommended by NICE and at least one of the American or European guidelines.

Data analysis

To standardise reporting, we used international classification systems. We described patient populations using the World Health Organization's International Statistical Classification of Diseases and Related Health Problems 10th Revision (WHO ICD-10) [34]. We classified medications using the WHO Anatomical Therapeutic Chemical (WHO ATC) classification system [35]. We used the disease definitions and relevant thresholds provided in the reviews, for example, the cut-off for reduced left ventricular ejection fraction in heart failure (i.e., 45%). When possible, we converted reported effect estimates into risk ratios (see Additional file 1: Table S2 for conversion methods) [36–39].

For significant effect estimates that underwent quality assessment, we calculated the number needed to treat to avoid one hospitalisation and the number needed to treat to cause one hospitalisation. For each estimate, we used the median control-group event rate from the RCTs in the meta-analysis [15, 33, 38–40]. When data on event rates were unclear or not reported by the review authors, we obtained the original RCTs and extracted the data.

We used Excel for data extraction and management. For the quantitative data analysis, we used STATA 14 [41]. The results are reported in accordance with PRISMA guidance [42].

Results

We screened 11,442 titles and abstracts and 1563 full text articles (Fig. 1). Of these, 140 systematic reviews met the inclusion criteria. Agreement between reviewers was good for both the title/abstract screen (kappa = 0.85, 95% confidence interval, CI 0.83 to 0.87) and full-text screen (kappa = 0.77, 95% CI 0.73 to 0.82). Complete references, detailed information and full AMSTAR results for each review are included in Additional file 1: Tables S3, S4 and S5.

Table 1 describes the summary characteristics of the 140 reviews. The median AMSTAR score for review quality was 8/11 (interquartile range 6 to 9). Review quality was most often downgraded because the review authors did not state their potential conflicts of interest (AMSTAR criterion 11).

The reviews included an underlying evidence base of 1968 unique RCTs (925,364 patients), of which 690 RCTs reported hospital admission outcomes for 577,604 patients. The number of RCTs underpinning the treatment comparisons ranged from 1 to 184 (median 3), with patient sample sizes ranging from 18 to 88,367 (median 1116). The reviews contained data on 100 unique medications tested in 47 patient populations (Additional file 1: Table S6). Altogether, 125 reviews (89%) examined therapies for patients with chronic diseases. Much of the evidence was for patients with circulatory diseases (53 reviews, 38%) or respiratory diseases (56 reviews, 40%). The most common conditions were heart failure (35 reviews, 25%), chronic obstructive pulmonary disease (COPD; 27 reviews, 19%), acute exacerbations of asthma (20 reviews, 14%) and chronic asthma (14 reviews, 10%). Hospital admissions were identified as a primary outcome in 61 of the reviews (44%). Seventy-eight reviews (56%) reported significantly fewer hospital admissions in intervention arms compared with control arms, while a small minority (8 reviews, 6%) reported significant increases because of the intervention.

Prioritised list of evidence- and guideline-based medications that significantly reduce emergency hospital admissions

From the 140 included reviews, we extracted 517 treatment comparisons that reported hospital admission outcomes (Fig. 2). All treatment comparisons are available in the online database supplement (Additional file 2: Database 1). Of the 517 comparisons, 159 had pooled effect estimates showing a statistically significant effect on hospital admissions. Using GRADE criteria, we identified high and moderate evidence for 28 medications that significantly reduced hospital admissions in 15 patient populations. Evidence summaries for all graded estimates showing a significant reduction in admissions are given in Additional file 1: Table S7.

Of the 28 medications with high- or moderate-quality evidence, 11 were supported by clinical guidelines from the United States, United Kingdom or Europe. Table 2 shows the evidence summaries for these therapies. These 11 medications were tested in 12 comparisons; aldosterone antagonists were tested in two different heart failure groups. Nine treatments were tested against a placebo and three against an active comparator.

There were seven treatments that reduced admissions from out-patient, day-procedure or community settings in patients with heart failure, stable coronary artery disease or stable COPD, while two treatments reduced admissions among patients with acute asthma in the

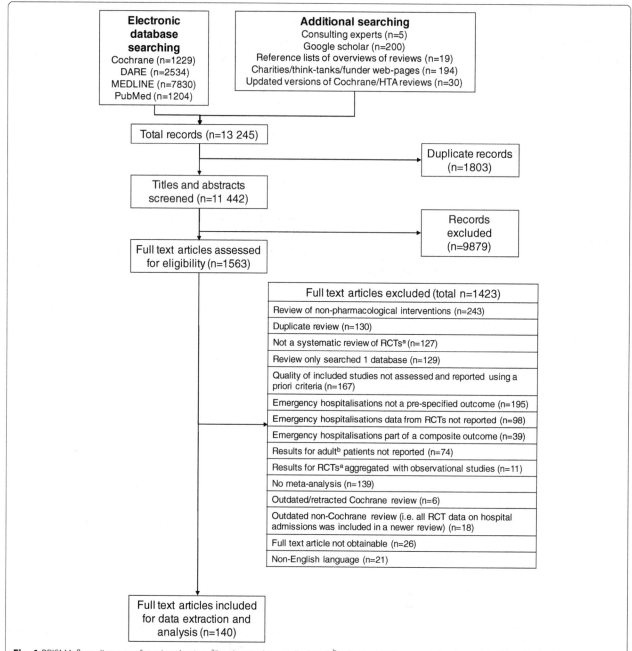

Fig. 1 PRISMA flow diagram of study selection. [a]Randomised controlled trial. [b]Individual RCTs were defined as adult if they had inclusion criteria of 16 years of age or older for participants. We considered results from a meta-analysis as adult if the included participants' mean age was 18 years or more across all included trials. RCT randomised controlled trial

emergency department, and two treatments reduced readmissions after index hospitalisation among patients with schizophrenia.

Information on the drugs, dosing, length of follow-up, ages and event rates from the RCTs that contributed data to the high- and moderate-quality effect estimates is listed in Additional file 1: Table S8. Information on the GRADE quality assessments for each estimate is presented in Additional file 1: Table S9.

Medications that increase admissions

While reviewing the evidence for medications that reduced admissions, we also identified high- and moderate-quality evidence for three therapies that significantly increased hospital admissions: cyclooxygenase-2 (COX-2) inhibitors in patients for whom non-steroidal anti-inflammatory drugs (NSAIDs) were indicated, intermittent antipsychotic drug therapy in patients with schizophrenia and fluticasone in patients with COPD (Table 3). Evidence summaries for

Table 1 Summary characteristics of included systematic reviews and the randomised controlled trial data captured by the reviews

Characteristic	Reviews n (%)
Review level information (n = 140)	
Cochrane reviews	49 (35)
Number of unique medications investigated[a]	100
Number of unique patient populations investigated[b]	47
Reviews focusing on medications for patients with chronic diseases	125 (89)
Patient population[c]	
Diseases of the respiratory system	56 (40)
Diseases of the circulatory system	53 (38)
Factors influencing health status and contact with health services[d]	8 (6)
Diseases of the digestive system	8 (6)
Mental and behavioural disorders	7 (5)
Diseases of the genitourinary system	5 (4)
Pregnancy, childbirth and puerperium	5 (4)
Endocrine, nutritional and metabolic diseases	5 (4)
Mixed patient populations	3 (2)
Multi-morbidity	2 (1)
Other[e]	4 (3)
Hospitalisation was a primary outcome	61 (44)
Review reported pooled effect estimates showing significant reductions in hospital admissions	78 (56)
AMSTAR score for review quality, median (IQR)	8 (6 to 9)
Review year of publication	
2010–2016	96 (69)
2000–2009	42 (30)
1991–1999	2 (1)
Randomised controlled trial (RCT) information	
Number of unique RCTs	1968
Number of unique patients	925,364
Number of unique RCTs reporting admissions data	690
Number of unique patients with admissions data	577,604
Number of patients per RCT reporting hospital admission outcomes, median (IQR)	190 (62 to 603)
Number of treatment comparisons reporting hospital admission outcomes	517

AMSTAR Assessing the Methodological Quality of Systematic Reviews, *IQR* interquartile range, *RCT* randomised controlled trial
[a]Unique at the level of pharmacological subgroup in the World Health Organization's Anatomical Therapeutic Chemical classification system
[b]Unique at the three-character coding level using the 10th revision of the World Health Organization's International Statistical Classification of Diseases and Related Health Problems (ICD-10)
[c]These specific classifications represent the summary level of coding in ICD-10
[d]For example, patients receiving day surgery
[e]Infection and parasitic disease (n = 1 review), diseases of the musculoskeletal system and connective tissue (n = 1 review), and diseases of the nervous system (n = 2 reviews)

graded estimates showing a significant increase in admissions are given in Additional file 1: Table S10. Information on the drugs, dosing, length of follow-up, ages and event rates from the RCTs that contributed data to the high- and moderate-quality effect estimates is listed in Additional file 1: Table S8. Information on the GRADE quality assessments for each estimate is presented in Additional file 1: Table S9.

Discussion

Summary of findings

We examined 140 reviews of 100 medications, and identified high- to moderate-quality evidence for 28 therapies that significantly reduced admissions in 15 different populations. Eleven of these therapies were supported by major clinical guidelines from the United States, the United Kingdom or Europe. We also identified high- and

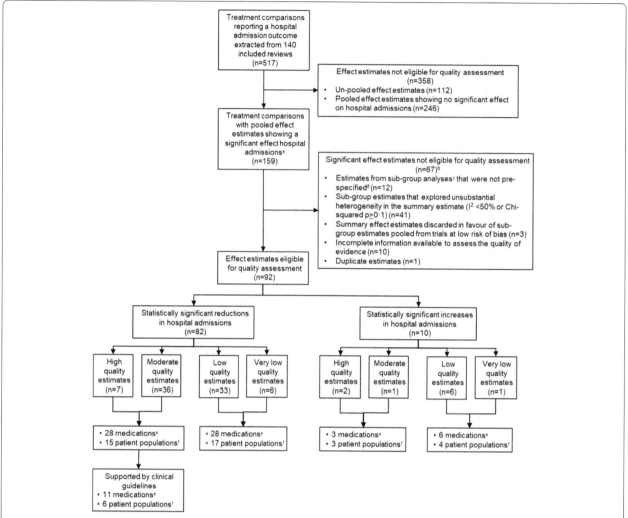

Fig. 2 Flow diagram of the process to identify effective medications supported by high- or moderate-quality evidence. [a]Statistically significant at the $p < 0.05$ level. [b]Estimates were for subgroup estimates that did not meet our criteria for quality assessment. [c]Subgroup or sensitivity analysis as defined by authors. [d]Pre-specified in the methods section of the review article. [e]Unique at the level of pharmacological subgroup in the World Health Organization's Anatomical Therapeutic Chemical classification system. [f]Unique at the three-character coding level using the World Health Organization's 10th revision of the International Statistical Classification of Diseases and Related Health Problems

moderate-quality evidence for three medications that increased admissions.

In the context of the literature

Previous reviews of interventions to reduce hospital admissions have focused on non-pharmacological initiatives [10, 43–45]. Our study, therefore, fills an important gap as the first systematic investigation of medications that affect hospital admissions. We mapped a large evidence base and prioritised therapies based on the quality of the evidence and support of clinical guidelines.

Our results complement a growing body of evidence about drug-related hospital admissions. Several systematic reviews of observational studies have shown that approximately 3% of all emergency hospitalisations are related to suspected adverse drug reactions and drug–drug interactions [46–51]. Drugs often associated with hospital admissions include antiplatelet drugs, diuretics, renin-angiotensin system blockers, NSAIDs and anticoagulants. However, the reviews have not considered the number of admissions these drugs help to avoid and therefore, have not provided evidence about their net effects on admissions. Our study complements this literature, as it shows a strong body of evidence supporting a beneficial reduction in admissions for renin-angiotensin system blockers [angiotensin-converting-enzyme (ACE) inhibitors and angiotensin II receptor blockers] and aldosterone receptor antagonists. We have also identified strong evidence for a harmful increase in cause-specific admissions due to heart failure from the use of COX2 inhibitors and pneumonia from the use of inhaled corticosteroids in COPD patients. Many of the other drugs

Table 2 Evidence- and guideline-based medications that reduce emergency hospital admissions

Author, Year[ID No.]	Patient population	Medication treatment	Control	Patients (RCTs)	Mean age[a]	Outcome and mean follow-up[b]	NNT (95% CI) RR (95% CI)	I²%	Quality of evidence[c]	Clinical guideline support America	UK	Europe
Reduces hospital admissions from out-patient, day-procedure or community settings												
Xie, 2016[8916a]	Heart failure with reduced left ejection fraction or left ventricular dysfunction	ACE inhibitors	Placebo	12,763 (5)	62 ± 4	HF hospitalisation at 32 months	NNT: 19 (16 to 25) RR: 0.71 (0.66 to 0.78)	0	Moderate	AHA, ACC	NICE	ESC
Xie, 2016[8916b]		Angiotensin-II receptor blockers	Placebo	9878 (4)	65 ± 2	HF hospitalisation at 26 months	NNT: 19 (14 to 30) RR: 0.77 (0.70 to 0.86)	30	Moderate	AHA, ACC	NICE	ESC
Xie, 2016[8916c]		Aldosterone antagonists	Placebo	11,477 (4)	65 ± 3	HF hospitalisation at 18 months	NNT: 22 (15 to 55) RR: 0.71 (0.57 to 0.88)	74	Moderate	AHA, ACC	NICE	ESC
Hood, 2014[3415]		Digoxin[d]	Placebo	7262 (4)	61 ± 3	Hospitalisation at 12 months	NNT: 28 (23 to 37) RR: 0.71 (0.64 to 0.77)	29	High	AHA, ACC	NICE	ESC
Le, 2016[8817a]	Heart failure with prior MI	Aldosterone antagonists	Placebo	15,786 (13)	63 ± 6	Hospitalisation at 15 months	NNT: 67 (39 to 233) RR: 0.93 (0.88 to 0.98)	35	Moderate	AHA, ACC	NICE	
Afilalo, 2007[100c]	Stable coronary artery disease	Intensive statin therapy	Moderate statin therapy	27,547 (4)	61 ± 2	HF hospitalisation at 41 months	NNT: 115 (84 to 189) RR: 0.73 (0.63 to 0.83)	4	Moderate	AHA, ACC	NICE	ESC; EAS
Kew, 2013[4002h]	Stable COPD	Long-acting beta 2 agonists	Placebo	3804 (7)	62 ± 2	COPD hospitalisation at 9 months	NNT: 77 (47 to 420) RR: 0.74 (0.57 to 0.95)	35	Moderate	ATS[e]	NICE	ESR[e]
Ni, 2014[8850a]		Long-acting muscarinic antagonists[f]	Placebo	5624 (10)	64 ± 3	COPD hospitalisation at 9 months	NNT: 106 (70 to 321) RR: 0.65 (0.47 to 0.88)	0	High	ATS	NICE	ESR
Reduces hospital admissions from the emergency department												
Edmonds, 2012[2159]	Acute asthma exacerbation	Early use of inhaled corticosteroids	Placebo	377 (5)	38 ± 8	Hospitalisation, Follow-up unclear	NNT: 7 (5 to 12) RR: 0.42 (0.25 to 0.67)	0	Moderate	ATS	NICE	
Rodrigo, 2005[6568a]		Anticholinergics	Beta 2 agonists	1556 (9)	18 to 55	Hospitalisation at ED discharge	NNT: 12 (8 to 26) RR: 0.68 (0.53 to 0.86)	14	Moderate	ATS	NICE	
Reduces readmissions after an index hospital admission												
Leucht, 2012[4508a]	Schizophrenia	Antipsychotic maintenance therapy	No maintenance or placebo	2090 (16)	38 ± 9	Rehospitalisation at 11 months	NNT: 5 (4 to 7) RR: 0.38 (0.27 to 0.55)	45	High	APA	NICE	EPA[g]
Kishimoto, 2013[4065a]		Second-generation antipsychotics	First-generation antipsychotics	2869 (12)	33 ± 6	Hospitalisation at 13 months	NNT: 17 (12 to 48) RR: 0.72 (0.58 to 0.90)	18	Moderate	APA	NICE	EPA[g]

ID No. identification number, *RCT* randomised controlled trial, *NNT* number needed to treat to avoid one emergency hospital admission, *RR* risk ratio, *CI* confidence interval, *ED* emergency department, *ACE* angiotensin-converting enzyme, *HF* heart failure, *COPD* chronic obstructive pulmonary disease, *MI* myocardial infarction, *NICE* National Institute for Health and Care Excellence, *ESC* European Society of Cardiology, *AHA* American Heart Association, *ACC* American College of Cardiology, *EAS* European Atherosclerosis Society, *ATS* American Thoracic Society, *ESR* European Respiratory Society, *APA* American Psychiatric Association, *EPA* European Psychiatric Association

[a] Means and standard deviations for patient ages in years. Mean of means and median ages in trials contributing to the pooled estimate. Not all included trials reported age in a form that could be averaged

[b] Mean length of follow-up across trials, unless otherwise specified. Mean of means, medians and total study durations reported in trials contributing to the pooled estimate. Not all included trials reported follow-up in a form that could be averaged. Rounded to the nearest whole month

[c] Moderate- or high-quality evidence according to the Grading of Recommendations Assessment, Development and Evaluation working group criteria

[d] For patients with normal sinus rhythm

[e] The ESR/ATS suggested in their joint 2012 guideline that long-acting beta 2 agonists are a clinically acceptable treatment for stable COPD. However, in their 2017 guideline on preventing exacerbations, they recommended monotherapy with long-acting muscarinic antagonists in preference to long-acting beta 2 agonists if the treatment goal is to prevent a future exacerbation. They indicated that this recommendation places less emphasis on symptomatic relief and that the differential effect on mortality or adverse events is unknown

[f] Aclidinium bromide. Four other meta-analyses with moderate-quality evidence examined other long-acting muscarinic antagonists (e.g. tiotropium) and reported similar effects

[g] The European Psychiatric Association has not published a clinical guideline for schizophrenia but has published a review of national guidelines across Europe and found significant agreement with respect to use of antipsychotic maintenance therapy and of second-generation antipsychotics

commonly associated with drug-related admissions did not appear in our study. Several reviews of RCTs focusing on antiplatelet drugs and anticoagulants were excluded, because they reported admissions as part of composite outcomes. The net effect of antiplatelet drugs and anticoagulants on hospital admissions is, therefore, not clear from the published systematic review literature.

Implications for practice

Policymakers and commissioners may use these results to prioritise quality measurement and improvement efforts. We have systematically identified a list of 11 evidence- and guideline-based treatments for five major chronic diseases: heart failure, stable coronary artery disease, COPD, asthma and schizophrenia. These diseases cause millions of hospital admissions each year globally [52–56] and account for about 5% of all emergency admissions in high-income countries [57–59]. Yet, there is evidence of significant variation in the prescribing of some these 11 therapies in the United States and Europe, including under-dosing and under-prescribing [60–62]. Therefore, improving utilisation of these medications could translate to substantial reductions in hospital admissions. Potential improvement targets include minimising gaps in prescribing, correcting over- and under-dosing, and improving patient adherence, although the specific target of any improvement initiatives should be driven by locally identified shortfalls in care.

The results of this study may be fed into existing mechanisms for tracking and improving clinical practices in health systems. Prescribing data for some of the 11 evidence- and guideline-based medications are currently monitored in several health systems, for example, use of ACE inhibitors, angiotensin II receptor blockers and beta blockers is currently measured as part of the UK Quality and Outcomes Framework, a pay-for-performance incentive structure that has demonstrably reduced prescribing gaps for these medications and improved prescribing efficiency for other medications [63–65]. All of the top 11 medications we identified could be considered for inclusion in these types of quality assurance and incentive structures. This pathway to optimising medication utilisation may be a feasible strategy to help reduce emergency hospital admissions.

For some of the therapies in this review, bridging treatment gaps and improving prescribing may result in immediate benefits and may rely only on a small number of stakeholders. For example, we found evidence that treating patients with acute exacerbations of asthma in the emergency department with inhaled corticosteroids or anticholinergics helped to avoid hospital admissions. Optimal utilisation of these medications could be achieved through direct efforts by emergency department physicians and hospital pharmacists.

However, many of the therapies in this review form part of ongoing chronic disease management, and beneficial effects occur after months of use. Optimal utilisation of these medications would require coordination of multiple stakeholders, including physicians in different specialties, home care or case management nurses, community pharmacists and patients.

We can estimate potential reductions in hospital admissions by combining the results of our study with data on existing treatment gaps and disease prevalence. For example, in studies of prescribing for heart failure in the United States and Europe, 13% of patients with reduced left ventricular ejection fractions who are eligible for treatment do not receive the first-line therapy [60, 66]. It has been estimated that 1.5% of people in developed countries have heart failure, of whom 40% have reduced ejection fractions [52, 67–69]. Therefore, about 400,000 Europeans and 250,000 Americans with heart failure and reduced ejection fractions are eligible for first-line therapy but are not receiving it [70]. Based on the numbers needed to treat and baseline hospitalisation event rates that we have reported for ACE inhibitors and angiotensin II receptor blockers, closing these treatment gaps could help to avoid approximately 28,000 (95% CI 24,000 to 37,000) hospital admissions in Europe and 18,000 (95% CI 15,000 to 24,000) admissions in the United States per year.

Our results also reinforce the dangers of prescribing COX2 inhibitors, particularly for patients at risk of cardiovascular disease, inhaled corticosteroids in patients with moderate to severe stable COPD, and intermittent antipsychotic drug therapy for patients with schizophrenia. It is, therefore, reassuring that the harms associated with the use of these drugs and steps to ensure that they are used appropriately, if at all, have been reported widely in clinical and government prescribing guidelines [71–73].

In addition to high- and moderate-quality evidence, this study identified 28 medications with low- and very low-quality evidence for reducing admissions. According to the GRADE working group, these estimates for reducing admissions are likely to change if additional research were conducted [18]. Therefore, given the uncertainty around the estimates of effects for these 28 medications, we would not recommend prioritising these for reducing emergency admissions. However, we recognise that the level of evidence required to act may vary depending on the circumstances, the stakeholders involved and the available evidence (which may change over time). If limited evidence is available and there is a pressing need to act, lower-quality evidence may be sufficient to justify cautious implementation of an intervention. Our prioritisation of medications with high- and moderate-quality evidence does not prevent stakeholders from using the low- and very low-quality evidence if

Table 3 Medications that increase emergency hospital admissions

Author, Year[ID No.]	Patient population	Medication treatment	Control	Patients (RCTs)	Mean age[a]	Outcome mean follow-up[b]	NNH (95% CI) RR (95% CI)	I²%	Quality of the evidence[c]
Increase hospital admissions from out-patient, day-procedure, or community settings									
Baigent, 2013[1653a]	Patients indicated for NSAID treatment	COX2-inhibitors	Placebo	88,367 (184)	Unclear	HF hospitalisation, Follow-up unclear	NNH: 3 (2 to 6) rr: 2.28 (1.62 to 3.20)[d]	Unclear	Moderate
Sampson, 2013[6806f]	Schizophrenia	Intermittent antipsychotic therapy	Maintenance antipsychotic therapy	661 (6)	35 ± 5	Hospitalisation at 21 months	NNH: 7 (4 to 15) RR: 1.58 (1.28 to 1.97)	19	High
Kew, 2014[4004z]	Moderate to severe stable COPD	Fluticasone	Placebo	16,338 (15)	64 ± 1	Pneumonia hospitalisation at 12 months	NNH: 164 (114 to 259) RR: 1.81 (1.51 to 2.17)	0	High

ID No. identification number, *RCT* randomised controlled trial, *NNH* number needed to treat to cause one emergency hospital admission, *RR* risk ratio, *CI* confidence interval, *NSAID* non-steroidal anti-inflammatory drugs, *COX2* Cyclooxygenase 2, *HF* heart failure, *rr* rate ratio, *COPD* chronic obstructive pulmonary disease

[a]Means and standard deviations for patient ages in years. Mean of means and median ages in trials contributing to the pooled estimate. Not all included trials reported age in a form that could be averaged

[b]Mean length of follow-up across trials, unless otherwise specified. Mean of means, medians and total study durations reported in trials contributing to the pooled estimate. Not all included trials reported follow-up in a form that could be averaged. Rounded to the nearest whole month

[c]Moderate- or high-quality evidence according to the Grading of Recommendations Assessment, Development and Evaluation working group criteria

[d]Rate ratio

justified in the context of their health-care settings; however, we recommend a robust evaluation to ensure resources are appropriately allocated to those interventions most likely to impact on practice.

Implications for research

Only 1% of the reviews examined the effect of medications in patients with multi-morbidity. Given the challenges of effective clinical management and high hospitalisation risk for patients with multiple diseases [47, 74], we need to identify which medication combinations most help multi-morbid patients to avoid hospitalisation.

Low- and very low-quality evidence indicates the need for high-quality research to increase confidence in the reliability of effect estimates. Some of the medications in this overview were supported by low- and very low-quality evidence, suggesting a need for additional high-quality research. Hospitalisations, however, are only one important patient and health system outcome. A larger set of core outcomes that reflect patient and health system priorities should be considered when establishing research priorities, including assessment of mortality, adverse events, quality of life and cost.

Similarly, there were 17 drugs with high- and moderate-quality evidence that were not supported by clinical guidelines. We did not record whether the medications had been evaluated. In formulating guidelines, the effect of an intervention on reducing emergency admissions would form only one of many criteria considered by multi-disciplinary panels of stakeholders. We would not recommend that drugs be included in guidelines or considered for inclusion solely because they reduce hospital admissions.

Researchers should consider reporting rates of hospital admissions, as opposed to ratio measures; 476 of the 517 (92%) effect estimates we reviewed were reported as odds or risk ratios. These are crude measures of hospitalisation, as they assess admission as a binary outcome: present or absent. These effect measures equate a patient who has had one admission during follow-up with a patient who has had five admissions. In patients with chronic diseases, such as heart failure or COPD, for which hospital admissions are common, rate-based measures may have greater utility in evaluating the effectiveness of interventions.

Strengths and limitations of the study

This study has three key strengths. First, it was comprehensive. We identified, analysed and synthesised information on nearly one million patients to identify the highest quality evidence for medications that affect emergency hospital admissions. Secondly, we minimised the impact of duplicate RCT evidence between reviews by excluding outdated reviews; every review we included has a unique set of hospital admission data. Thirdly, we classified all patient populations using ICD-10 and therapies using WHO ATC. This helped to homogenise and simplify the data, which was heterogeneously reported in the systematic reviews. When possible, we also converted quantitative data to comparable measures and units (i.e. risk ratios for estimates and months for follow-up duration). This will enable users of our review to navigate and interpret this large body of evidence.

This study has some limitations. First, although we extracted and reported all effect estimates, we have conducted only quality assessments on significant estimates. While it may be useful for decision makers to know the quality of evidence for all tested interventions, our aim was to support decision-making by identifying and prioritising therapies for which an effect has been demonstrated. All the estimates are listed in the online database (Additional file 2). Secondly, we planned to examine secondary outcomes, such as mortality and cost; however, feasibility concerns emerged during the conduct of the review. Therefore, we analysed only our primary outcome, hospital admissions. To provide information about other outcomes, we have extracted and presented conclusions from the abstract of each review. Furthermore, medications that were supported by high- or moderate-quality evidence were cross-referenced with clinical guidelines to identify those for which the overall balance of benefit to harm was judged to be acceptable by key health-care stakeholders. Thirdly, we excluded reviews that reported hospital admissions only as part of a composite end point. We may, therefore, have excluded potentially valuable therapies. However, by excluding composite outcomes, we can be confident that the effective therapies we identified have a significant effect on hospital admissions. Fourthly, we analysed clinical guidelines from at least one national organisation in the UK, Europe or America and identified support for 11 of the medications in this overview. However, it is possible that there are other relevant clinical guidelines that we did not analyse that support additional medications from this study. Readers of the overview may combine the findings with relevant clinical guidelines in their field to identify additional medications that may be considered for quality measurement and improvement to reduce hospital admissions. Fifthly, our GRADE ratings of indirectness were assessed by generalist clinicians and it is possible that clinical specialists (e.g. cardiologists) may have different opinions regarding the comparability of certain subgroups of patients and interventions. Finally, we planned to include reviews in all languages; however, feasibility concerns emerged during the conduct of the review and as a result we included only reviews published in English. Therefore, we may have missed effective therapies examined in non-English reviews.

Conclusions

We identified 11 medications supported by strong evidence and clinical guidelines that could be considered in quality monitoring and improvement strategies to help reduce emergency hospital admission rates. The findings are relevant to health systems with a large burden of chronic disease and those managing increasing pressures on acute health-care services.

Acknowledgments
We would like to thank Dr Karen Kearley, Clinical Director for Research and Development on the Oxfordshire clinical commissioning group, and Dr Raj Bajwa, clinical general practice chair of the Chiltern clinical commissioning group, who provided input on the methods and framing of this manuscript so that it may better inform health-care decision-making. The opinions expressed in this study are those of the authors and not necessarily those of the NIHR, the Department of Health or the NHS.

Funding
This was an unfunded study. NB was funded by a Clarendon Scholarship, a Goodger and Schorstein Scholarship, and the National Institute for Health Research School for Primary Care Research.

Authors' contributions
NB, CH, IO, NR, DN and KM contributed to the design of the study. NB, CH, IO, NR, DN, KM, DC, BF, AT, JL, RF, BS, JO, OH, BN and SS contributed to the acquisition and analysis of data. The data was interpreted by NB, CH, IO, BF, DC, DN and KM. The manuscript was drafted by NB, CH, DC and KM, and was critically revised for important content by all authors. All authors approved the final version of the manuscript to be published. All authors agreed to be accountable for all aspects of the work.

Competing interests
All authors have completed the uniform disclosure form of the International Committee of Medical Journal Editors at www.icmje.org/coi_disclosure.pdf and declare the following. They have not had any support from any organisation for the submitted work. They have not had any financial relationship with any organisations that might have an interest in the submitted work in the previous 3 years. There have been no other relationships or activities that could appear to have influenced the submitted work. One of our co-authors (CH) was an author of a study included in this review (Neuraminidase inhibitors for preventing and treating influenza in healthy adults and children). This did not influence the current submitted work.

Author details
Nuffield Department of Primary Care Health Sciences, University of Oxford, Radcliffe Observatory Quarter, Woodstock Road, Oxford OX2 6GG, United Kingdom. [2]Centre for Evidence-Based Medicine, University of Oxford, Oxford, United Kingdom . [3]Faculty of Medicine, University of British Columbia, Vancouver, Canada. [4]Faculty of Public Health and Policy, London School of Hygiene and Tropical Medicine, London, United Kingdom. [5]The Health Foundation, London, United Kingdom. [6]Department of Critical Care Medicine, University of Calgary, Calgary, Canada. [7]Snyder Institute for Chronic Diseases, University of Calgary, Calgary, Canada. [8]Bodelian Libraries, University of Oxford, Oxford, UK.

References
1. Kohn LT, Donaldson MS, Institute of Medicine, CJM. To Err Is Human: Building a Safer Health System. Washington, DC: National Academy Press; 2000.
2. Burke JP. Infection control - a problem for patient safety. N Engl J Med. 2003;348(7):651–6. https://doi.org/10.1056/NEJMhpr020557.
3. Klevens RM, Edwards JR, Richards CL Jr, et al. Estimating health care-associated infections and deaths in U.S. hospitals, 2002. Public Heal Rep. 2007;122(2):160–6. http://www.ncbi.nlm.nih.gov/pubmed/17357358
4. Kaier K, Mutters NT, Frank U. Bed occupancy rates and hospital-acquired infections-should beds be kept empty? Clin Microbiol Infect. 2012;18(10): 941–5. https://doi.org/10.1111/j.1469-0691.2012.03956.x.
5. Forero R, Hillman KM, McCarthy S, Fatovich DM, Joseph AP, Richardson DB. Access block and ED overcrowding: Short Report. Emerg Med Australas. 2010;22(2):119–35. https://doi.org/10.1111/j.1742-6723.2010.01270.x.
6. National Audit Office Department of Health. Emergency Admissions to Hospital: Managing the Demand. 2013. http://www.nao.org.uk/wp-content/uploads/2013/10/10288-001-Executive-Summary.pdf.
7. Department of Health. Department of Health Annual Report and Accounts. 2016;16:2015–16. https://assets.publishing.service.gov.uk/government/uploads/system/uploads/attachment_data/file/539602/DH_Annual_Report_Web.pdf.
8. British Broadcasting Corporation. Hospital admissions in England reach new high. 2016. http://www.bbc.co.uk/news/health-37924167. Accessed 1 Aug 2017.
9. National Health Service England. A&E Attendances and Emergency Admissions 2016–17. England Time Series. 2017. https://www.england.nhs.uk/statistics/statistical-work-areas/ae-waiting-times-and-activity/statistical-work-areasae-waiting-times-and-activityae-attendances-and-emergency-admissions-2016-17/. Accessed 1 Aug 2017.
10. Purdy S, Alyson H, Rebecca T, Mala M, Dyfed H, Peter B, Glyn Ee SP. Interventions to Reduce Unplanned Hospital Admission: A Series of Systematic Reviews. Bristol: University of Bristol; 2012.
11. Leppin AL, Gionfriddo MR, Kessler M, et al. Preventing 30-Day Hospital Readmissions: A Systematic Review and Meta-analysis of Randomized Trials. JAMA Intern Med. 2014; https://doi.org/10.1001/jamainternmed.2014.1608.
12. Xie W, Zheng F, Song X, Zhong B, Yan L. Renin-angiotensin-aldosterone system blockers for heart failure with reduced ejection fraction or left ventricular dysfunction: Network meta-analysis. Int J Cardiol. 2016;205:65–71. https://doi.org/10.1016/j.ijcard.2015.12.010.
13. Becker L, Oxman A. Overviews of reviews. Cochrane Handbook for Systematic Reviews of Interventions Version 5.1.0. 2011. http://training.cochrane.org/handbook.
14. Bobrovitz N, Onakpoya I, Roberts N, Mahtani K, Heneghan C. An overview of systematic reviews of interventions to reduce unplanned hospital admissions among adults. PROSPERO 2014 CRD42014014779 Available from: http://www.crd.york.ac.uk/PROSPERO/display_record.php?ID=CRD42014014779.
15. Bobrovitz N, Onakpoya I, Roberts N, Heneghan C, Mahtani KR. Protocol for an overview of systematic reviews of interventions to reduce unscheduled hospital admissions among adults. BMJ Open. 2015;5(8):1–7. https://doi.org/10.1136/bmjopen-2015-008269.
16. National Health Service data model and dictionary service. Data dictionary. 2017. http://www.datadictionary.nhs.uk/data_dictionary/attributes/a/add/admission_method_de.asp. Accessed 1 June 2014.
17. Shea BJ, Hamel C, Wells GA, et al. AMSTAR is a reliable and valid measurement tool to assess the methodological quality of systematic reviews. J Clin Epidemiol. 2009;62(10):1013–20. https://doi.org/10.1016/j.jclinepi.2008.10.009.
18. Schünemann H, Brożek J, Guyatt G, Oxman A. GRADE Handbook: Handbook for grading the quality of evidence and the strength of recommendations using the GRADE approach. 2013. http://gdt.guidelinedevelopment.org/app/handbook/handbook.html#h.9rdbelsnu4iy. Accessed 1 June 2014.
19. Office for National Statistics. United Kingdom population mid-year estimate. 2017. https://www.ons.gov.uk/peoplepopulationandcommunity/populationandmigration/populationestimates/timeseries/ukpop/pop.
20. Higgins JPT, Green S (editors). Cochrane Handbook for Systematic Reviews of Interventions Version 5.1.0 [updated March 2011]. The Cochrane Collaboration, 2011. Available from http://handbook.cochrane.org.
21. Guyatt GH, Oxman AD, Schünemann HJ, Tugwell P, Knottnerus A. GRADE guidelines: a new series of articles in the Journal of Clinical Epidemiology. J Clin Epidemiol. 2011;64(4):380–2. https://doi.org/10.1016/j.jclinepi.2010.09.011.
22. National Institute for Health and Care Excellence. NICE Guidance. 2017. https://www.nice.org.uk/guidance. Accessed 1 Aug 2017.
23. National Institute for Health and Care Excellence. Developing NICE Guidelines: The Manual. 2014. https://www.nice.org.uk/Media/Default/About/what-we-do/our-programmes/developing-NICE-guidelines-the-manual.pdf.
24. Ponikowski P, Voors AA, Anker SD, et al. 2016 European Society of Cardiology Guidelines for the diagnosis and treatment of acute and chronic heart failure. Eur Heart J. 2016;37(27):2129–2200m. https://doi.org/10.1093/eurheartj/ehw128.
25. Montalescot G, Sechtem U, Achenbach S, et al. 2013 European Society of Cardiology guidelines on the management of stable coronary artery disease. Eur Heart J. 2013;34(38):2949–3003. https://doi.org/10.1093/eurheartj/eht296

26. Reiner Ž, Catapano AL, De Backer G, et al. European Society of Cardiology/European Atherosclerosis Society Guidelines for the management of dyslipidaemias. Eur Heart J. 2011;32(14):1769–818. https://doi.org/10.1093/eurheartj/ehr158.
27. Yancy CW, Jessup M, Bozkurt B, et al. 2013 ACCF/AHA guideline for the management of heart failure: Executive summary: A report of the American college of cardiology foundation/american heart association task force on practice guidelines. J Am Coll Cardiol. 2013;62(16):1495–539. https://doi.org/10.1016/j.jacc.2013.05.020.
28. Fihn SD, Blankenship JC, Alexander KP, et al. 2014 ACC/AHA/AATS/PCNA/SCAI/STS Focused Update of the Guideline for the Diagnosis and Management of Patients With Stable Ischemic Heart Disease: A Report of the American College of Cardiology /American Heart Association Task Force on Practice Cardiovascul, vol. 130; 2014. https://doi.org/10.1161/CIR.00000000000.
29. Yancy CW, Jessup M, Bozkurt B, Butler J, Casey DE Jr, Colvin MM, Drazner MH, Filippatos GS, Fonarow GC, Givertz MM, Hollenberg SM, Lindenfeld J, Masoudi FA, PE MB, Peterson PN, Stevenson LWWC. 2017 ACC/AHA/HFSA Focused Update of the 2013 ACCF/AHA Guideline for the Management of Heart Failure: A Report of the American College of Cardiology/American Heart Association Task Force on Clinical Practice Guidelines and the Heart Failure Society; 2017. https://doi.org/10.1161/CIR.0000000000000509.
30. Wedzicha JA, Calverley PMA, Albert RK, et al. Prevention of COPD exacerbations: a European Respiratory Society/American Thoracic Society guideline. Eur Respir J. 2017;50(3):1602265. https://doi.org/10.1183/13993003.02265-2016.
31. Schatz M, Kazzi AAN, Brenner B, et al. Managing Asthma Exacerbations in the Emergency Department: Summary of the National Asthma Education and Prevention Program Expert Panel Report 3 Guidelines for the Management of Asthma Exacerbations. Proc Am Thorac Soc. 2009;6(4):353–6. https://doi.org/10.1513/pats.P09ST1.
32. Gaebel W, Weinmann S, Sartorius N, Rutz W, McIntyre JS. Schizophrenia practice guidelines: international survey and comparison. Br J Psychiatry J Ment Sci. 2005;187:248–55.
33. Dixon LB, Perkins DO, Mcintyre JS. Treatment of Patients With Schizophrenia Second Edition. Psychiatr Serv. 2004;161:i-iv+1-56. https://doi.org/10.1037/0003-066X.57.12.1052.
34. World Health Organisation. International Statistical Classification of Disease and Related Health Problems Version 10. 2016. http://apps.who.int/classifications/icd10/browse/2016/en. Accessed 1 June 2015.
35. World Health Organisation Collaborating Centre for Drug Statistics Methodology. Anatomical Therapeutic Chemical classification index. Oslo; 2016. https://www.whocc.no/atc_ddd_index/. Accessed 1 June 2015
36. The Cochrane Collaboration. Chapter 11.5.5 Statistical considerations in "Summary of findings" tables. Cochrane Handbook for Systematic Reviews of Interventions. 2011. http://training.cochrane.org/handbook.
37. Zhang J, Yu KF. What's the relative risk? A method of correcting the odds ratio in cohort studies of common outcomes. JAMA. 1998;280(19):1690–1. https://doi.org/10.1001/jama.280.19.1690.
38. The Centre for Evidence-Based Medicine. Number Needed to Treat (NNT). 2012. http://www.cebm.net/number-needed-to-treat-nnt/. Accessed 1 June 2014.
39. Newcombe RG, Bender R. Implementing GRADE: calculating the risk difference from the baseline risk and the relative risk. Evid Based Med. 2014;19(1):6–8. https://doi.org/10.1136/eb-2013-101340.
40. Newcombe RG. MOVER-R confidence intervals for ratios and products of two independently estimated quantities. Stat Methods Med Res. 2013 https://doi.org/10.1177/0962280213502144.
41. StataCorp. Stata Statistical Software: Release 14. 2015.
42. Moher D, Liberati A, Tetzlaff J, Altman DG, Grp P. Preferred Reporting Items for Systematic Reviews and Meta-Analyses: The PRISMA Statement (Reprinted from Annals of Internal Medicine). Phys Ther. 2009;89(9):873–80. https://doi.org/10.1371/journal.pmed.1000097.
43. Thomas R, Huntley A, Mann M, et al. Specialist clinics for reducing emergency admissions in patients with heart failure: a systematic review and meta-analysis of randomised controlled trials. Heart. 2013;99(4):233–9. https://doi.org/10.1136/heartjnl-2012-302313.
44. Coon J, Martin A, Abdul-Rahman A, et al. Interventions to reduce acute paediatric hospital admissions: A systematic review. Arch Dis Child. 2012;97(Suppl 1):A99. https://doi.org/10.1136/archdischild-2012-301885.234.
45. Prieto-Centurion V, Markos MA, Ramey NI, et al. Interventions to reduce rehospitalizations after chronic obstructive pulmonary disease exacerbations: A systematic review. Ann Am Thorac Soc. 2014;11(3):417–24. https://doi.org/10.1513/AnnalsATS.201308-254OC.
46. Pedros C, Formiga F, Corbella X, Arnau J. Adverse drug reactions leading to urgent hospital admission in an elderly population: Prevalence and main features. Eur J Clin Pharmacol. 2016;72(2):219–26. https://doi.org/10.1007/s00228-015-1974-0.
47. Al Hamid A, Ghaleb M, Aljadhey H, Aslanpour Z. A systematic review of hospitalization resulting from medicine-related problems in adult patients. Br J Clin Pharmacol. 2014;78(2):202–17. https://doi.org/10.1111/bcp.12293.
48. Wilbur K, Hazi H, El-Bedawi A. Drug-Related Hospital Visits and Admissions Associated with Laboratory or Physiologic Abnormalities-A Systematic-Review. PLoS One. 2013;8(6) https://doi.org/10.1371/journal.pone.0066803.
49. Kongkaew C, Noyce PR, Ashcroft DM. Hospital Admissions Associated with Adverse Drug Reactions: A Systematic Review of Prospective Observational Studies. Ann Pharmacother. 2008;42(7):1017–25. https://doi.org/10.1345/aph.1L037.
50. Lester D. Theories of attempted suicide: Should they differ from theories of completed suicide? Clin Neuropsychiatry. 2009;6(5):188–91. https://doi.org/10.1002/pds.
51. Howard RL, Avery AJ, Slavenburg S, et al. Which drugs cause preventable admissions to hospital? A systematic review. Br J Clin Pharmacol. 2007;63(2):136–47. https://doi.org/10.1111/j.1365-2125.2006.02698.x.
52. Mozaffarian D, Benjamin E, Go A, et al. Heart Disease and Stroke Statistics-2016 Update: A Report from the American Heart Association. Circulation. 2016;133(4):e38–360.
53. Wier L, Elixhauser A, Pfuntner A, Au D. Overview of Hospitalizations among Patients with COPD, 2008: Statistical Brief #106. Healthc Cost Util Proj Stat Briefs. 2011;February:1–11.
54. U.S. Department of Health & Human Services. Asthma Hospital Inpatient Discharges. 2010. https://www.cdc.gov/asthma/most_recent_data.htm.
55. Tran D, Ohinmaa A, Thanh N, et al. The current and future financial burden of hospital admissions for heart failure in Canada: a cost analysis. Can Med Assoc J open. 2016;4(3):365–70. https://doi.org/10.9778/cmajo.20150130.
56. Venkatesh AK, Dai Y, Ross JS, et al. Variation in U.S. Hospital Emergency Department Admission Rates by Clinical Condition. Med Care. 53(3):237–44. https://doi.org/10.1097/MLR.0000000000000261. Variation
57. Health and Social Care Information Centre. Hospital Episode Statistics, Admitted Patient Care - England, 2014-15. 2015. http://content.digital.nhs.uk/catalogue/PUB19124. Accessed 1 Aug 2017.
58. Hospital N, Medical A, Survey C. National Hospital Ambulatory Medical Care Survey : 2013 Emergency Department Summary Tables. 2013.
59. Australian Institutes of Health and Welfare. Admitted patient care 2014–15: Australian hospital statistics. 2016. https://www.aihw.gov.au/reports/hospitals/ahs-2014-15-admitted-patient-care/contents/table-of-contents . Accessed 1 Aug 2017.
60. Chin KL, Skiba M, Tonkin A, et al. The treatment gap in patients with chronic systolic heart failure: a systematic review of evidence-based prescribing in practice. Heart Fail Rev. 2016;21(6):1–23. https://doi.org/10.1007/s10741-016-9575-2.
61. Price D, West D, Brusselle G, et al. Management of COPD in the UK primary-care setting: an analysis of real-life prescribing patterns. Int J Chron Obstruct Pulmon Dis. 2014. p. 889–905.
62. British Society for Heart Failure, NICOR H. British Society for Heart Failure National Heart Failure Audit. 2017.
63. Doran T, Kontopantelis E, Valderas JM, et al. Effect of financial incentives on incentivised and non-incentivised clinical activities: longitudinal analysis of data from the UK Quality and Outcomes Framework. BMJ. 2011;342:d3590. https://doi.org/10.1136/bmj.d3590.
64. Bennie M, Godman B, Bishop I, Campbell S. Multiple initiatives continue to enhance the prescribing efficiency for the proton pump inhibitors and statins in Scotland. Expert Rev Pharmacoeconomics Outcomes Res. 2012; 12(1):125–30.
65. Kendrick T, Stuart B, Newell C, Geraghty AWA, Moore M. Did NICE guidelines and the Quality Outcomes Framework change GP antidepressant prescribing in England? Observational study with time trend analyses

2003–2013. J Affect Disord. 2015;186:171–7. https://doi.org/10.1016/j.jad.2015.06.052.
66. National Institute for Health and Care Excellence. Chronic heart failure in adults: management. Clinical guideline. 2014. nice.org.uk/guidance/cg108.
67. Task A, Members F, Ponikowski P, et al. 2016 ESC Guidelines for the diagnosis and treatment of acute and chronic heart failure The Task Force for the diagnosis and treatment of acute and chronic heart failure of the European Society of Cardiology (ESC) Developed with the special contribution; 2016. p. 2129–200. https://doi.org/10.1093/eurheartj/ehw128.
68. Grigorian L, Barge E, Bassante P. Heart failure in patients with preserved and deteriorated left ventricular ejection fraction. Heart. 2005;91:489–95. https://doi.org/10.1136/hrt.2003.031922.
69. Redfield MM. Trends in Prevalence and Outcome of Heart Failure with Preserved Ejection Fraction; 2017. p. 251–9.
70. The world bank group. Population totals. 2017. http://data.worldbank.org/indicator/SP.POP.TOTL.
71. Medicines and Healthcare products Regulatory Agency. Cox-2 Selective Inhibitors and Non-Steroidal Anti-Inflammatory Drugs' (NSAIDs): Cardiovascular Safety. 2015. https://www.gov.uk/government/publications/cox-2-selective-inhibitors-and-non-steroidal-anti-inflammatory-drugs-nsaids-cardiovascular-safety.
72. National Institute for Health and Care Excellence. Chronic obstructive pulmonary disease in over 16s: diagnosis and management. 2010. https://www.nice.org.uk/guidance/cg101/resources/chronic-obstructive-pulmonary-disease-in-over-16s-diagnosis-and-management-pdf-35109323931589. Accessed 20 July 2008.
73. National Institute for Health and Care Excellence. Psychosis and schizophrenia in adults: prevention and management. Clinical guideline [CG178]. 2014. https://www.nice.org.uk/guidance/cg178/chapter/1-recommendations.
74. Payne R, Abel G, Guthrie B, Mercer S. The effect of physical multimorbidity, mental health conditions and socioeconomic deprivation on unplanned admissions to hospital: a retrospective cohort study. Can Med Assoc J. 2013;185(5):E221–E228.

Epidemiological and genomic determinants of tuberculosis outbreaks in First Nations communities in Canada

Alexander Doroshenko[1*], Caitlin S. Pepperell[2], Courtney Heffernan[3], Mary Lou Egedahl[3], Tatum D. Mortimer[2], Tracy M. Smith[2], Hailey E. Bussan[2], Gregory J. Tyrrell[4] and Richard Long[3]

Abstract

Background: In Canada, tuberculosis disproportionately affects foreign-born and First Nations populations. Within First Nations' peoples, a high proportion of cases occur in association with outbreaks. Tuberculosis transmission in the context of outbreaks is thought to result from the convergence of several factors including characteristics of the cases, contacts, the environment, and the pathogen.

Methods: We examined the epidemiological and genomic determinants of two well-characterized tuberculosis outbreaks attributed to two super-spreaders among First Nations in the province of Alberta. These outbreaks were associated with two distinct DNA fingerprints (restriction fragment-length polymorphisms or RFLPs 0.0142 and 0.0728). We compared outbreak isolates with endemic isolates not spatio-temporally linked to outbreak cases. We extracted epidemiological variables pertaining to tuberculosis cases and contacts from individual public health records and the provincial tuberculosis registry. We conducted group analyses using parametric and non-parametric statistical tests. We carried out whole-genome sequencing and bioinformatic analysis using validated protocols.

Results: We observed differences between outbreak and endemic groups in the mean number of total and child-aged contacts and the number of contacts with new positive and converted tuberculin skin tests in all group comparisons ($p < 0.05$). Differences were also detected in the proportion of cases with cavitation on a chest radiograph and the mean number of close contacts in selected group comparisons ($p < 0.02$). A phylogenetic network analysis of whole-genome sequencing data indicated that most outbreak and endemic strains were closely related to the source case for the 0.0142 fingerprint. For the 0.0728 fingerprint, the source case haplotype was circulating among endemic cases prior to the outbreak. Genetic and temporal distances were not correlated for either RFLP 0.0142 ($r^2 = -0.05$) or RFLP 0.0728 ($r^2 = 0.09$) when all isolates were analyzed.

Conclusions: We found no evidence that endemic strains acquired mutations resulting in their emergence in outbreak form. We conclude that the propagation of these outbreaks was likely driven by the combination of characteristics of the source cases, contacts, and the environment. The role of whole-genome sequencing in understanding mycobacterial evolution and in assisting public health authorities in conducting contact investigations and managing outbreaks is important and expected to grow in the future.

Keywords: Tuberculosis, Outbreak, Whole-genome sequencing, First nations

---

* Correspondence: adoroshe@ualberta.ca
[1]Division of Preventive Medicine, Department of Medicine, Faculty of Medicine and Dentistry and School of Public Health, University of Alberta, Edmonton, Canada
Full list of author information is available at the end of the article

Background

Tuberculosis (TB) remains a disease of major public health importance worldwide. According to the World Health Organization, there were 10.4 million incident cases of TB worldwide in 2016, most of which occur in developing countries [1]. While the incidence rate of TB in Canada is relatively low (4.6 per 100,000 in 2015), the decrease in the number of cases is slow, and minority groups, particularly foreign-born persons and indigenous peoples, are disproportionately affected [2]. This is especially true in the Canadian Prairies, including the provinces of Manitoba, Saskatchewan, and Alberta, which account for over 50% of the cases of TB among indigenous peoples in Canada [3]. Within indigenous groups, a high proportion of cases occur in connection with outbreaks [4].

Transmission of TB in the context of outbreaks is complex and is thought to result from the convergence of several factors including: (1) a highly infectious source case whose diagnosis may have been delayed, (2) a large number of susceptible contacts, and (3) an environment suitable for transmission [5]. More recently, variation among strains of *Mycobacterium tuberculosis* (MTB), which could, for example, lead to differences in transmissibility or disease progression, has been postulated as an additional explanatory factor [6]. As recently as 2012, the Public Health Agency of Canada emphasized the need to develop or enhance strategies that address TB prevention and control in high-risk settings and to conduct a TB-related program evaluation [7]. Understanding how transmission of TB occurs, as well as how infection progresses to active TB disease, particularly within high-risk settings such as outbreaks, is important for developing more effective prevention and control strategies.

DNA fingerprinting techniques (restriction fragment-length polymorphism or RFLP, mycobacterial interspersed repetitive units or MIRU, and spoligotyping) and molecular epidemiology now complement conventional epidemiology and are often used to understand TB transmission events better [8]. In recent years, whole-genome sequencing (WGS) has been increasingly used to investigate MTB outbreaks [9]. Findings from these investigations suggest that WGS may be superior to conventional genotyping for pathogen tracing and characterizing TB outbreaks at higher resolution, as well as helping to detect *super-spreaders* [10]. The discriminatory power of WGS compared to conventional genotyping methods may result in the detection of sub-clusters and the discovery of greater heterogeneity of previously defined outbreaks [10, 11]. With the decrease in the cost of WGS, its role in characterizing historical isolates of MTB is growing.

The relative contributions of pathogen versus source case, contacts, and the environment in propagating outbreaks in First Nations communities in Canada are unknown. In this study, we used conventional and molecular epidemiological tools to examine epidemiological and genomic determinants of two well-characterized outbreaks of TB among Alberta First Nations. This setting offers a unique opportunity to identify the potential role of subtle genetic variation among MTB strains in producing outbreaks, as our molecular epidemiological analysis had previously shown that the outbreaks traced to MTB RFLP types that had circulated in these communities in endemic form. The objectives of this study were (1) to explore and describe WGS characteristics and potential DNA changes between outbreak and endemic strains of MTB with the same DNA fingerprint and (2) to understand the relative contributions of pathogen versus source case, contacts, and the environment in the propagation of First Nations outbreaks. We postulated that bacterial genetic changes could potentially be associated with outbreak behavior against a stable background of circulating endemic MTB strains. Conversely, a lack of genetic change or similarity of strains from outbreak and endemic cases would suggest a greater role for the source case, contacts, or the environment in the propagation of an outbreak.

Methods
Settings and selection of study cases

In Alberta, all incident TB cases are reported to Alberta Health Services under the provisions of the Public Health Act [12]. All cases are recorded in the provincial TB registry (Integrated Public Health Information System or iPHIS) and all mycobacteriology testing in the province is performed in the Provincial Laboratory for Public Health (ProvLab). Since 1991, all MTB isolates from culture-positive cases have been archived in ProvLab. ProvLab also performs molecular typing on all TB isolates, generating a RFLP pattern that allows isolates to be linked to, and clustered with, other cases in the province. All outbreaks in First Nations communities are investigated by the Provincial TB Program and First Nations and Inuit Health Branch (Health Canada). In the context of outbreak management, Canadian TB standards define the initial active TB case from which the process of contact investigation begins as an *index case*, the person who was judged to be the original source of infection for secondary cases or contacts as a *source case* (who may or may not be the same as the index case), and any persons identified as being exposed to an active case of disease as *contacts*. Household contacts and those contacts with whom exposure was considered to be equivalent to that of a household setting (even if it occurred in a community setting) are considered to be close contacts and given priority for public health management [13]. Furthermore, an outbreak is defined in the Canadian TB standards as two or more identified contacts diagnosed as secondary cases of active TB in the course of contact investigation *or* two or more cases occurring within 1 year of each other and discovered to be linked, with the linkage recognized outside of contact investigation [13].

In 1992 and 1998, there were two epidemiologically defined TB outbreaks in two unrelated and spatially distinct First Nations' communities in northern Alberta. The outbreaks were reported as such in contemporaneous government records [14, 15] and later in the peer-reviewed literature [4]. They were characterized as related to transmission from two highly infectious smear-positive, HIV-seronegative adult source cases, who had an intense cough. The outbreaks were associated with two unique RFLP types: 0.0142 and 0.0728. Each source case was associated with RFLP-specific clusters of 17 (type 0.0142) and 10 (type 0.0728) secondary cases, respectively, which were diagnosed within 12 months of the diagnosis of the presumptive source case.

From 1991 to 2013, there were also 6 and 40 endemic cases (defined as not meeting the above outbreak definition) of RFLP 0.0142 and 0.0728, respectively. Among those, one (RFLP 0.0142) and 14 (RFLP 0.0728) were smear-positive pulmonary cases. They were considered to have the potential to cause an outbreak but none of them resulted in outbreaks. The remaining 5 and 26 endemic cases of the 0.0142 and 0.0728 strains, respectively, were pulmonary smear-negative and non-pulmonary TB cases and were deemed non-infectious. Non-pulmonary cases included two cases of tuberculous lymphadenitis, one case of pleural TB, one case of central nervous system TB, and one case of disseminated TB. All isolates were susceptible to first-line anti-tuberculous medications. In total, 75 cases recorded in the TB registry were included in the study and were classified into four groups: outbreak source cases as determined by public health authorities (group 1a), secondary outbreak cases (group 1b), endemic potential source cases that did not cause an outbreak (group 2a), and endemic non-infectious cases (group 2b) (Table 1).

Conventional epidemiological and statistical analysis

The provincial TB registry and individual public health records on outbreak and endemic cases of RFLP types 0.0142 and 0.0728 were examined retrospectively. We abstracted and derived the following epidemiological variables pertaining to characteristics of cases and contacts: age of case, presence of cavitation on chest radiograph, number of total and close contacts per case, number of child-aged contacts (<15 years old) per case, and the number of new positive tuberculin skin tests (TSTs) and TST conversions among contacts. Individuals in group 1b were secondary TB cases of individuals in group 1a and also regarded as contacts of those in group 1a. As transmission was judged to have occurred from a source case, the contacts of those in group 1b were different individuals to the contacts of those in group 1a. We also examined a place of residence of TB cases to determine whether they were on- or off-reserve at the time of diagnosis. Reserve areas are defined by the Canadian Indian Act [16]. Reserve status was determined based on individual reporting and was characterized as "yes" when a case reported a reserve as their usual place of residence or where they lived most of the time. We examined the season during which TB was diagnosed among cases, since winter in the Canadian Prairies is long and leads to increased indoor activities, potentially increasing the risk of transmission particularly in crowded living conditions. In the context of our northern Canadian climate, the season was defined as warm or cold [17]. Aggregate census data by the community of residence of cases was used to assess housing density and mean household income.

Reserve status, season, housing density, and household income were used as proxy measures of the physical and social environment in which cases lived. The distributions of continuous data variables (age; numbers of total, close, and child-age contacts; and numbers of new TST positive tests and TST conversions) were tested for normality by a Shapiro–Wilk test. For variables displaying a normal distribution, we also checked the distribution of the residuals. We conducted group comparisons separately and sequentially to determine the difference in epidemiological factors between outbreak and endemic cases. Specifically, to compare infectious cases that led to an outbreak against infectious cases that did not lead to an outbreak, we compared groups 1a and 2a. To evaluate the impact of less infectious cases on potential transmission, we included group 2b. And finally, to determine whether any secondary cases identified in group 1b could act as secondary source cases, we examined all four groups. Our three- and four-group analyses included global comparisons between all respective groups. We computed the mean, standard deviation, median, and minimum and maximum for normally distributed variables; the mean, median, minimum and maximum, and interquartile range for non-normally distributed variables; and proportions and percentages for categorical variables. We used one-way ANOVA or Kruskal–Wallis tests to examine group differences for continuous variables that were or were not normally distributed, respectively. A Fisher's exact test was used to examine group differences for categorical variables. For group comparisons, we combined both RFLP types. We performed adjustments for

Table 1 Summary of outbreak and endemic cases (RFLP types 0.0142 and 0.0728) in First Nations communities in Alberta Canada, 1991–2013

RFLP type	Outbreak cases		Endemic cases	
	Group 1a	Group 1b	Group 2a	Group 2b
0.0142	1	17	1	5
0.0728	1	10	14	26

RFLP restriction fragment-length polymorphism

multiple comparisons using a Benjamini–Hochberg procedure with a false discovery rate of 0.1 [18]. Furthermore, we separately examined group differences while excluding non-pulmonary cases from group 2b, as contact tracing may not be necessary under these circumstances. Statistical analyses were performed using STATA version 14.0 [19].

Whole-genomic sequencing and bioinformatics

We sought every MTB isolate with each of the two described RFLP types using WGS to compare outbreak isolates to isolates not epidemiologically linked to outbreaks but with the same RFLP type. All available isolates from these two outbreaks and RFLP-matched endemic isolates were retrieved from the Alberta ProvLab archives and sent to the University of Wisconsin–Madison for WGS, which was performed on 67 isolates. WGS was not performed on eight cases (four from group 1b, one from group 2a, and three from group 2b) as seven isolates from cases reported in the TB registry were unavailable and one isolate did not yield DNA for sequencing.

Bacterial strains and growth conditions
MTB isolates were identified by the ProvLab by standard MTB isolation and identification assays. Isolates were stored at -70 °C until required. To perform genomic DNA sequencing, MTB strains were retrieved from storage at -70 °C and thawed. Then, 100 μl of each strain was inoculated into 10 ml of Middlebrook 7H9 broth (HiMedia) containing 0.2% w/v glycerol, 10% v/v OADC supplement (oleic acid, albumin, D-glucose, and catalase; Becton Dickinson) and 0.05% w/v Tween-80, and incubated at 37 °C with shaking for 3–5 weeks.

DNA extraction
Once cultures reached OD_{600} ~ 1, gDNA for WGS was isolated by following the Qiagen Genomic DNA Handbook protocol (08/2001) for bacteria using a Qiagen Genomic-tip 20/G. Briefly, cultures were transferred to 50 ml Falcon tubes containing ~35 3-mm glass beads and placed on a shaker overnight to break up clumps. Cultures were then pelleted at 3780 g for 10 min at 4 °C and re-suspended in Buffer B1. From this point, we followed the "Sample Preparation and Lysis Protocol for Bacteria" and "Protocol for Isolation of Genomic DNA from Blood, Cultured Cells, Tissue, Yeast, or Bacteria."

Whole-genome sequencing
Library preparation was performed using a modified Nextera protocol as described by Baym et al. [20] with a reconditioning PCR step with fresh primers and polymerase for an additional five PCR cycles to minimize chimeras and a two-step bead-based size selection with a target fragment size of 650 bp. Libraries were submitted to the University of Wisconsin–Madison Biotechnology Center. The quality and quantity of the finished libraries were assessed using an Agilent DNA High Sensitivity chip (Agilent Technologies, Santa Clara, CA) and Qubit dsDNA HS Assay Kit, respectively. Libraries were standardized to 2 μM. For all samples, paired-end 250-bp sequencing was performed using HiSeq v1.5 SBS chemistry on an Illumina HiSeq 2500 sequencer. Images were analyzed using the Illumina Pipeline, version 1.8.2. Our raw WGS data have been deposited in the Sequence Read Archive of the National Center for Biotechnology Information (accession PRJNA390065).

Reference-guided assembly and variant calling
The quality of reads was checked with FastQC [21]. Reads were trimmed to remove adapters and low-quality bases using Trim Galore v 0.2.6 [22]. We mapped reads to H37Rv (NC_000962.3) using the BWA-MEM v 0.7.7 algorithm [23]. We used GATK v 2.8.1 [24] for indel realignment and variant calling. Structural variants were identified using Pindel v 0.2.5b6 [25]. We created single-nucleotide polymorphism (SNP) alignments from variant calls produced by reference-guided assembly as described above. SNPs falling in repetitive regions of the MTB genome (i.e., PE/PPE genes) and SNPs that corresponded to a gap or an ambiguous call in other isolates were removed. The alignment for RFLP types 0.0142 and 0.0728 contained 13 and 168 total SNPs, respectively, after filtering. Alignments of SNPs specific to the individual RFLP types and a VCF of all SNPs are available at FigShare (https://doi.org/10.6084/m9.figshare.5101039).

We used networks to visualize the relationships between bacterial isolates. In a network, multiple lineages can descend from a single node, and nodes may be connected in a multitude of ways without conforming to a bifurcating structure. We used the methods implemented in PopART to create median joining networks from SNP alignments [26] and to visualize genetic distances between isolates for each RFLP type.

Results

Descriptive epidemiology of outbreak and endemic cases
The distribution of outbreak and endemic cases of RFLP types 0.0142 and 0.0728 over time is shown in Fig. 1. For comparison, public health authorities in Alberta received 3450 notifications of TB between 1991 and 2013 and 619 of those notifications were cases among indigenous peoples (personal communication with the TB control program in Alberta). Outbreak and endemic cases belonging to the 0.0142 RFLP type occurred over a shorter interval (during 5 out of the 23 years we analyzed), while cases belonging to the 0.0728 RFLP type were more evenly spread over time (occurring in 17 out of the 23 years under observation). Most cases in the

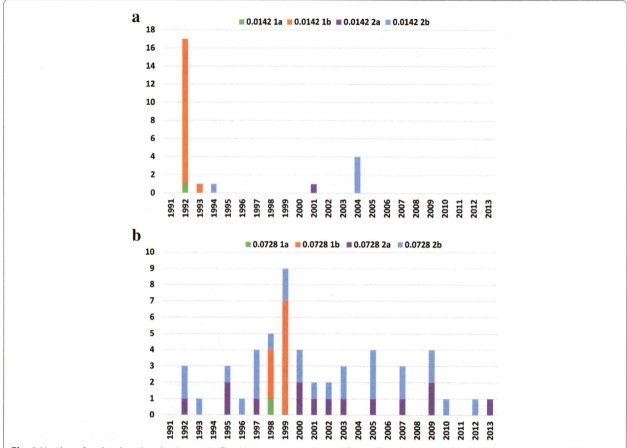

Fig. 1 Number of outbreak and endemic cases in First Nations communities in Alberta, Canada, 1991–2013. **a** RFLP type 0.0142 and **b** RFLP type 0.0728. RFLP restriction fragment-length polymorphism

1992 outbreak occurred during a single calendar year, while in the 1998 outbreak they occurred over two calendar years. Other than outbreak years 1992 and 1998, for which most cases were reported, there were five other years when at least four endemic cases (cases from groups 2a and 2b for both RFLP types) occurred (in 1997, 2000, 2004, 2005, and 2009). There were a greater number of 0.0728 RFLP type smear-positive cases, which could have potentially led to outbreaks compared to similar cases belonging to the 0.0142 RFLP type. Despite this apparent differential outbreak potential, we observed only one outbreak for each RFLP type.

A statistical summary of selected case, contact, and environmental attributes and group comparisons are shown in Tables 2 and 3, respectively. Among the continuous variables, only the age of cases had a normal distribution ($p = 0.095$). When comparing infectious source cases that led to outbreaks with infectious cases that did not result in outbreaks (groups 1a versus 2a), there were significant differences in the mean number of total contacts per case and the mean number of new TST positive tests among contacts ($p < 0.05$). Differences remained statistically significant when only child-age contacts and TST conversions among contacts were compared. In a three-group comparison (adding group 2b), there were also statistically significant differences in the proportion of cases with cavitation on a chest radiograph and the mean number of close contacts per case. These differences had a higher level of statistical significance when we compared all four groups ($p < 0.001$). Statistically significant differences in the age distribution of cases and in the proportions of cases living on a reserve and those who were diagnosed during the winter months were only detected in the all-group comparison ($p < 0.007$). Adjustments for multiple comparisons did not materially alter our inferences (Additional file 1: Table S1). Furthermore, excluding the five cases of non-pulmonary TB in group 2b from the analysis (in the three- and four-group comparisons) did not alter our inference about statistical group differences. Aggregate census data on community-based household income revealed there was a minimal variation in mean household income in reserve communities, ranging from CAD$ 26,048 to 29,726 per annum. The range of household income for non-reserve communities was much higher, from

Table 2 Summary statistics of outbreak and endemic cases of tuberculosis due to RFLP types 0.0142 and 0.0728 in Alberta First Nations communities, 1991–2013

	Group 1a (n = 2)	Group 1b (n = 27)	Group 2a (n = 15)	Group 2b (n = 31)
Age, years				
Mean (standard deviation)	25 (4.2)	21.4 (15.9)	37.7 (13.4)	44.4 (21.9)
Median	25	21	44	40
Minimum to maximum	22–28	0–59	18–56	1–92
Percentage of cases with cavitation on chest radiograph	100	0	57.1[#]	3.3
Number of total contacts per case				
Mean	811.5[§]	3.2	106	18.5
Median	811.5	0	51	6
Minimum to maximum	488–1135	0–34	10–672	0–189
75% –25% interquartile range	647	1	79	9
Number of close contacts per case				
Mean	72[§]	1.9	47.7	9.4
Median	72	0	17	5
Minimum to maximum	69–75	0–18	0–465	0–80
75% – 25% interquartile range	6	0	29	10
Number of child-age[†] contacts per case				
Mean	27	0.7	3.9	2.2
Median	27	0	2	1
Minimum to maximum	26–28	0–8	0–23	0–17
75% – 25% interquartile range	2	0	5	3
Number of new TST positive tests among contacts				
Mean	15.5	0.2	1.8	0.3
Median	15.5	0	1	0
Minimum to maximum	13–18	0–2	0–13	0–2
75% – 25% interquartile range	5	0	2	0
Number of TST conversions among contacts				
Mean	14.5	0.1	1.9	0.3
Median	14.5	0	1	0
Minimum to maximum	12–17	0–2	0–20	0–1
75% – 25% interquartile range	5	0	1	0
Percentage of diagnoses made during cold season	100	92.5	46.7	38.7
Percentage of cases living on reserve	100	25.9	73.3	48.4

[#]Adjusted for one missing value
[†]Children were defined as being aged under 15 years
[§]An entire community was screened as part of the contact investigation in one of the outbreaks described
RFLP restriction fragment-length polymorphism, *TST* tuberculin skin test

CAD$ 46,697 to 57,085 per annum [27]. The estimates for housing density on a reserve ranged from 1.3 to 1.5 persons per room and 2.58 persons per bedroom [27].

Phylogenetic relationships between endemic and outbreak isolates

Isolates with the two different RFLP types had an average of 148 single-nucleotide differences between them (Fig. 2). In comparisons of isolates of the same RFLP type, there is a bimodal distribution of pairwise differences, which could represent a closely related group of strains from the outbreak versus a more diverse collection of endemic strains. However, these peaks do not correspond to comparisons between outbreak and endemic strains. SNP distances within outbreak-associated isolates and between outbreak and endemic strains are similar (Fig. 3). We compared

Table 3 Group comparisons between outbreak and endemic cases of tuberculosis due to RFLP types 0.0142 and 0.0728 in Alberta First Nations communities, 1991–2013

	Two-group comparison (groups 1a and 2a) p values	Three-group comparison (groups 1a, 2a and 2b) p values	Four-group comparison (all groups) p values
Age of cases, years	0.2127*	0.2733*	0.0001*
Proportion of cases with cavitation on chest radiographs	0.559¶	0.0001¶	<0.0001¶
Mean number of total contacts per case	0.0369**	0.0001**	0.0001**
Mean number of close contacts per case	0.0522**	0.0126**	0.0001**
Mean number of child-age contacts per case	0.0239**	0.0202**	0.0004**
Mean number of new TST positive tests among contacts	0.0241**	0.0027**	0.0007**
Mean number of new TST conversions among contacts	0.0417**	0.0001**	0.0001**
Proportion of diagnoses made during cold season	0.265¶	0.35¶	<0.0001¶
Proportion of cases living on reserve	0.574¶	0.128¶	0.007¶

RFLP restriction fragment-length polymorphism, *TST* tuberculin skin test
*One-way ANOVA test
**Kruskal–Wallis test (adjusted for ties)
¶Fisher's exact test

single-nucleotide and structural variants between outbreak and endemic strains for each RFLP type and found that no variants were unique to the outbreak-associated isolates, suggesting that the outbreaks were not due to unique bacterial adaptations.

A network analysis of RFLP type 0.0142 strains indicated that measurable evolution occurred over the course of the outbreak (up to six SNPs), although most of the outbreak and endemic strains are closely related to the source case (one SNP distance) (Fig. 3). These analyses also demonstrated that the genomic regions examined can remain stable over long periods: strains that differed by a single SNP appeared up to 9 years after the diagnosis of the source case (Fig. 4).

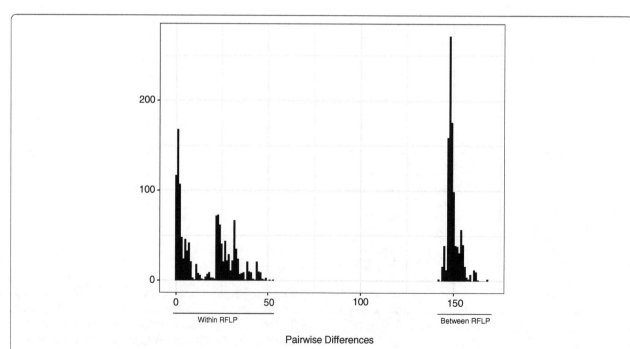

Fig. 2 Pairwise single-nucleotide differences between isolates. SNP distances between every pair of isolates in the data set were calculated. Pairwise comparisons of isolates classified as different RFLP types have a peak at 148 differences. In comparisons among isolates with the same RFLP type, we observe a bimodal distribution of pairwise differences. This bimodal distribution reflects the structure within RFLP 0.0728, which is more genetically diverse than RFLP 0.0142. RFLP restriction fragment-length polymorphism, SNP single-nucleotide polymorphism

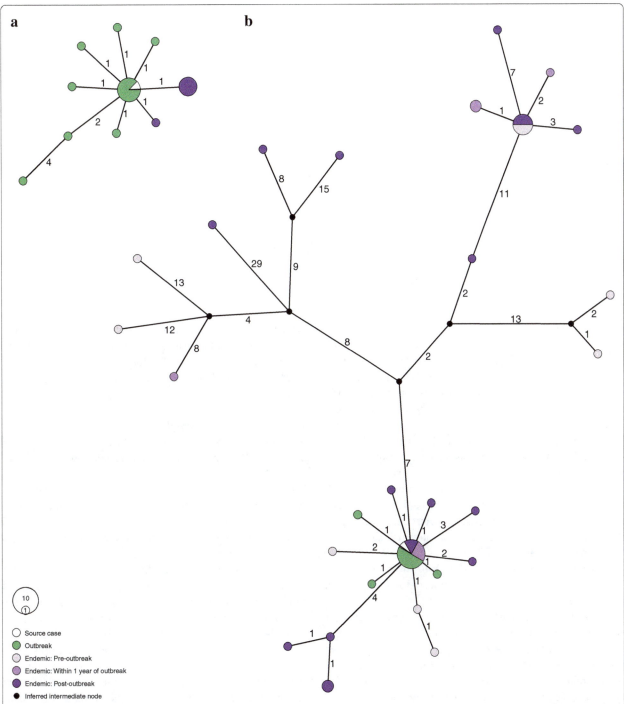

Fig. 3 Median joining network of *Mycobacterium tuberculosis* haplotypes based on single-nucleotide polymorphisms for **a** RFLP 0.0142 and **b** RFLP 0.0728. The nodes are colored according to the outbreak and endemic classifications of the isolates. Edges are labeled according to the number of SNPs between the nodes. The size of a node is scaled based on the number of isolates with an identical sequence. The source cases for each outbreak are white (corresponding to group 1a). Secondary cases from each outbreak are green (corresponding to group 1b). Endemic cases occurring prior to the beginning of the outbreak are light purple (corresponding to group 2a). Endemic cases occurring within 1 year of outbreak cases are medium purple. Endemic cases occurring after the outbreak are dark purple (the latter two corresponding to group 2b). Black nodes are intermediate nodes inferred by the median joining algorithm. There are no isolates from endemic cases prior to the outbreak for RFLP 0.0142. Outbreak cases have 0–6 differences from the source case in RFLP 0.0142 and 0–1 differences from the source case in RFLP 0.0728. RFLP restriction fragment-length polymorphism, SNP single-nucleotide polymorphism

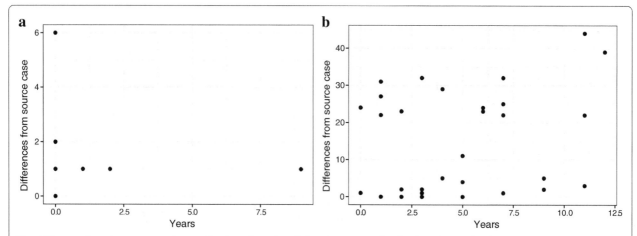

Fig. 4 Distances from the source case for two *Mycobacterium tuberculosis* strains associated with tuberculosis outbreaks: **a** RFLP 0.0142 and **b** RFLP 0.0728. The x-axis shows the time interval between diagnosis in the source case and identification of a case with an identical RFLP type (temporal distance), while the y-axis shows the number of single-nucleotide differences between *Mycobacterium tuberculosis* isolates associated with the two cases (genetic distance). These distances are not linearly correlated. RFLP restriction fragment-length polymorphism

Endemic strains that were closely related to the source of the type 0.0728 outbreak appeared before, during, and after the outbreak (Fig. 3). Unlike type 0.0142, type 0.0728 outbreak strains were all closely related to each other (i.e., within one SNP). Strains identical to the source appeared up to 5 years after the outbreak, and a strain that differed at three positions appeared 11 years later, indicating that the genomic fingerprint could remain stable over years for this genetic background, as well as for type 0.0142 (Fig. 4).

Two distinct lineages of endemic pre-outbreak MTB strains evolved from the source case haplotype, suggesting that the source haplotype was circulating prior to the outbreak of type 0.0728. The network also shows that genetically distant MTB isolates (e.g., 44 SNPs distant from the source case) share the same RFLP type. These genetically distant strains appeared before, during, and after the outbreak.

Phylogenetic relationships among our isolates are not well represented by a bifurcating tree (maximum likelihood trees contained 6–9 nodes with bootstrap support less than 50% dispersed throughout the trees), so instead we estimated median joining networks for both RFLP types (Fig. 3). This also precluded using root-to-top regression to estimate the substitution rate. Instead, we performed a linear regression of the temporal and genetic distances of isolates from the source case to look for evidence of a molecular clock (Fig. 4). Genetic and temporal distances did not appear to be correlated for either RFLP 0.0142 ($r^2 = -0.05$) or RFLP 0.0728 ($r^2 = 0.09$) when all MTB isolates were analyzed. If a SNP threshold of 5, as described by Walker et al. [11], were used to define linked cases, the r^2 values are 0.08 and 0.42, respectively. This indicates that the temporal signal in type 0.0728 genomic data is obscured when more distantly related MTB strains are included in the analysis. Restricting the analysis to closely related strains produces a slope of 0.36 SNPs per year.

Discussion

In this study, we analyzed MTB genomic data combined with epidemiological data to address the question of whether TB outbreaks in First Nations communities resulted from genetic changes in endemic strains or from the characteristics of cases, contacts, or the environment. Enhanced transmissibility or virulence could emerge periodically because of ongoing evolution of endemic MTB strains, which could contribute to outbreaks of TB. MTB population genetic data from Western Canadian First Nations communities were ideally suited to investigate this hypothesis. The bacterial population consists of a small number of well-defined lineages of MTB [28, 29] and the epidemiology of TB in these communities is characterized by endemic disease punctuated by rare but explosive outbreaks or micro-epidemics [4]. Lee et al. demonstrated that a recent large outbreak in a Nunavik community involved the expansion of endemic clones of MTB, which was associated with an epidemiologic amplification, leading to a multipronged outbreak affecting >5% of the population in a small village [30]. A further in-depth analysis of WGS data is suggesting that widespread MTB infection in this region is more likely due to an environment conducive to TB transmission than a particularly well-adapted strain [31]. Lau et al. found that the rate of infection and disease among close contacts of patients with typical radiographic findings was much greater in comparison to contacts of cases with atypical chest radiographs, suggesting a primary role of case characteristics in transmitting

TB [32]. Furthermore, the role of a highly infectious case in a poorly ventilated home or other restricted indoor environment was suggested as a condition for high TB infection and re-infection and consequently for outbreaks [33].

In our study, we found that there were no outbreak variants (SNPs or structural variants) common to outbreak strains but missing from endemic strains. Our results indicate that the two outbreaks likely grew out of endemic diversity: circulating endemic strains differed from the outbreak strain by 0–1 SNP for the two RFLP types. In settings with a stable endemic strain population, it may, therefore, be difficult to differentiate outbreak cases from endemic cases based on WGS alone.

Walker et al. estimated the rate of naturally occurring genetic changes identified by WGS to be 0.5 SNPs per genome per year. They also found that most epidemiologically linked cases were separated by fewer than five SNPs, suggesting a threshold of genetic changes that may signify a cluster or outbreak occurrence [11]. Bryant et al. similarly estimated a rate of 0.3 substitutions per genome per year, but they noted that the r^2 values were low [34]. In analyzing the entire population of strains belonging to each of the RFLP types, we found little evidence of a molecular clock ($r^2 = -0.05$–0.09). However, after applying the threshold from Walker et al. to the type 0.0728 strains, we found a correlation between genetic and temporal distances as has been reported previously and a slope of 0.36 that is concordant with previous evolutionary rate estimates [34, 35]. RFLP type 0.0728 comprises MTB strains that are relatively distantly related (based on SNP distance), suggesting that the sample includes sub-populations that have diverged over long timescales (i.e., we are sampling across ancestral diversity). Larger samples and phylogeny-based inference may be needed to detect a temporal signal in the whole population. MTB rate variation related to clinical latency could also obscure temporal signals in the genomic data [36].

Our results argue against a model in which adaptation of MTB is a primary driver of TB outbreaks. The epidemiological data in our study point to outbreaks being driven by the combination of characteristics of the source cases, contacts, and the environment as postulated by Grzybowski [5]; however, we cannot definitively state which of these attributes individually played a more important role in the propagation of the outbreaks. In our two-group comparison (1a versus 2a), the difference in the proportions of cases with cavities on chest radiographs and in the mean number of close contacts did not reach statistical significance. However, this is more likely due to the smaller sample size and less balanced groups rather than being clinically insignificant. With a larger sample (three-group comparisons), these differences became statistically significant; however, cases in group 2b were considered less infectious. Finally, there were only a small number of secondary cases (i.e., cases in group 1b) who had their own contacts convert their TSTs or had a new positive TST without documented conversion. This argues against the possibility that these secondary TB cases acted as significant secondary sources. A high rate of disease progression among contacts could also result from a particularly aggressive MTB strain but, as noted above, our results do not support this. An alternative explanation is that the source cases had an intense cough and an unusually high bacterial burden and produced aerosols that delivered a large or repeated inoculum to their contacts [37]. It is also plausible that environmental conditions contributed to these outbreaks. However, census data on housing density do not show changes in association with the outbreaks and simply may not be granular enough to detect differences among households that propagated outbreaks versus those where transmission was limited. The season of TB diagnosis may be affected by the poor access to care and that other respiratory conditions are investigated before TB is considered during the winter season. A recent study by Acuna-Villaorduna et al. [38] emphasized the importance of obtaining information on proximity of exposure using simple qualitative terms. It is important that public health authorities collect reliable data on the intensity of coughing and the proximity of exposure in TB outbreak investigations.

Our study has several limitations. Molecular fingerprinting (i.e., RFLP typing) of MTB isolates in Alberta started in 1990. Therefore, we do not have molecular data on TB cases that could be related to the two RFLP types of interest in this study prior to that time. We cannot, therefore, definitively say that there were no endemic cases of RFLP type 0.0142 prior to the 1992 outbreak. The presence of endemic cases of RFLP type 0.0728 before and after the 1998 outbreak and their distribution over time suggests that endemic cases of RFLP type 0.0142 did exist prior to the 1992 outbreak and our haplotype network suggests that this was indeed the case. The retrospective nature of our study limited our ability to obtain data of sufficient completeness or granularity on all symptoms and co-morbidities among cases as well as the environment of affected communities to allow for a more comprehensive analysis of these contributions to TB outbreak propagation. Also, in small closely knit communities, all community members can be listed as contacts of a single source case, i.e., attributed to just one individual (as occurred with one of our source cases) even though the contacts can be multi-directional. Our statistical analysis of conventional epidemiological data was affected by the small number of observations in group 1a, which in turn was restricted by the number of source cases associated with the two outbreaks we studied. This limitation can potentially be overcome by studying similar outbreaks in other jurisdictions. Finally, since we used short-read technology to sequence the isolate genomes, we were unable to identify variants within repetitive regions of the genome such as PE/PPE genes, which could contain variants unique to the outbreak strains.

We found that while WGS offers improved resolution of transmission networks relative to other molecular typing techniques, our results show that distinguishing outbreak strains from an endemically circulating bacterial population can be challenging using WGS alone. It can be argued, based on our WGS findings, that our endemic strains could simply be an unrecognized part of an outbreak or secondary outbreaks. We believe, however, that the spatio-temporal differences between our outbreak and endemic strains are substantial (endemic cases were scattered among multiple northern and relatively isolated communities over a period of up to 23 years) and argue against this assertion. Moreover, outbreaks usually come to the attention of public health authorities after cases linked by conventional spatio-temporal characteristics are reported. At that time, opportunities for public health preventive measures to limit outbreak propagation (contact tracing, finding secondary cases, TST/QFT testing, and latent TB treatment) are optimal. The further in time and space cases of TB are from the epicenter of an outbreak (regardless of whether they can be linked by WGS or not), the more challenging it is to establish that transmission indeed occurred at the time of the initial event rather than as a result of remote infection.

Conclusions
The role of WGS in understanding mycobacterial evolution and in assisting public health authorities in conducting contact investigations and managing outbreaks is important and expected to grow in the future. In our study, we did not find evidence to support the hypothesis that endemic strains of MTB acquired mutations resulting in their emergence in outbreak form. In this setting, we found that the propagation of TB outbreaks appeared to be driven by the combination of characteristics of the source cases, contacts, and possibly the environment. Preventive measures should concentrate on prompt diagnosis and effective management of cases and identification of contacts. There is a strong need to collect, prospectively and in finer detail, data relating to symptoms among cases, the environment, and socio-economic factors affecting First Nations communities.

Abbreviations
ANOVA: Analysis of variance; CAD: Canadian dollar; iPHIS: Integrated Public Health Information System; MIRU: Mycobacterial interspersed repetitive units; MTB: *Mycobacterium tuberculosis*; ProvLab: Provincial Laboratory for Public Health; RFLP: Restriction fragment-length polymorphism; SNP: Single-nucleotide polymorphism; TB: Tuberculosis; TST: Tuberculin skin test; WGS: Whole-genome sequencing

Acknowledgements
The authors would like to thank the staff at the ProvLab at the University of Alberta for providing the isolates used for sequencing, the University of Wisconsin Biotechnology Center DNA Sequencing Facility for providing sequencing facilities and services, and the staff and trainees at the Alberta Health Services TB program and TB Program Evaluation and Research Unit for assisting with obtaining public health records.

Funding
This study was funded through start-up funds provided by the University of Alberta to AD. This material is also based upon work supported by the National Science Foundation Graduate Research Fellowship Program under grant DGE-1256259 to TDM. Any opinions, findings, and conclusions or recommendations expressed in this material are those of the authors and do not necessarily reflect the views of the National Science Foundation. TDM is also supported by a National Institutes of Health National Research Service Award (T32 GM07215). CSP is supported by the National Institutes of Health (R01AI113287).

Authors' contributions
RL and AD conceptualized and designed this study. GJT provided the mycobacterial isolates. CSP, TDM, TMS, and HEB performed the WGS and bioinformatic analysis. CH and MLE summarized the epidemiological data. AD performed the statistical analysis and wrote the first version of the manuscript. CSP and TDM wrote the section of the manuscript pertaining to WGS. All authors contributed to developing the methodology for this study and critically reviewed and approved the manuscript.

Competing interests
The authors declare that they have no competing interests.

Author details
[1]Division of Preventive Medicine, Department of Medicine, Faculty of Medicine and Dentistry and School of Public Health, University of Alberta, Edmonton, Canada. [2]Departments of Medicine (Infectious Diseases) and Medical Microbiology & Immunology, School of Medicine and Public Health, University of Wisconsin–Madison, Madison, USA. [3]Department of Medicine, Faculty of Medicine and Dentistry and TB Program Evaluation and Research Unit, University of Alberta, Edmonton, Canada. [4]Department of Laboratory Medicine and Pathology, University of Alberta, Provincial Laboratory for Public Health, Alberta Health Services, Edmonton, Canada.

References
1. World Health Organization. Global tuberculosis report 2017. Geneva: WHO; 2017. http://www.who.int/tb/publications/global_report/en/. Accessed 29 Dec 2017.
2. Gallant V, Duvvuri V, McGuire M. Tuberculosis in Canada – Summary 2015. Can Commun Dis Rep 2017; 43(3/4). http://www.phac-aspc.gc.ca/publicat/ccdr-rmtc/17vol43/dr-rm43-3-4/ar-04-eng.php. Accessed 29 Dec 2017.
3. Long R, Hoeppner V, Orr P, Ainslie M, King M, Abonyi S, et al. Marked disparity in the epidemiology of tuberculosis among aboriginal peoples on the Canadian prairies: the challenges and opportunities. Can Respir J. 2013; 20(4):223–30.
4. Long R, Whittaker D, Russell K, Kunimoto D, Reid R, Fanning A, et al. Pediatric tuberculosis in Alberta first nations (1991-2000): outbreaks and the protective effect of bacille Calmette-Guerin (BCG) vaccine. Can J Public Health. 2004;95(4):249–55.
5. Grzybowski S. A small epidemic of tuberculosis. Am Rev Tuberc. 1957;75(3):432–41.
6. Valway SE, Sanchez MP, Shinnick TF, Orme I, Agerton T, Hoy D, et al. An outbreak involving extensive transmission of a virulent strain of Mycobacterium tuberculosis. N Engl J Med. 1998;338(10):633–9.

7. Public Health Agency of Canada. Guidance for Tuberculosis Prevention and Control Programs in Canada. Ottawa: Public Health Agency of Canada; 2012. http://www.phn-rsp.ca/pubs/gtbpcp-oppctbc/pdf/Guidance-for-Tuberculosis-Prevention-eng.pdf. Accessed 29 Dec 2017
8. Centers for Disease Control and Prevention. Guide to the application of genotyping to tuberculosis prevention and control. 2012 http://www.cdc.gov/tb/programs/genotyping/Chap3/3_CDCLab_1Science.htm. Accessed 29 Dec 2017.
9. Roetzer A, Diel R, Kohl TA, Ruckert C, Nubel U, Blom J, et al. Whole genome sequencing versus traditional genotyping for investigation of a Mycobacterium tuberculosis outbreak: a longitudinal molecular epidemiological study. PLoS Med. 2013;10(2):e1001387.
10. Gardy JL, Johnston JC, Ho Sui SJ, Cook VJ, Shah L, Brodkin E, et al. Whole-genome sequencing and social-network analysis of a tuberculosis outbreak. N Engl J Med. 2011;364(8):730–9.
11. Walker TM, Ip CLC, Harrell RH, Evans JT, Kapatai G, Dedicoat MJ, et al. Whole-genome sequencing to delineate *Mycobacterium tuberculosis* outbreaks: a retrospective observational study. Lancet Infect Dis. 2013;13(2): 137–46.
12. Province of Alberta. Public Health Act. Revised Statutes of Alberta 2000 Chapter P-37 Edmonton 2016. http://www.qp.alberta.ca/documents/acts/p37.pdf . Accessed 29 Dec 2017.
13. Public Health Agency of Canada. The Lung Association. Canadian Thoracic Society. Canadian Tuberculosis Standards, 7th Edition. Ottawa. 2014. https://www.canada.ca/en/public-health/services/infectious-diseases/canadian-tuberculosis-standards-7th-edition/edition-22.html. Accessed 29 Dec 2017.
14. Alberta Health. Tuberculosis services annual report. Edmonton: Alberta Health; 1992.
15. Health Canada. TB in First Nations communities. Ottawa: Health Canada; 1999. http://publications.gc.ca/collections/Collection/H35-4-7-1999E.pdf . Accessed 11 July 2018.
16. Justice Canada. Indian Act (R.S.C., 1985, c. I-5). Ottawa: Justice Canada; 2017. http://laws-lois.justice.gc.ca/PDF/I-5.pdf. Accessed 29 Dec 2017.
17. Environment Canada. Historical Climate Data. Ottawa. http://climate.weather.gc.ca. Accessed 29 Dec 2017.
18. Benjamini Y, Hochberg Y. Controlling the false discovery rate: a practical and powerful approach to multiple testing. J R Stat Soc Series B Stat Methodol. 1995;B57:289–300.
19. Juul S, Frydenberg M. An introduction to Stata for health researchers. 4th ed. College Station: Taylor & Francis; 2014.
20. Baym M, Kryazhimskiy S, Lieberman TD, Chung H, Desai MM, Kishony R. Inexpensive multiplexed library preparation for megabase-sized genomes. PLoS One. 2015;10:e0128036.
21. Babraham Bioinformatics. FastQC. http://www.bioinformatics.babraham.ac.uk/projects/fastqc. Accessed 29 Dec 2017.
22. Babraham Bioinfomatics.Trim Galore! http://www.bioinformatics.babraham.ac.uk/projects/trim_galore. Accessed 29 Dec 2017.
23. Li H. Aligning sequence reads, clone sequences and assembly contigs with BWA-MEM. http://arxiv.org/abs/1303.3997. Accessed 29 Dec 2017.
24. DePristo MA, Banks E, Poplin R, Garimella KV, Maguire JR, Hartl C, et al. A framework for variation discovery and genotyping using next-generation DNA sequencing data. Nat Genet. 2011;43(5):491–8.
25. Ye K, Schulz MH, Long Q, Apweiler R, Ning Z. Pindel: a pattern growth approach to detect break points of large deletions and medium sized insertions from paired-end short reads. Bioinformatics. 2009;25:2865–71.
26. Leigh JW, Braynt D. Popart: full-feature software for haplotype network construction. Methods Ecol Evol. 2015;6:1110–6.
27. Statistics Canada. Community Profile Archives. http://www12.statcan.gc.ca. Accessed 29 Dec 2017.
28. Pepperell C, Hoeppner VH, Lipatov M, Wobeser W, Schoolnik GK, Feldman MW. Bacterial genetic signatures of human social phenomena among M. tuberculosis from an aboriginal Canadian population. Mol Biol Evol. 2010; 27(2):427–40.
29. Pepperell CS, Granka JM, Alexander DC, Behr MA, Chui L, Gordon J, et al. Dispersal of Mycobacterium tuberculosis via the Canadian fur trade. Proc Natl Acad Sci U S A. 2011;108(16):6526–31.
30. Lee RS, Radomski N, Proulx JF, Manry J, McIntosh F, Desjardins F, et al. Re-emergence and amplification of tuberculosis in the Canadian Arctic. J Infect Dis. 2015;211(12):1905–14.
31. Lee RS, Radomski N, Proulx JF, Levade I, Shapiro BJ, McIntosh F, et al. Population genomics of Mycobacterium tuberculosis in the Inuit. Proc Natl Acad Sci U S A. 2015;112(44):13609–14.
32. Lau A, Barrie J, Winter C, Elamy AH, Tyrrell G, Long R. Chest radiographic patterns and the transmission of tuberculosis: implications for automated systems. PLoS One. 2016;11(4):e0154032.
33. Long R, Lau A. How RG Ferguson's groundbreaking studies influenced our understanding of tuberculosis reinfection: where to next? Intl J Tuberc Lung Dis. 2016;20(10):1285–7.
34. Bryant JM, Schürch AC, van Deutekom H, Harris SR, de Beer JL, de Jager V, et al. Inferring patient to patient transmission of Mycobacterium tuberculosis from whole genome sequencing data. BMC Infect Dis. 2013;13:110.
35. Eldholm V, Monteserin J, Rieux A, Lopez B, Sobkowiak B, Ritacco V, et al. Four decades of transmission of a multidrug-resistant mycobacterium tuberculosis outbreak strain. Nat Commun. 2015;6:e16644.
36. Weinert LA, Depledge DP, Kundu S, Gershon AA, Nichols RA, Balloux F, et al. Rates of vaccine evolution show strong effects of latency: implications for varicella zoster virus epidemiology. Mol Biol Evol. 2015;32(4):1020–8.
37. Jones-López EC, White LF, Kirenga B, Mumbowa F, Ssebidandi M, Moine S, et al. Cough aerosol cultures of Mycobacterium tuberculosis: insights on TST / IGRA discordance and transmission dynamics. PLoS One. 2015;10(9): e0138358.
38. Acuna-Villaorduna C, Jones-Lopez EC, Fregona G, Marques-Rodrigues P, Gaeddert M, Geadas C, et al. Intensity of exposure to pulmonary tuberculosis determines risk of tuberculosis infection and disease. Eur Respir J. 2018;51:1701578. https://doi.org/10.1183/13993003.01578-2017.

Specific microRNA signatures in exosomes of triple-negative and HER2-positive breast cancer patients undergoing neoadjuvant therapy within the GeparSixto trial

Ines Stevic[1], Volkmar Müller[2], Karsten Weber[3], Peter A. Fasching[4], Thomas Karn[5], Frederic Marmé[6], Christian Schem[7], Elmar Stickeler[8], Carsten Denkert[9], Marion van Mackelenbergh[10], Christoph Salat[11], Andreas Schneeweiss[12], Klaus Pantel[1], Sibylle Loibl[3], Michael Untch[13] and Heidi Schwarzenbach[1*]

Abstract

Background: The focus of this study is to identify particular microRNA (miRNA) signatures in exosomes derived from plasma of 435 human epidermal growth factor receptor 2 (HER2)-positive and triple-negative (TN) subtypes of breast cancer (BC).

Methods: First, miRNA expression profiles were determined in exosomes derived from the plasma of 15 TNBC patients before neoadjuvant therapy using a quantitative TaqMan real-time PCR-based microRNA array card containing 384 different miRNAs. Forty-five miRNAs associated with different clinical parameters were then selected and mounted on microRNA array cards that served for the quantification of exosomal miRNAs in 435 BC patients before therapy and 20 healthy women. Confocal microscopy, Western blot, and ELISA were used for exosome characterization.

Results: Quantification of 45 exosomal miRNAs showed that compared with healthy women, 10 miRNAs in the entire cohort of BC patients, 13 in the subgroup of 211 HER2-positive BC, and 17 in the subgroup of 224 TNBC were significantly deregulated. Plasma levels of 18 exosomal miRNAs differed between HER2-positive and TNBC subtypes, and 9 miRNAs of them also differed from healthy women. Exosomal miRNAs were significantly associated with the clinicopathological and risk factors. In uni- and multivariate models, miR-155 ($p = 0.002$, $p = 0.003$, respectively) and miR-301 ($p = 0.002$, $p = 0.001$, respectively) best predicted pathological complete response (pCR).

Conclusion: Our findings show a network of deregulated exosomal miRNAs with specific expression patterns in exosomes of HER2-positive and TNBC patients that are also associated with clinicopathological parameters and pCR within each BC subtype.

Keywords: MicroRNAs, Exosomes, Breast cancer, Triple negative, HER2-positive, Pathological complete response, Neoadjuvant therapy

---

* Correspondence: h.schwarzenbach@uke.de
[1]Department of Tumor Biology, University Medical Center Hamburg-Eppendorf, Martinistraße 52, 20246 Hamburg, Germany
Full list of author information is available at the end of the article

Background

Breast cancer (BC) comprises several subtypes that are in clinical routine defined by estrogen receptor (ER), progesterone receptor (PR), and human epidermal growth factor receptor 2 (HER2) status. Each BC subtype exhibits varied responses to different therapeutic regimens. Triple-negative (TNBC) and HER2-positive tumors are associated with a worse prognosis, a more aggressive clinical outcome, and a higher risk for relapse than luminal-like tumors that are positive for hormone receptors [1].

Since particular microRNA (miRNA) signatures are associated with BC subtypes and aggressiveness, as well as patient response to drug therapy and clinical outcome [2, 3], they open up new approaches for the development of non-invasive diagnostic and therapeutic tests. The deregulated expression of miRNAs in cancer may among others be caused by their frequent location in fragile chromosomal regions harboring DNA amplifications, deletions or translocations [4]. As evolutionary conserved family, these small non-coding RNA molecules inhibit post-transcriptionally gene expression by binding to complementary sequences in the 3′ untranslated-region (3′UTR) of their target mRNAs [5]. MiRNAs circulate highly stable in human blood [6]. They are released into the blood circulation either passively by apoptosis and necrosis or actively by exosomes from multiple cell types [7, 8]. The process of sorting and packaging of miRNAs into exosomes depends on the cell origin, and is selective, favoring certain miRNAs for exosomal cargo to others [9, 10]. Exosomes are small membrane vesicles in size of 30–100 nm [11]. They can mediate cell-to-cell communication by transferring proteins, lipids, and nucleic acids between donor and recipient cells, resulting possibly in modulation of the recipient cells. It is assumed that tumor-derived exosomes can transform normal, wild-type cells into malignant cells [12, 13]. In this manner, they stimulate cellular signaling and regulate metabolic functions and homeostasis of hematopoietic cells [14, 15]. MiRNAs derived from cancer-associated exosomes have been implicated in supporting or restraining tumor growth, conferring drug resistance, promoting recurrence, and preparing a metastatic niche [10]. Considering their biologic relevance, strategies to interfere with loading or delivery of exosomal oncogenic miRNAs might be used as a therapeutic approach.

Currently, TNBC is a focus of intense research since treatment options beyond chemotherapy are urgently required. In contrast, many options for HER2-positive patients exist but the optimal combination strategies are unclear, and clarifying the mechanisms of resistance is required. In both settings, it is important to improve the insights into the biology of tumor progression in the context of therapy. Neoadjuvant treatment strategies offer short-term results of treatment efficacy by evaluation of pathological complete response (pCR). Since this response is associated with long-term outcome, the treatment strategy is now used for the clinical evaluation of treatment strategies in BC patients.

In this study, we determined the expression of miRNA profiles in circulating exosomes of BC patients before neoadjuvant therapy within a randomized phase II neoadjuvant GeparSixto trial using quantitative TaqMan real-time PCR-based microRNA array cards. We detected a significant difference in the exosomal miRNA patterns between TNBC and HER2-positive patients. The packaging of particular miRNAs in exosomes was associated with clinicopathological and risk factors, and predicted pCR.

Methods
Study populations

Within the multicenter GeparSixto trial from August 2011 to December 2012, BC patients were randomized to receive 18 weeks of neoadjuvant treatment with paclitaxel (80 mg/m^2/week) and non-pegylated liposomal doxorubicin (20 mg/m^2/week) with or without addition of carboplatin (AUC 2.0–1.5/week) [16]. Hormone-receptor status, HER2 status, and Ki67 expression were centrally confirmed prior to randomization. Plasma samples of 211 HER2-positive and 224 TNBC patients were collected directly before neoadjuvant therapy. After therapy, plasma samples of 4 HER2-positive and 5 TNBC patients were available. Median age of BC patients was 47 years and ranged from 21 to 78 years. Detailed patient characteristics are summarized in Table 1 (categorial variables) and Additional file 1: Table S1 (continuous variables). During 2016, plasma samples were collected from 20 healthy women with no history of cancer and in good health based on self-report (median age 55, range 47 to 69). Regarding blood processing, uniform management concerning the specific described protocols was performed. Blood collection and experiments were performed in compliance with the Helsinki Declaration and were approved by the ethics committee (Ethik-Kommission der Ärztekammer Hamburg, Hamburg). Plasma samples from 435 BC patients and 20 healthy women were analyzed with different techniques as described below, and sample flow is depicted in Fig. 1.

Verification of hemolysis in plasma samples

To avoid quantifying exosomal miRNAs in hemolytic plasma samples that may influence our results, we performed hemoglobin measurements by spectral analysis [17]. In 7 ml of whole blood, red blood cells were lysed by erythrocyte lysis buffer (containing 0.3 M sucrose, 10 mM Tris pH 7.5, 5 mM $MgCl_2$ and 1% Triton X100). A dilution series (1:1, 1:3, 1:4, 1:6, 1:8, 1:10, 1:12, 1:14,

Table 1 Breast cancer patient characteristics (categorial variables)

Parameters		All BC patients analyzed in this study	HER2-positive patients	TNBC patients	All BC patients in GeparSixto trial	p value*
Total		435 (100.0%)	211 (100.0%)	244 (100.0%)	588 (100.0%)	
Subtype	HER2-positive patients	211 (48.5%)	Subgroups of all BC patients analyzed in this study		273 (46.4%)	0.0909
	TNBC patients	224 (51.5%)			315 (53.6%)	
Age	< 50	249 (57.2%)	120 (56.9%)	129 (57.6%)	341 (58.0%)	0.5684
	≥ 50	186 (42.8%)	91 (43.1%)	95 (42.4%)	247 (42.0%)	
Lymph node metastasis	N0	240 (56.1%)	106 (50.7%)	134 (61.2%)	338 (58.7%)	0.0333
	N+	188 (43.9%)	103 (49.3%)	85 (38.8%)	238 (41.3%)	
	Missing	7	2	5	12	
Tumor size	T1–2	365 (84.3%)	167 (79.9%)	198 (88.4%)	499 (85.2%)	0.3570
	T3–4	68 (15.7%)	42 (20.1%)	26 (11.6%)	87 (14.8%)	
	Missing	2	2	0	2	
Grading	G1–2	151 (34.7%)	93 (44.1%)	58 (25.9%)	207 (35.2%)	0.6944
	G3	284 (65.3%)	118 (55.9%)	166 (74.1%)	381 (64.8%)	
Lymphocyte predominant breast cancer	pos.	108 (25.1%)	44 (21.4%)	64 (28.6%)	142 (24.4%)	0.5825
	neg.	322 (74.9%)	162 (78.6%)	160 (71.4%)	439 (75.6%)	
	Missing	5	5	0	7	
Therapy arm	PM	222 (51.0%)	109 (51.7%)	113 (50.4%)	293 (49.8%)	0.3478
	PMCb	213 (49.0%)	102 (48.3%)	111 (49.6%)	295 (50.2%)	
Pathological complete response (pCR)	Yes	223 (51.3%)	113 (53.6%)	110 (49.1%)	296 (50.3%)	0.4540
	No	212 (48.7%)	98 (46.4%)	114 (50.9%)	292 (49.7%)	

PM non-carboplatin treatment arm, *PMCb* carboplatin treatment arm
*Characteristics of patients were compared between patients with analyzed samples and all patients of GeparSixto study (modified intend-to-treat population) using Fisher's exact tests

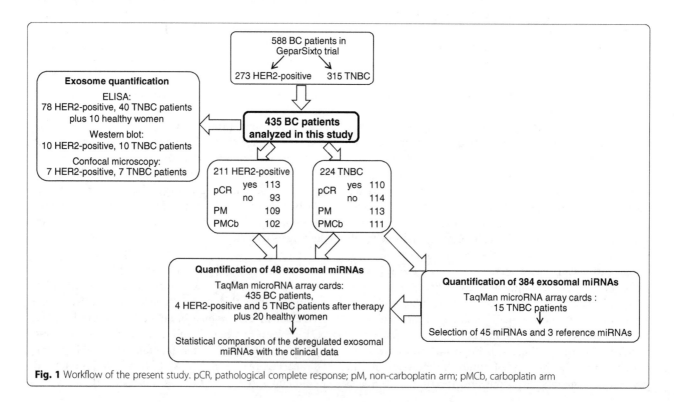

Fig. 1 Workflow of the present study. pCR, pathological complete response; pM, non-carboplatin arm; pMCb, carboplatin arm

1:18, 1:20) of lysed red blood cells in plasma was prepared that served as a standard curve for the measurement of hemolysis in all plasma samples. Fifty microliters of each plasma sample (standard and plasma of interest) was measured in duplicates on a Microplate reader (Tecan, Männerdorf, Switzerland). Absorbance peaks at 414, 541, and 576 nm were indicative for free hemoglobin, with the highest peak at 414 nm. The higher the absorbance in samples is, the higher is the degree of hemolysis. The average values and standard deviations were calculated from the duplicates (see Additional file 1: Figure S1).

Isolation of total exosomes from plasma

Total exosomes were isolated by ExoQuick (BioCat, Heidelberg, Germany) according to the manufacturer's instructions. Briefly, 550 µl of plasma, removed from cells and debris by two centrifugation steps at 3000g for 15 min, was incubated with 120 µl ExoQuick exosome precipitation solution at 4 °C, for 30 min. Following centrifugation at 1500g for 30 min, the exosomes were precipitated and then resuspended in 50 µl PBS (phosphate-buffered saline) buffer (Life Technologies, Darmstadt, Germany).

Visualization of exosomes using confocal microscopy

The isolated exosomes were labeled by the Exo-GLOW Exosome Labeling Kits (System Biosciences, Palo Alto, California, USA). Five hundred-microliter resuspended exosomes and 50 µl Exo-Red in PBS were incubated at 37 °C for 10 min. The labeling reaction was stopped with 100 µl ExoQuick-TC reagent at 4 °C for 30 min. After centrifugation for 3 min at 14,000 rpm, the labeled exosome pellet was resuspended in 500 µl PBS and monitored under a confocal microscope Leica sp5 with a 63x magnification using the 1.4 oil objective lens (Leica Microsystems, Wetzlar, Germany).

ELISA

Exosomes were quantified by the Exosome Antibodies & ELISA Kit (System Biosciences), which is specific for the exosomal protein CD63. For performing ELISA, 400 µl plasma was purified from fibrin by adding 4 µl thrombin (BioCat, Heidelberg, Germany) at a final concentration of 5 U/ml. Following exosome extraction by ExoQuick, 50 µl exosome resuspension in duplicate and CD63 protein standards (undiluted, diluted 1:2, 1:4, 1:8, 1:16, 1:32 and 1:64) were added to the micro-titer plate (Tecan). The absorbance at 450 nm of the samples was measured on a spectrophotometric plate reader (Tecan), and the amounts of CD63 protein were calculated according to the exosome protein standard curve.

Western blot

To calculate the adequate protein amounts for carrying out a Western blot, the protein concentrations were at first measured with the DC Protein Assay Kit (BioRad, Munich, Germany) at a wavelength of 650 nm on a spectrophotometric plate reader (Tecan). A standard curve of 0, 0.625, 1.25, 2.5, 5, and 10 mg/ml BSA (bovine serum albumin; Sigma Aldrich Chemie, Munich, Germany) was applied by the double-dilution method. Five microliters of exosomes, exosome supernatant, and BSA (Sigma Aldrich Chemie) standard protein samples, all solved in RIPA buffer (Merck, Darmstadt, Germany), were added to 96-well plates according to the manufacturer's instructions. The protein concentrations were then calculated according to a linear equation by applying the regression method.

Exosomes were lysed in RIPA buffer (Merck) and PBS (Life Technologies), and 30 µg of proteins from exosomes and exosome supernatant were electrophoretically separated and blotted onto a PVDF membrane (Millipore, Billerica, USA) which was subsequently incubated with antibodies specific for CD63 (ABGENT, San Diego, California, USA), CD81 (Invitrogen, Darmstadt, Germany) and AGO2 (TAKARA BIO INC, Shiga, Japan) overnight. Detection of the proteins was carried out using peroxidase-conjugated secondary antibodies (Dako, Glostrup, Denmark) and the chemiluminescence ECL detection solution (Sigma-Aldrich, St. Louis, MO, USA).

Extraction of miRNAs and conversion into cDNA

MiRNAs were extracted from 50 µl exosomes resuspended in 150 µl lysis buffer by using the TaqMan microRNA ABC Purification Kit (Thermo Fisher Scientific, Darmstadt, Germany) according to the manufacturer's recommendations. The extracted miRNAs were immediately reverse transcribed into cDNA using a modified protocol of TaqMan MicroRNA Reverse Transcription kit (Thermo Fisher Scientific). The 15-µl reaction containing 6 µl Custom RT primer pool, 0.3 µl 100 mM dNTPs with dTTP, 3 µl 50 U/µl MultiScribe Reverse Transcriptase, 1.5 µl 10× RT buffer, 0.19 µl 20 U/µl RNase Inhibitor (Thermo Fisher Scientific), and 4 µl extracted RNA was carried out at 16 °C for 30 min, 42 °C for 30 min, and 85 °C for 5 min on a MJ Research PTC-200 Peltier Thermal Cycler (Global Medical Instrumentation, Ramsey, Minnesota, USA). The cDNA samples were stored at − 20 °C for future use.

Preamplification of miRNAs

To increase the input cDNA, a preamplification step of cDNA was included. Five-microliter cDNA was preamplified in a 25-µl reaction containing 12.5-µl TaqMan PreAmp Master Mix and 3.75-µl Custom PreAmp Primer Pool (Thermo Fisher Scientific). PCR was run on a MJ

Research PTC-200 Peltier Thermal Cycler (Global Medical Instrumentation): 1 cycle at 95 °C for 10 min, 55 °C for 2 min, and 72 °C for 2 min; 16 cycles at 95 °C for 15 s and 60 °C for 4 min; and a terminal cycle 99.9 °C for 10 min. To avoid false-positive data (e.g., primer dimer formation or unspecific PCR products), a negative control without any templates was included from the starting point of all experiments.

MiRNA expression profiling

To identify differentially expressed miRNAs, real-time TaqMan PCR was at first carried out by using the TaqMan microRNA array Human Pool A cards containing 384 different miRNAs (Thermo Fisher Scientific), and plasma samples from 15 TNBC patients treated with/without chemotherapy and with/without pathological response (pCR). Subsequently, microRNA array cards (Thermo Fisher Scientific) mounted with the 45 most significantly deregulated miRNAs derived from the above array card and 2 endogenous reference miRNAs (miR-92a and miR-484) as well as 1 exogenous control miRNA (cel-miR-39) for data normalization were quantified in plasma of 435 BC patients and 20 healthy women by real-time TaqMan PCR. To carry out real-time TaqMan PCR, the protocol of Thermo Fisher Scientific was modified as followed: The 112.5-μl PCR reaction containing 56.25-μl TaqMan Universal Master Mix II and 2-μl preamplification product was loaded on the array cards. PCR was run on a 7300 HT 384 block (Applied Biosystems): 1 cycle at 95 °C for 10 min and 40 cycles at 95 °C for 15 s, 60 °C for 1 min.

Following 45 miRNAs were selected: snRNU6, let-7g, miR-16, miR-20a, miR-27a, miR-27b, miR-30c, miR-99b, miR-106b, miR-125b, miR-128a, miR-143, miR-145, miR-148a, miR-150, miR-152, miR-155, miR-181a, miR-185, miR-193b, miR-199a-3p, miR-202, miR-301, miR-324-3p, miR-328, miR-335, miR-340, miR-365, miR-370, miR-374, miR-376a, miR-376c, miR-382, miR-410, miR-422a, miR-423-5p, miR-433, miR-489, miR-511, miR-598, miR-628-5p, miR-652, miR-660, miR-744, miR-891a.

As tested by the Genorm Algorithm software, miR-92a and miR-484 provided evidence to be the most suitable reference miRNAs for data normalization.

Data normalization and statistical analyses

The statistical analyses were performed using the Thermo Fisher Scientific Analysis Software, Relative Quantification Analysis Module, version 3.1 (https://www.thermofisher.com/de/de/home/cloud.html), SPSS software package, version 22.0 (SPSS Inc. Chicago, Illinois, USA) and Statistical Programing Language R, version 3.3.2 (R Core Team 2016, Vienna, Austria).

All raw real-time PCR data were imported into the Thermo Fisher Scientific Analysis Software. First, the amplification curves were manually checked due to their shape of the curve. If a curve was atypical, the Cq value was omitted from the analysis. Second, Cq values with a Cq confidence score below 0.95 were discarded. The Cq confidence score was calculated according to the algorithm implemented in the Thermo Fisher Scientific Analysis Software and describes how likely it is that an obtained Cq value actually comes from a proper amplification curve by assessing the quality of the exponential phase of the respective curve.

The cleaned data were calculated and evaluated by the ΔCq method as follows: ΔCq = value Cq (miRNA of interest) – mean value Cq (reference miR-92a and miR-484). Surprisingly, snRNU6 was not detectable in most plasma samples and could not be used as a normalizer. According to the Genorm Algorithm software, most suitable reference miRNA were miR-92a and miR-484 for data normalization. Thus, normalization of miRNAs of interest was performed with these reference miRNAs [18]. Exogenous cel-miR-39 which was spiked in the plasma samples served as a control for the isolation process.

The Thermo Fisher Scientific Analysis software was used for performing hierarchical clustering (heat map) and Volcano plots. For the heat map, distances between samples and assays were calculated using unsupervised hierarchical clustering based on the ΔCq values and Pearson's correlation. Clustering method was average linkage. The Volcano plot displays the p value versus the fold change for each target in the patient group of interest (BC patient group, HER2-positive or TNBC subgroups) relative to a reference group (healthy group or even HER2-positive subgroup). Here, ΔΔCq was calculated as mean ΔCq (miRNA of interest in the group of interest) – mean of ΔCq (miRNA of interest in the reference group). Then, the relative quantification (Rq or gene expression fold change) was calculated as $2^{-(\Delta\Delta Cq)}$. ΔCq values were used to calculate p values using unpaired two-tailed student t test, and assuming unequal variances. Subsequently, the relative expression data (Rq) and p values adjusted for multiple testing by Benjamini and Hochberg method were log2 and log10-transformed, respectively, and plotted as a volcano plot.

Box plots for the ELISA values of exosomes and data of miRNAs, as well as receiver operating characteristic (ROC) curves, were carried out by the SPSS (version 22) software. For nonparametric comparisons of two dependent and independent variables, miRNA levels before and after therapy and differences in group levels were compared by Wilcoxon and Mann-Whitney U tests, respectively.

Fisher's exact and Mann-Whitney U tests were carried out for categorial variables (Table 1) and continuous variables (see Additional file 1: Table S1), respectively. Differences of miRNA levels among the (sub)-groups were calculated using the two-tailed Student t test (Table 2). Associations between miRNA levels and dichotomous clinical variables were analyzed by calculating the difference of mean ΔCq values among clinical groups and using an unpaired Student's t test (Table 3).

Correlations between miRNA levels and continuous clinical variables are presented by Pearson's correlation coefficients (see Additional file 1: Table S2). No multiple test correction was applied to the p values in Table 3 and Additional file 1: Table S2. The dependency of pCR on miRNA levels, represented by ΔCq values, was estimated from logistic regression models: For each miRNA

Table 2 Significantly deregulated exosomal miRNAs in plasma of HER2-positive and TNBC patients

miRNAs	All patients analyzed in this study vs. Healthy women	HER2-positive patients vs. Healthy women	TNBC patients vs. Healthy women	TNBC patients vs. Her2-positive patients
	p-value (fold change)			
let-7g	-	-	-	p=0.020 (1.3)
miR-16	-	-	-	p=0.023 (0.8)
miR-27a	p=0.020 (1.7)	p=0.004 (1.9)	-	p=0.009 (0.8)
miR-27b	p=0.010 (2.3)	p=0.001 (2.8)	p=0.021 (1.9)	p<0.0001 (0.7)
miR-30c	p=0.040 (0.7)	p=0.032 (0.7)	p=0.035 (0.7)	-
miR-128a	-	-	p=0.048 (1.6)	-
miR-143	-	-	-	p<0.0001 (0.6)
miR-145	-	-	p=0.036 (1.6)	-
miR-148a	-	-	-	p<0.0001 (2.0)
miR-150	p=0.020 (0.6)	p=0.007 (0.5)	p=0.028 (0.6)	-
miR-152	p=0.010 (1.9)	p=0.005 (1.9)	p=0.004 (1.9)	-
miR-199a-3p	p=0.010 (3.9)	p=0.005 (3.9)	p=0.005 (3.9)	-
miR-202	-	-	-	p=0.0001 (2.4)
miR-324-3p	-	-	p=0.040 (2.3)	-
miR-328	-	p=0.035 (1.6)	-	-
miR-335	-	-	p=0.028 (2.5)	p<0.0001 (1.8)
miR-340	p=0.040 (3.0)	p=0.039 (2.7)	p=0.017 (3.3)	-
miR-365	-	p=0.005 (1.9)	-	p<0.0001 (0.6)
miR-370	-	-	-	p=0.023 (1.5)
miR-376a	p=0.040 (2.6)	-	p=0.011 (3.0)	-
miR-376c	-	-	p=0.006 (2.1)	p<0.0001 (1.6)
miR-382	-	-	p=0.011 (2.7)	p<0.0001 (1.7)
miR-410	p=0.030 (2.1)	p=0.023 (2.1)	p=0.017 (2.2)	-
miR-422a	-	p=0.011 (0.2)	-	p<0.0001 (3.0)
miR-423-5p	-	-	p=0.036 (1.5)	-
miR-433	-	-	p=0.025 (2.3)	p=0.001 (1.5)
miR-489	-	-	-	p=0.007 (1.6)
miR-598	p=0.040 (2.8)	p=0.028 (2.8)	p=0.028 (2.8)	-
miR-628	-	p=0.049 (0.15)	-	p<0.0001 (2.6)
miR-652	-	-	-	p<0.0001 (1.9)
miR-891a	-	-	-	p=0.0001 (2.7)

Cells filled with "-" denote insignificant correlations
Exosomal miRNAs levels which are deregulated in one or both subgroups and additionally differ between the two subgroups of HER2-positive and TNBC patients are marked in grey

Table 3 Significant associations between the plasma levels of exosomal miRNAs and clinicopathological/risk parameters (categorical variables)

Clinical/risk factors	miRNAs*	All BC patients p(t test)**	HER2-positive patients p(t test)**	TNBC patients p(t test)**
Age (< 50, ≥ 50)	miR-20a	0.011	–	–
	miR-30c	–	–	0.038
	miR-99b	0.006	–	0.002
	miR-106b	0.024	–	–
	miR-145	0.015	–	0.040
	miR-150	0.008	–	0.015
	miR-185	0.035	–	–
	miR-202	0.046	–	–
	miR-301	0.019	0.032	–
	miR-891a	0.007	–	0.010
Nodal status (N0, N+)	miR-16	–	0.023	–
	miR-328	–	0.019	–
	miR-660	–	0.016	–
Tumor size (T1–2, T3–4)	miR-185	–	0.040	–
	miR-199a-3p	0.034	–	–
	miR-374	–	–	0.030
	miR-376a	–	0.004	–
	miR-382	0.031	0.014	–
	miR-410	–	0.038	–
	miR-433	–	0.037	–
	miR-628-5p	–	0.041	–
Grading (G1–2, G3)	miR-16	0.033	–	–
	miR-20a	0.024	–	0.032
	miR-30c	–	–	0.023
	miR-155	–	–	0.038
	miR-193b	–	–	0.028
	miR-422a	–	0.010	–
	miR-628-5p	–	0.005	–
Lymphocyte predominant breast cancer (neg, pos)	miR-148a	0.036	–	–
	miR-335	0.048	–	–
	miR-652	–	0.040	–
	miR-891a	0.050	0.022	–

Cells filled with "–" denote insignificant correlations
*Only miRNAs are listed which significantly correlate with the clinical parameter in one of the (TNBC and HER2-positive) patient subgroups and/or all patients
**p(t test), Student's t test

and each subgroup (all patients, HER2-positive patients, TNBC patients, and patients in the treatment arm), a univariate model as well as a multivariate model including the covariables age (continuous), nodal status (N0 vs. N+), tumor size (T1–2 vs. T3–4), and grading (G1–2 vs. G3) were calculated, and the odd ratio with the 95% confidence interval and the associated Wald p value for the miRNA are presented (Table 4). A p value < 0.05 was considered as statistically significant. All p values are two-sided.

Results

Higher levels of exosomes in the blood circulation of BC patients

First, we analyzed the exosomes by confocal microscopy, Western blot, and ELISA (Fig. 1). To visualize the

Table 4 Logistic regression models for pCR with *p* values, odds ratio, and confidence intervals

miRNAs	Patients Model	All BC patients		HER2-positive patients		TNBC patients	
		Univariate	Multivariate	Univariate	Multivariate	Univariate	Multivariate
miR-20a	All	–	–	–	–	–	–
	In PM	–	–	–	–	–	–
	In PMCb	$p = 0.020$ 1.39 (1.05–1.84)	$p = 0.019$ 1.41 (1.06–1.89)	–	–	–	–
miR-27b	All	–	–	$p = 0.035$ 1.30 (1.02–1.65)	$p = 0.050$ 1.28 (1.00–1.63)	–	–
	In PM	–	–	–	–	–	–
	In PMCb	$p = 0.038$ 1.27 (1.01–1.59)	$p = 0.030$ 1.30 (1.03–1.64)	–	–	–	–
miR-99b	All	$p = 0.103$ 1.14 (0.97–1.34)	$p = 0.039$ 1.19 (1.01–1.41)	–	–	–	–
	In PM	–	–	–	–	–	–
	in PMCb	–	–	–	–	–	–
miR-155	All	$p = 0.002$ 1.25 (1.08–1.44)	$p = 0.003$ 1.24 (1.08–1.44)	$p = 0.049$ 1.24 (1.00–1.53)	$p = 0.035$ 1.26 (1.02–1.56)	$p = 0.013$ 1.29 (1.05–1.57)	$p = 0.018$ 1.29 (1.04–1.58)
	In PM	$p = 0.033$ 1.26 (1.02–1.55)	$p = 0.049$ 1.24 (1.00–1.53)	–	–	–	–
	In PMCb	$p = 0.032$ 1.24 (1.02–1.51)	$p = 0.023$ 1.27 (1.03–1.55)	–	–	–	–
miR-193b	All	$p = 0.039$ 1.13 (1.01–1.26)	$p = 0.055$ 1.12 (1.00–1.26)	$p = 0.010$ 1.26 (1.06–1.50)	$p = 0.012$ 1.26 (1.05–1.51)	–	–
	In PM	–	–	–	–	–	–
	In PMCb	–	–	–	–	–	–
miR-301	All	$p = 0.002$ 1.25 (1.08–1.44)	$p = 0.001$ 1.27 (1.10–1.46)	$p = 0.013$ 1.30 (1.06–1.60)	$p = 0.011$ 1.32 (1.07–1.64)	–	–
	In PM	$p = 0.040$ 1.22 (1.01–1.48)	$p = 0.028$ 1.25 (1.02–1.52)	–	–	–	–
	In PMCb	$p = 0.020$ 1.28 (1.04–1.57)	$p = 0.022$ 1.29 (1.04–1.6)	$p = 0.012$ 1.53 (1.10–2.12)	$p = 0.016$ 1.51 (1.08–2..12)	–	–
miR-365	All	–	–	–	–	–	–
	In PM	–	–	$p = 0.052$ 1.35 (1.00–1.81)	$p = 0.038$ 1.39 (1.02–1.90)	–	–
	In PMCb	–	–	–	–	–	–
miR-423-5p	All	$p = 0.048$ 1.19 (1.00–1.42)	$p = 0.064$ 1.18 (0.99–1.41)	–	–	–	–
	In PM	–	–	–	–	–	–
	In PMCb	–	–	–	–	–	–
miR-511	All	–	–	–	–	–	–
	In PM	–	–	–	–	–	–
	In PMCb	–	–	–	–	$p = 0.239$ 0.90 (0.76–1.07)	$p = 0.043$ 0.78 (0.62–0.99)
miR-628-5p	All	–	–	–	–	$p = 0.024$ 0.81 (0.67–0.97)	$p = 0.017$ 0.79 (0.65–0.96)
	In PM	–	–	–	–	–	–
	In PMCb	–	–	–	–	–	–
miR-660	All	–	–	$p = 0.044$ 1.35 (1.01–1.80)	$p = 0.027$ 1.40 (1.04–1.89)	–	–
	In PM	–	–	–	–	–	–
	In PMCb	–	–	–	–	–	–

Table 4 Logistic regression models for pCR with p values, odds ratio, and confidence intervals *(Continued)*

miRNAs	Patients Model	All BC patients		HER2-positive patients		TNBC patients	
		Univariate	Multivariate	Univariate	Multivariate	Univariate	Multivariate
miR-891a	All	$p = 0.063$ 1.07 (1.00–1.15)	$p = 0.036$ 1.08 (1.01–1.16)	–	–	–	–
	In PM	–	–	–	–	–	–
	In PMCb	–	–	–	–	–	–

Cells filled with "–" denote insignificant miRNA contributions to the models. MiRNAs which do not show significant contributions in any population were omitted. For each miRNA variable and each patient group, a univariate as well as a multivariate model with the covariables of age, nodal status, tumor size, and grading were calculated

The odds ratio with the 95% confidence interval and the associated Wald p value for the miRNAs are presented

PM non-carboplatin treatment arm, *PMCb* carboplatin treatment arm

exosomes by confocal microscopy, we stained them in plasma of 14 BC patients and healthy women with Exo-Red. As exemplarily shown in the wide-field fluorescence image, the labeled exosomes from a healthy woman, a BC patient, and supernatant are little red dots due to their sizes below the diffraction limit. Some more exosomes can be seen in the plasma of a BC patient than in a healthy woman. In the supernatant, we can also detect a few exosomes, but the level is very low (Fig. 2a). However, it should be kept in mind that these images show only one frame of the pool of exosomes and one time point. The extraction of exosomes from 20 BC patients was also verified on a Western Blot using antibodies specific for the exosomal markers CD63 and CD81, as well as for AGO2. The AGO2-specific antibody recognized cell-free miRNAs bound to AGO2 protein (103-kDa band) in the exosome supernatant, but did not detect AGO2 in the non-lysed exosome pellet. These findings show that the exosome fraction may be pure and devoid of cell-free miRNAs. However, they do not exclude that exosomes may still contain traces of contaminations of cell-free AGO2-bound miRNAs that due to the sensitivity of the Western blot were not detectable. As expected in lysed exosomes, AGO2 protein could be detected; however, its

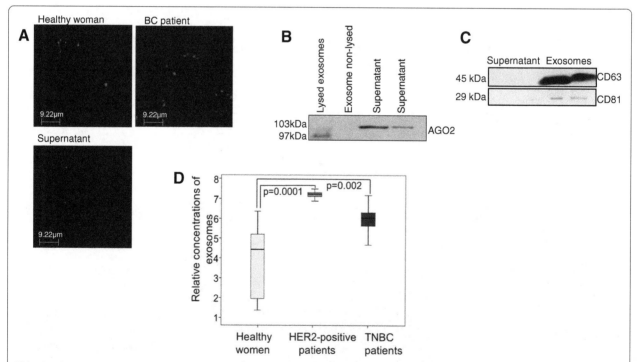

Fig. 2 Verification and quantification of exosomes. Exosomes were precipitated from plasma of a healthy woman, a BC patient and supernatant by the agglutinating agent ExoQuick. Exosomes labeled by ExoRed are visible as red dots under the confocal microscope using 63x magnification with a scale bar presented in the picture (**a**). The extraction of exosomes from BC patients was also verified by Western blot using antibodies specific for the exosome proteins CD63 and CD81, and the miRNA-associated AGO2 protein. The Western blot shows a representative example of the supernatant, lysed and non-lysed exosomes where AGO2 protein was detected in lysed exosomes and supernatant (**b**). A further Western blot shows exosomes and supernatant, while in exosomes CD63 and CD81 proteins were identified (**c**). The box plot compares the exosome levels in the plasma of healthy women ($n = 10$), HER2-positive patients ($n = 78$), and TNBC patients ($n = 40$) as measured by an ELISA coated with CD63 antibodies (**d**)

band was at size of around 97 kDa and lower than its bands in the supernatant (Fig. 2b). This discrepancy can possibly be explained due to the fact that supernatant was differently treated and not lysed, and a high concentration of other proteins and contaminants are still available which could produce a shift in size. As described by the company, the AGO2-specific antibody recognizes a band at size of 103 kDa which is detected in the supernatant. Moreover, Sharma et al. showed that the band is at size of 97 kDa corresponding to our findings in the lysed exosomes [19]. However, further analyses have to be carried out to explain this inconsistency. As visible by the 45 and 29 kDa-bands, CD63- and CD81-specific antibodies recognized the non-lysed exosomes in the pellet, respectively, but did not detect any exosomes in the exosome supernatant (Fig. 2c). In contrast to the wide-field fluorescence images that show some exosomes in the supernatant and not in Western blot, these findings indicate that Western blot is not sensitive enough. We also quantified circulating exosomes from plasma of 78 HER2-positive and 40 TNBC patients using an ELISA coated with antibodies against the exosomal marker CD63, and compared their exosome levels with those of 10 healthy women. The exosome levels were significantly higher in HER2-positive ($p = 0.0001$) and TNBC patients ($p = 0.002$) than in healthy women, indicating an excessive, active secretion of exosomes in BC patients. Although the exosome levels were higher in HER2-positive patients than in TNBC patients, the difference between these two levels was not significant ($p = 0.086$, Fig. 2d).

Different exosomal miRNA signatures in HER2-positive and TNBC patients

Following the qualitative and quantitative analyses of exosomes, we determined the miRNA expression profiles in exosomes derived from plasma of 15 TNBC patients before neoadjuvant therapy using a quantitative TaqMan real-time PCR-based microRNA array card containing 384 different miRNAs (Fig. 1). The patient group included 8 patients treated with carboplatin, (4 with pCR and 4 without pCR), and 7 patients from the non-carboplatin arm (4 with pCR and 3 without pCR). We aimed to select from the panel of 384 miRNAs those exosomal miRNAs which are most differentially expressed between the respective subgroups defined by pCR and treatment arm. While the plasma levels of only one exosomal miRNA (miR-199a, $p = 0.036$) differed between patients with and without pCR, the levels of 4 exosomal miRNAs (miR-125, $p = 0.029$; miR-193b, $p = 0.029$; miR-365, $p = 0.029$; miR-370, $p = 0.016$) differed according to the treatment arm (data not shown). These 5 miRNAs and 40 additional miRNAs that were significantly associated with other clinical parameters (tumor size, nodal status, grading) were selected and mounted (together with two references and one exogenous control miRNA) on 48-microRNA array cards, and further analyzed in plasma from 435 BC patients before treatment and 20 healthy women (Fig. 1). The complete list of miRNAs of this 48-microRNA array card is described in the "Methods" section. The ΔCq values of all 45 miRNAs vs. the mean of references miR-92a and miR-484 among all 455 samples were median-centered and clustered by unsupervised hierarchical clustering based on average linkage and Pearson's correlation as distance metric. The resulting heatmap shows conspicuously an integrated dark green color of some columns on left side referring to the mean levels of exosomal miRNAs detected in plasma of healthy women suggesting there is no change in their miRNA expression in contrast to the patients. The color scale under the heat map represents ΔCq from the median of all data (see Additional file 1: Figure S2).

The volcano plots with the log2 fold changes plotted on the x-axis and the negative log10 p values plotted on the y-axis show all down- (left side) and upregulated (right side) plasma levels of exosomal miRNAs in BC patients. As shown in Fig. 4, the plots compare the expression levels of exosomal miRNA in plasma of all 435 BC patients (A) and the subgroups of 211 HER2-positive BC (B) and 224 TNBC patients (C) with those of 20 healthy women, as well as the levels between TNBC and HER2-positive BC patients (D). Compared with healthy women, we identified 8 up- (red dots) and 2 downregulated (green dots), 9 up- and 4 downregulated and 15 up- and 2 downregulated exosomal miRNAs in the entire cohort of BC patients (A), and in the subgroups of HER2-positive BC (B) and TNBC patients (C), respectively. The levels of 18 exosomal miRNAs differed between TNBC and HER2-positive BC patients, whereby 5 and 13 miRNAs were higher and lower in HER2-positive than in TNBC patients (D), respectively (Fig. 3).

Table 2 summarizes the significant results with the adjusted p values and fold changes of miRNAs as derived from volcano plots (Fig. 3). From 45 miRNAs, 30 exosomal miRNAs were either differentially expressed in the subgroups of HER2-positive and TNBC patients, or in all BC patients compared with those of healthy women. Of particular interest are the relative differences of exosomal miRNA levels between HER2-positive and TNBC patients. From the 18 exosomal miRNAs, whose levels differed significantly between HER2-positive and TNBC patient subgroups, 9 miRNAs were also deregulated in one or both subgroups compared with healthy women (Table 2).

With respect to the subgroup, the significant differences between TNBC and HER2-positive patients were reflected by AUC values of 0.737, 0.655, and 0.759 for miR-335, miR-422a, and miR-628, respectively. To

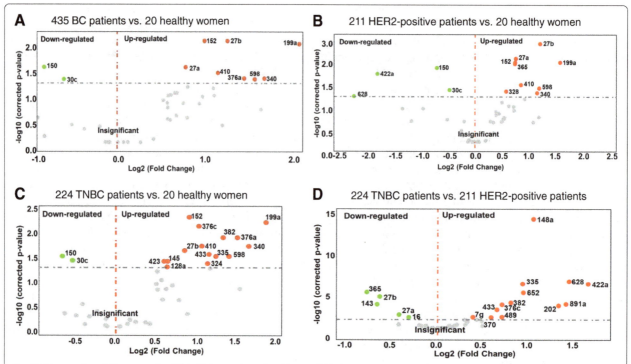

Fig. 3 Volcano plot of 45 exosomal miRNAs. Volcano plots of *p* values vs fold changes compare the expression of exosomal miRNAs in 435 BC (**a**), 211 HER2-positive (**b**), and 224 TNBC patients (**c**) with that of 20 healthy women, as well as between HER2-positive and TNBC patients (**d**). The grey dashed line refers to the threshold value corresponding to a corrected *p* value of *p* = 0.05. Significantly downregulated exosomal miRNAs are shown as green dots, significantly upregulated exosomal miRNAs as red dots. Grey dots represent non-significant changes. *p* values are calculated by the Student *t* test and corrected according to the Benjamini and Hochberg method

improve the discrimination, the concentrations of exosomal miR-335 and miR-628 as well as miR-335, miR-422a, and miR-628 were combined by logistic regression. The combined scores of these exosomal miRNAs could discriminate between TNBC and HER2-positive patients with a sensitivity of 65% and 68% and a specificity of 84% and 81%, respectively (these numbers may be biased towards higher values, because the scores were fitted on the same data). Sensitivities and specificities were determined at the highest Youden index (sensitivity + specificity − 1) (see Additional file 1: Figure S3).

Exosomal miRNA levels after neoadjuvant therapy

Plasma samples from only 9 BC (4 HER2-positive and 5 TNBC) patients were available directly after neoadjuvant therapy before surgery (Fig. 1). To obtain information on changes in the plasma levels induced by the therapy, we compared the levels of exosomal miRNAs after therapy with those before therapy, and those of healthy women. Only 4 miRNAs (miR-27a, miR-155, miR-376a, and miR-376c) significantly changed their levels after therapy. Since the levels of the other miRNAs hardly differed between before and after therapy, the box plot and the table (*p* values) only show the dynamics of these 4 miRNAs (Fig. 4). Although the data are not representative because of the small number of BC patients, they nevertheless show that the decrease in the levels of 4 exosomal miRNAs to normal (healthy) levels after therapy may be affected by neoadjuvant therapy (Fig. 4). Unfortunately, the cohort of 9 BC patients was too small to result in a robust statistical evaluation.

Associations of exosomal miRNA levels with the established risk factors

Table 3 (categorial variables) and Additional file 1: Table S2 (continuous variables) summarize the significant correlations between the exosomal miRNA levels and the clinicopathological risk parameters of BC patients. Strikingly, the levels of miRNAs in both subgroups (HER2-positive and TNBC) displayed a different preference to correlate with clinicopathological parameters: With only one exception (miR-152 and stromal lymphocytes, see Additional file 1: Table S2), no miRNA correlated with a clinical parameter, such as nodal status, tumor size, grading, lymphocyte predominant BC, Ki67 expression, and intratumoral lymphocytes, in both subgroups. In particular, the levels of exosomal miR-16 (*p* = 0.23), miR-328 (*p* = 0.19), and miR-660 (*p* = 0.016) were associated with lymph node status in HER2-positive patients (Table 3). Accordingly, the levels of exosomal miR-16 were lower in TNBC than in HER2-positive

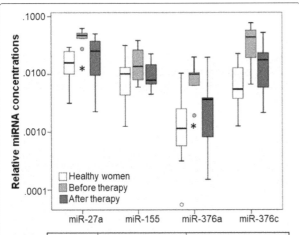

Fig. 4 Exosomal miRNA levels before and after neoadjuvant therapy. The box blot shows the plasma levels of exosomal miRNAs of 9 BC patients before and after neoadjuvant therapy and 20 healthy women. p values comparing the expression levels before and after therapy, and between patients and healthy women are indicated in the table below the blot. Cells filled with "-" denote insignificant correlations

patients ($p = 0.023$), while those of miR-328 were only upregulated in HER2-positive patients compared to healthy patients ($p = 0.035$, Table 2). In the subgroup of TNBC patients, only the levels of exosomal miR-374 were associated with higher tumor size, whereas in HER2-positive BC patients, the levels of 6 exosomal miRNAs (miR-185, miR-376a, miR-382, miR-410, miR-433, and miR-628) were associated with the tumor size (Table 3). These findings show the heterogeneity of both BC subtypes that is reflected by the subtype-specific miRNA expression or packaging of miRNAs into exosomes or both, and the relationship of these unique exosomal miRNA patterns with the diverse clinical parameters.

Associations of exosomal miRNA levels with pCR and treatment arm

Finally, univariate as well as multivariate (with covariables age, nodal status, tumor size and grading) logistic regression models for pCR were carried out in all patients and in the subgroups defined by TNBC patients, HER2-positive patients, and patients in the carboplatin (pMCb) and non-carboplatin (pM) arm. Table 4 contains the unit odds ratio with 95% confidence interval and the corresponding Wald p value for the miRNA variable in each model; model results are only reported if the uni- or multivariate model showed a significant contribution of the miRNA to the model, and only miRNAs contributing to all or the single subgroups are reported. At the beginning of our study quantifying exosomal miRNAs in plasma of 8 patients treated with carboplatin (4 with pCR and 4 without pCR), and 7 patients from the non-carboplatin arm (4 with pCR and 3 without pCR) using the microRNA array containing 384 different miRNAs, we detected that the plasma levels of miR-199a ($p = 0.036$) differed between patients with and without pCR, and the levels of miR-125 ($p = 0.029$), miR-193b ($p = 0.029$), miR-365 ($p = 0.029$) and miR-370 ($p = 0.016$) differed according to the treatment arm (data not shown). Now, in uni- and multivariate models comprising our large cohort of 435 patients including the single subgroups, the levels of exosomal miR-199a and the other 4 miRNAs did not correlate with pCR and the treatment arm, respectively, any more, suggesting that our starting patient cohort of 15 patients was too small to establish a significance of these exosomal miRNAs with pCR or treatment arm. In addition, the concentrations of no single miRNA in our set of 45 exosomal miRNAs were associated with the treatment arm, indicating that this set of miRNAs measured in pretreatment plasma samples cannot predict the treatment arm. However, 12 miRNAs could predict pCR in uni- or multivariate models comprising all patients or the single subgroups. Strikingly, the levels of miR-155 most significantly predicted pCR in uni- ($p = 0.002$) and multivariate model ($p = 0.003$) comprising all patients, as well as HER2-positive patients and TNBC patients (Table 4). This exosomal miRNA was also significantly downregulated in the 9 patients after therapy (Fig. 4; $p = 0.023$). Furthermore, the levels of miR-301 were also most significantly associated with pCR in uni- ($p = 0.002$) and multivariate model ($p = 0.001$) comprising all patients, as well as HER2-positive patients. Both the levels of miR-155 and miR-301 correlated somewhat better with pCR in the PMCb than PM arm (Table 4), indicating an improved response to carboplatin-based therapy.

Discussion

Molecular classification of BC into HER2-positive and TNBC tumors is essential for optimal use of current therapies and for development of new drugs. Of interest is that exosomes participate in cell-to-cell communication between cancer cells and normal host cells, and thus, are crucial components for regulation of the tumor microenvironment [20]. In this regard, investigation of the involvement of exosomal miRNAs of these tumors could provide new diagnostic/prognostic biomarkers and therapeutic target molecules, apart from a better understanding of tumor growth processes. In the current study, we identified miRNA signatures in exosomes specific to discriminate between HER2-positive and TNBC patients, indicating the different biology in these subgroups. Strikingly, different exosomal miRNA patterns were associated with the clinicopathological characteristics within the respective subgroups. As far as we know, this is the first study that measured a panel of 45 miRNAs in exosomes derived from a large cohort of 435 BC patients.

As we recently reported for ovarian cancer patients [21], we found that BC patients also had an excessive, active secretion of exosomes into their blood circulation. Although the levels of exosomes were somewhat higher in HER2-positive than TNBC patients, the difference was not significant. These findings suggest that a high secretion of exosomes may be a general feature of cancer patients. However, the exosomes differed in their content within both subgroups. Namely, we detected differently expressed miR-27a/b, miR-335, miR-365, miR-376c, miR-382, miR-422a, miR-433, and miR-628 in exosomes of either HER2-positive or TNBC patients compared with healthy women. This subtype-specific distribution of miRNAs in exosomes may indicate both, a different miRNA expression pattern and a selective exosomal packaging process. Based on the ability of exosomes to communicate between cells, the detection of these miRNA panels in exosomes may be superior to the detection of cell-free miRNAs in plasma or serum. To date, the presence of these miRNAs has not yet been described in BC-derived exosomes.

In our study, we detected that in comparison with healthy women, the levels of exosomal miR-27a were only significantly upregulated in HER2-positive patients (but not in TNBC patients), whereas the levels of miR-27b were upregulated in both subtypes, but with a significantly higher exosomal occurrence in HER2-positive patients. MiR-27a was reported to activate the Wnt/β-catenin signaling pathway to promote the proliferation, migration, and invasion of BC cells [22]. So far, an association of miR-27a with HER2-positive BC has not been described. However, in contrast to our data an association of this miRNA with TNBC was revealed in a meta-analysis, but its quantification was carried out in tumor tissues and not in exosomes [23]. These findings possibly point to a selective packaging of miRNAs in exosomes independent of their expression levels. Conversely, our findings on the higher levels of exosomal miR-27b in HER2-positive patients are supported and complemented by the data by Jin et al. [24] showing that HER2 stimulated miR-27b expression through the AKT/NF-κB signaling cascade. We also detected that the levels of exosomal miR-27b predict pCR in HER2-positive patients, indicating its narrow association with HER2-positive tumors. Despite the conventional role of miR-335 to act as a tumor suppressor in BC [25], our data demonstrate its significantly increased occurrence in exosomes from TNBC patients. Nevertheless,

Martin et al. [26] reported that miR-335 may also act in an oncogenic way in BC, to repress genes involved in the ERα signaling pathway, and consequently, to enhance resistance to the growth inhibitory effects of tamoxifen. Contrary to our findings that show significantly upregulated levels of exosomal miR-365 in the subgroup of HER2-positive (but not in TNBC), miR-365 was reported to be downregulated and act as a tumor suppressor in BC. Kodahl et al. [27] showed that its expression levels were lower in serum of ER-positive BC patients than healthy controls, whereas we show that its levels in HER2-positive patients who do not express ER were increased. In addition, miR-365 was also described to be oncogenic. Overexpression of miR-365 promoted cell proliferation and invasion through targeting ADAMTS-1 (a disintegrin and metalloproteinase with thrombospondin motifs) in BC cells [28]. In our study, significantly higher levels of exosomal miR-376c and miR-382 were observed in TNBC patients, but not in HER2-positive BC patients. Upregulated levels of miR-376c [29] and miR-382 [30] were also detected in plasma and serum of BC patients (regardless of the subtypes), respectively, by two previous studies. In BC, miR-382 targeted and repressed the Ras GTPase superfamily member RERG (Ras-related and estrogen-regulated growth inhibitor), to attenuate the inhibitory effects of RERG on the oncogenic Ras/ERK pathway. Thereby, miR-382 promoted BC cell viability, clonogenicity, survival, migration, invasion and in vivo tumorigenesis/metastasis [31]. Contrary, for example in oral squamous cancer, miR-376c seems to have tumor suppressive functions. Its overexpression in these cancer cells suppressed fission, proliferation, migration and invasion and induced cell apoptosis via targeting the transcription factor HOXB7 [32]. Finally, we found that the levels of exosomal miR-422a were downregulated in HER2-positive BC patients, whereas the levels of exosomal miR-433 were upregulated in TNBC patients, but till now, quantitative data on these miRNAs have not been published for BC patients. It was reported that in BC stem cells, upregulation of miR-422a attenuated microsphere formation, proliferation, and tumor formation via suppressing the PLP2 (Proteolipid protein 2) expression [33]. Moreover, miR-433 repressed Rap1a, a small G protein of the Ras guanosine triphosphatase (GTPase) superfamily that activates the MAPK signaling pathway, and thus repressed cell migration and proliferation and induced apoptosis in BC [34]. In addition, miR-433 targeted AKT3 in BC [35]. These findings highlight miR-422a and miR-433 as tumor suppressor genes.

Not only the miRNA patterns in exosomes differed between HER2-positive and TNBC patients, but they were also specifically associated with different clinicopathological parameters within the subgroups. For example, we identified a particular set of exosomal miRNAs (miR-16, miR-328, and miR-660) to be associated with lymph node status only in the subgroup of HER2-positive BC patients, but not in TNBC patients. In addition, we detected that miR-660 predicted pCR to neoadjuvant therapy in HER2-positive patients. Shen et al. already showed the potential of miR-660 as a therapeutic target for clinical treatment of BC, and its role as a regulator of proliferation, migration, and invasion of human BC cells [36]. Moreover, our present findings on the association of the levels of exosomal miR-16 with lymph node status are substantiated by our previous data [37], demonstrating such an association with cell-free miR-16 in plasma. Thus, our findings indicate a possible role of miR-16 in the development of lymph node metastases in BC. In the subgroup of TNBC patients, we discovered that only the levels of exosomal miR-374 were associated with a higher tumor size, whereas the levels of 6 exosomal miRNAs (miR-185, miR-376a, miR-382, miR-410, miR-433, and miR-628) showed such an association in HER2-positive BC patients. In addition, we revealed that miR-376a, those exosome-free plasma levels, are also upregulated in BC [29] displayed a dynamic presence in exosomes. Aside from miR-376a, three further miRNAs (miR-27a, miR-155, and miR-376c) were also downregulated to normal levels after neoadjuvant therapy, suggesting that these miRNAs may be released from the primary tumor into the blood to some extent, and their changes may directly reflect cancer status. Especially, miR-155 is a well-known miRNA with both tumor suppressive and oncogenic character, targeting, e.g., HER2 [38] and the transcription factor FOXO3a [39, 40] in BC, respectively. Along with miR-27a, there is also an association of miR-155 with the decreased expression of FOXO3a which is paralleled with the increased expression of RUNX2 [41].

In neoadjuvant settings, the early identification of non-responding BC is crucial to avoid ineffective treatments. In particular for aggressive TNBC and HER2-positive BC subtypes, achievement of pCR correlates with improved long-term outcome [16, 42]. Here, we show for the first time that the levels of exosomal miR-155 in all BC patients and their subgroups, as well as exosomal miR-301 with the exception of triple-negative BC patients most significantly predicted pCR to neoadjuvant therapy. This information could be used for treatment stratification considering alternative treatment options. However, to introduce exosomal miR-155 and miR-301 as predictive markers, further prospective studies are necessary to confirm their predictive value. Particularly, the quantification of these exosomal miRNAs in a large cohort of plasma samples before, during, and after chemotherapy is required. Since miR-301 regulates the PTEN/Akt and NFκB signaling pathways that are important in the progression of BC [43, 44], and binds to estrogen receptor 1 mRNA leading to estrogen independence of BC [45], miR-301 may be an early therapeutic target molecule in BC.

To summarize, our findings suggest that certain miRNAs are selectively enriched in exosomes of HER2-positive and TNBC patients and are also associated with the clinicopathological parameters and pCR within the BC subtypes. Exosomal miRNAs may reflect the characteristics of their parental cells and, therefore, may offer a tumor-related profile. Recently, we found that the majority of miRNAs detectable in plasma is concentrated in exosomes [2]. However, it is of note to mention that the plasma exosome population is a heterogeneous mixture of cancer and normal (wild type) exosomes, and may be derived from all cells types, especially from blood cells. This, of course, compromises the tumor specificity of the identified exosomal miRNA signatures. Therefore, methods to selectively enrich cancer exosomes from plasma or serum have to be advanced. Unfortunately, tumor-associated exosome markers allowing such an enrichment are poorly defined. In addition, our unpublished data show that the proportion of tumor-derived exosomes is small in comparison with normal, wild-type exosomes impeding the isolation of low-abundant miRNAs. However, the extensive secretion of exosomes in BC patients triggered by the tumor points to that the tumor also communicates with wild-type exosomes. Thus, we should keep in mind that not only exosomes derived from the primary tumor or metastases may be eligible for cancer personalized diagnostics, but also exosomes derived from other organs that are affected by tumor burden [46].

Although our results show a different packaging of miRNAs into exosomes, and exosomal miRNAs as future diagnostic markers and therapeutic molecules, there are some aspects that may limit our study. Our analyses were carried out by miRNA array cards. We did not verify them by single real-time PCR assays, since the number of miRNAs was too high, and the population size too large in our study. However, our previous analyses in an independent cohort before starting the current study showed that the data were nearly congruent applying miRNA array cards and single real-time PCR analyses. In addition, the number of plasma samples collected directly after neoadjuvant therapy was too low, to make a statistical conclusion on the impact of therapy on the miRNA expression levels. However, the strength of our study is the number of miRNAs analyzed and the size of our patient population before neoadjuvant therapy.

Conclusion

Our data demonstrate differentially expressed and packaged miRNA sets in BC exosomes that could serve as potentially diagnostic and therapeutic markers for BC. These specific exosomal miRNA profiles that exclusively reflect HER2-positive and TNBC as well as the different stages of BC may provide insight into the exosome biology for monitoring the disease. Further analyses are planned to analyze the significantly deregulated exosomal miRNAs in a higher number of plasma samples collected after treatment as well as in follow-up studies. Finally, a detailed investigation on their association with pCR and treatment arms is required.

Additional file

Additional file 1: Figure S1. Levels of free hemoglobin were measured in plasma samples by spectrophotometry at wavelengths from 350 to 650 nm. A dilution series of lysed red blood cells in plasma was prepared (below the chart). The degree of hemolysis was determined based on the optical density (OD) at 414 nm (absorbance peak of free hemoglobin, called Soret band), with additional peaks at 541 and 576 nm. Samples were classified as being hemolysed if the OD at 414 exceeded 0.25. The integrated curve of BC plasma samples comprises values from 0.08 to 0.20 indicating that the samples were non-hemolysed. **Figure S2.** Hierarchical cluster is shown by heat map of median centered ΔCq values of exosomal miRNAs (in rows) derived from plasma samples of 435 BC patients before treatment and 20 healthy women (in columns). The red and green colors indicate that the ΔCq values are below (relatively high expression) and above (relatively low expression levels) the median of all ΔCq values in the study, respectively. Bottom: clustering of samples. Left: clustering of probes. The scale bar provides information on the degree of regulation. The 5 clinically relevant miRNAs derived from the microRNA array cards containing 384 different miRNAs are indicated by a red arrow. **Figure S3.** Exosomal miRNAs differ between HER2-positive and TNBC patients. ROC analyses show the profiles of sensitivity and specificity of exosomal miR-335, miR-422a, and miR-628 and their combinations to distinguish TNBC from HER2-positive BC patients. The table below the ROC shows the summarization of sensitivities and specificities of exosomal miR-335, miR-422a, miR-628, and their combinations. **Table S1.** Patient characteristics at the time of primary diagnosis of breast cancer (continuous variables). **Table S2.** Significant associations between the plasma levels of exosomal miRNAs and clinicopathological risk parameters (continuous variables).

Abbreviations

3'UTR: 3' Untranslated-region; ADAMTS-1: A disintegrin and metalloproteinase with thrombospondin motifs; AUC: Area under the curve; BC: Breast cancer; ER: Estrogen receptor; HER2: Human epidermal growth factor receptor 2; miRNA: MicroRNA; pCR: Pathological complete response; pM: Non-carboplatin arm; pMCb: Carboplatin arm; PR: Progesterone receptor; RERG: Ras-related and estrogen-regulated growth inhibitor; ROC: Receiver operating characteristic; TNBC: Triple-negative breast cancer

Acknowledgements

We thank Ms. Bettina Steinbach for her excellent technical assistance, Dr. Antonio Virgilio Failla for microscopy, and Dr. Tanja Zeller's lab for using the PCR block. We are also grateful to Dr. Christian Pick (Thermo Fisher Scientific), who helped us to carry out the statistical evaluation of our data. We also thank Prof. Dr. Hans Joachim Seitz for his kind assistance during the stay of Ines Stevic.

Funding

This work was supported by the Wilhelm Sander Stiftung, Munich, Germany, and Walter Schulz-Stiftung, Planegg/Martinsried, Germany.

Authors' contributions

IS performed experiments. HS, IS, and VM designed the study. PAF, TK, FM, CS, ES, CD, MM, CS, AS, SL, and MU provided the plasma samples and clinical data. HS, IS, and KW analyzed and interpreted the measured data. HS and IS wrote and revised the manuscript. HS, KW, VM, IS, and KP reviewed the manuscript. KW performed the statistics. HS supervised the study. All authors read and approved the final manuscript.

Competing interests

The authors declare that they have no competing interests.

Author details

Department of Tumor Biology, University Medical Center Hamburg-Eppendorf, Martinistraße 52, 20246 Hamburg, Germany. Department of Gynecology, University Medical Center Hamburg-Eppendorf, Hamburg, Germany. [3]GBG Forschungs GmbH, Neu-Isenburg, Germany. Department of Gynecology and Obstetrics, University Hospital Erlangen, Comprehensive Cancer Center Erlangen-EMN, Friedrich-Alexander University Erlangen-Nuremberg, Erlangen, Germany. [5]University Women's Hospital, Frankfurt, Germany. [6]Center for Gynecological Oncology at University Women's Hospital, Heidelberg, Germany. [7]Mammazentrum Hamburg, Hamburg, Germany. [8]Universitätsklinikum Aachen, Aachen, Germany. [9]Charite Berlin, Institute of Pathology and German Cancer Consortium (DKTK), Partner Site, Berlin, Germany. [10]Universitätsklinikums Schleswig-Holstein Kiel, Kiel, Germany. [11]Hämatoonkologische Schwerpunktpraxis, Munich, Germany. [12]Universitätsklinikum Heidelberg, Heidelberg, Germany. [13]Helios Kliniken Berlin-Buch, Berlin, Germany.

References

1. Strehl JD, Wachter DL, Fasching PA, Beckmann MW, Hartmann A. Invasive breast cancer: recognition of molecular subtypes. Breast Care (Basel). 2011; 6(4):258–64.
2. Eichelser C, Stuckrath I, Muller V, Milde-Langosch K, Wikman H, Pantel K, et al. Increased serum levels of circulating exosomal microRNA-373 in receptor-negative breast cancer patients. Oncotarget. 2014;5(20):9650–63.
3. Schwarzenbach H. Circulating nucleic acids as biomarkers in breast cancer. Breast Cancer Res. 2013;15(5):211.
4. Calin GA, Sevignani C, Dumitru CD, Hyslop T, Noch E, Yendamuri S, et al. Human microRNA genes are frequently located at fragile sites and genomic regions involved in cancers. Proc Natl Acad Sci U S A. 2004; 101(9):2999–3004.
5. Bartel DP. MicroRNAs: target recognition and regulatory functions. Cell. 2009;136(2):215–33.
6. Mitchell PS, Parkin RK, Kroh EM, Fritz BR, Wyman SK, Pogosova-Agadjanyan EL, et al. Circulating microRNAs as stable blood-based markers for cancer detection. Proc Natl Acad Sci U S A. 2008;105(30):10513–8.
7. Stroun M, Lyautey J, Lederrey C, Olson-Sand A, Anker P. About the possible origin and mechanism of circulating DNA apoptosis and active DNA release. Clin Chim Acta. 2001;313(1–2):139–42.
8. Turchinovich A, Weiz L, Langheinz A, Burwinkel B. Characterization of extracellular circulating microRNA. Nucleic Acids Res. 2011;39(16):7223–33.
9. Pant S, Hilton H, Burczynski ME. The multifaceted exosome: biogenesis, role in normal and aberrant cellular function, and frontiers for pharmacological and biomarker opportunities. Biochem Pharmacol. 2012;83(11):1484–94.
10. Schwarzenbach H. The clinical relevance of circulating, exosomal miRNAs as biomarkers for cancer. Expert Rev Mol Diagn. 2015;15(9):1159–69.
11. Simpson RJ, Lim JW, Moritz RL, Mathivanan S. Exosomes: proteomic insights and diagnostic potential. Expert Rev Proteomics. 2009;6(3):267–83.
12. Valadi H, Ekstrom K, Bossios A, Sjostrand M, Lee JJ, Lotvall JO. Exosome-mediated transfer of mRNAs and microRNAs is a novel mechanism of genetic exchange between cells. Nat Cell Biol. 2007;9(6):654–9.
13. Chen X, Liang H, Zhang J, Zen K, Zhang CY. Horizontal transfer of microRNAs: molecular mechanisms and clinical applications. Protein Cell. 2012;3(1):28–37.
14. Lee TH, D'Asti E, Magnus N, Al-Nedawi K, Meehan B, Rak J. Microvesicles as mediators of intercellular communication in cancer--the emerging science of cellular 'debris. Semin Immunopathol. 2011;33(5):455–67.
15. Howcroft TK, Zhang HG, Dhodapkar M, Mohla S. Vesicle transfer and cell fusion: Emerging concepts of cell-cell communication in the tumor microenvironment. Cancer Biol Ther. 2011;12(3):159–64.
16. von Minckwitz G, Schneeweiss A, Loibl S, Salat C, Denkert C, Rezai M, et al. Neoadjuvant carboplatin in patients with triple-negative and HER2-positive early breast cancer (GeparSixto; GBG 66): a randomised phase 2 trial. Lancet Oncol. 2014;15(7):747–56.

17. Kirschner MB, Kao SC, Edelman JJ, Armstrong NJ, Vallely MP, van Zandwijk N, et al. Haemolysis during sample preparation alters microRNA content of plasma. PLoS One. 2011;6(9):e24145.
18. Schwarzenbach H, da Silva AM, Calin G, Pantel K. Data Normalization Strategies for MicroRNA Quantification. Clin Chem. 2015;61(11):1333–42.
19. Sharma NR, Wang X, Majerciak V, Ajiro M, Kruhlak M, Meyers C, et al. Cell type- and tissue context-dependent nuclear distribution of human Ago2. J Biol Chem. 2016;291(5):2302–9.
20. Zhao L, Liu W, Xiao J, Cao B. The role of exosomes and "exosomal shuttle microRNA" in tumorigenesis and drug resistance. Cancer Lett. 2015;356(2 Pt B):339–46.
21. Meng X, Muller V, Milde-Langosch K, Trillsch F, Pantel K, Schwarzenbach H. Diagnostic and prognostic relevance of circulating exosomal miR-373, miR-200a, miR-200b and miR-200c in patients with epithelial ovarian cancer. Oncotarget. 2016;7(13):16923–35.
22. Kong LY, Xue M, Zhang QC, Su CF. In vivo and in vitro effects of microRNA-27a on proliferation, migration and invasion of breast cancer cells through targeting of SFRP1 gene via Wnt/beta-catenin signaling pathway. Oncotarget. 2017;8(9):15507–19.
23. Lu L, Mao X, Shi P, He B, Xu K, Zhang S, et al. MicroRNAs in the prognosis of triple-negative breast cancer: a systematic review and meta-analysis. Medicine (Baltimore). 2017;96(22):e7085.
24. Jin L, Wessely O, Marcusson EG, Ivan C, Calin GA, Alahari SK. Prooncogenic factors miR-23b and miR-27b are regulated by Her2/Neu, EGF, and TNF-alpha in breast cancer. Cancer Res. 2013;73(9):2884–96.
25. Bertoli G, Cava C, Castiglioni I. MicroRNAs: new biomarkers for diagnosis, prognosis, therapy prediction and therapeutic tools for breast cancer. Theranostics. 2015;5(10):1122–43.
26. Martin EC, Conger AK, Yan TJ, Hoang VT, Miller DF, Buechlein A, et al. MicroRNA-335-5p and -3p synergize to inhibit estrogen receptor alpha expression and promote tamoxifen resistance. FEBS Lett. 2017;591(2):382–92.
27. Kodahl AR, Lyng MB, Binder H, Cold S, Gravgaard K, Knoop AS, et al. Novel circulating microRNA signature as a potential non-invasive multi-marker test in ER-positive early-stage breast cancer: a case control study. Mol Oncol. 2014;8(5):874–83.
28. Li M, Liu L, Zang W, Wang Y, Du Y, Chen X, et al. miR365 overexpression promotes cell proliferation and invasion by targeting ADAMTS-1 in breast cancer. Int J Oncol. 2015;47(1):296–302.
29. Cuk K, Zucknick M, Madhavan D, Schott S, Golatta M, Heil J, et al. Plasma microRNA panel for minimally invasive detection of breast cancer. PLoS One. 2013;8(10):e76729.
30. Mar-Aguilar F, Mendoza-Ramirez JA, Malagon-Santiago I, Espino-Silva PK, Santuario-Facio SK, Ruiz-Flores P, et al. Serum circulating microRNA profiling for identification of potential breast cancer biomarkers. Dis Markers. 2013;34(3):163–9.
31. Ho JY, Hsu RJ, Liu JM, Chen SC, Liao GS, Gao HW, et al. MicroRNA-382-5p aggravates breast cancer progression by regulating the RERG/Ras/ERK signaling axis. Oncotarget. 2017;8(14):22443–59.
32. Wang K, Jin J, Ma T, Zhai H. MiR-376c-3p regulates the proliferation, invasion, migration, cell cycle and apoptosis of human oral squamous cancer cells by suppressing HOXB7. Biomed Pharmacother. 2017;91:517–25.
33. Zou Y, Chen Y, Yao S, Deng G, Liu D, Yuan X, et al. MiR-422a weakened breast cancer stem cells properties by targeting PLP2. Cancer Biol Ther. 2018;19(5):436–44.
34. Zhang T, Jiang K, Zhu X, Zhao G, Wu H, Deng G, et al. miR-433 inhibits breast cancer cell growth via the MAPK signaling pathway by targeting Rap1a. Int J Biol Sci. 2018;14(6):622–32.
35. Hu X, Wang J, He W, Zhao P, Ye C. MicroRNA-433 targets AKT3 and inhibits cell proliferation and viability in breast cancer. Oncol Lett. 2018;15(3):3998–4004.
36. Shen Y, Ye YF, Ruan LW, Bao L, Wu MW, Zhou Y. Inhibition of miR-660-5p expression suppresses tumor development and metastasis in human breast cancer. Genet Mol Res. 2017;16(1).
37. Stuckrath I, Rack B, Janni W, Jager B, Pantel K, Schwarzenbach H. Aberrant plasma levels of circulating miR-16, miR-107, miR-130a and miR-146a are associated with lymph node metastasis and receptor status of breast cancer patients. Oncotarget. 2015;6(15):13387–401.
38. He XH, Zhu W, Yuan P, Jiang S, Li D, Zhang HW, et al. miR-155 downregulates ErbB2 and suppresses ErbB2-induced malignant transformation of breast epithelial cells. Oncogene. 2016;35(46):6015–25.
39. Kong W, He L, Coppola M, Guo J, Esposito NN, Coppola D, et al. MicroRNA-155 regulates cell survival, growth, and chemosensitivity by targeting FOXO3a in breast cancer. J Biol Chem. 2010;285(23):17869–79.
40. Yamamoto M, Kondo E, Takeuchi M, Harashima A, Otani T, Tsuji-Takayama K, et al. miR-155, a modulator of FOXO3a protein expression, is underexpressed and cannot be upregulated by stimulation of HOZOT, a line of multifunctional Treg. PLoS One. 2011;6(2):e16841.
41. Jurkovicova D, Magyerkova M, Sestakova Z, Copakova L, Bella V, Konecny M, et al. Evaluation of expression profiles of microRNAs and two target genes, FOXO3a and RUNX2, effectively supports diagnostics and therapy predictions in breast cancer. Neoplasma. 2016;63(6):941–51.
42. von Minckwitz G, Loibl S, Untch M, Eidtmann H, Rezai M, Fasching PA, et al. Survival after neoadjuvant chemotherapy with or without bevacizumab and everolimus for HER2-negative primary breast cancer (GBG 44-GeparQuinto)dagger. Ann Oncol. 2014;25(12):2363–72.
43. Shi W, Gerster K, Alajez NM, Tsang J, Waldron L, Pintilie M, et al. MicroRNA-301 mediates proliferation and invasion in human breast cancer. Cancer Res. 2011;71(8):2926–37.
44. Ma F, Zhang J, Zhong L, Wang L, Liu Y, Wang Y, et al. Upregulated microRNA-301a in breast cancer promotes tumor metastasis by targeting PTEN and activating Wnt/beta-catenin signaling. Gene. 2014;535(2):191–7.
45. Lettlova S, Brynychova V, Blecha J, Vrana D, Vondrusova M, Soucek P, et al. MiR-301a-3p suppresses estrogen signaling by directly inhibiting ESR1 in ERalpha positive breast cancer. Cell Physiol Biochem. 2018;46(6):2601–15.
46. Roccaro AM, Sacco A, Maiso P, Azab AK, Tai YT, Reagan M, et al. BM mesenchymal stromal cell-derived exosomes facilitate multiple myeloma progression. J Clin Invest. 2013;123(4):1542–55.

Healthcare costs and utilization associated with high-risk prescription opioid use: a retrospective cohort study

Hsien-Yen Chang[1,2,3], Hadi Kharrazi[1,3], Dave Bodycombe[1,3], Jonathan P. Weiner[1,3] and G. Caleb Alexander[2,4,5*]

Abstract

Background: Previous studies on high-risk opioid use have only focused on patients diagnosed with an opioid disorder. This study evaluates the impact of various high-risk prescription opioid use groups on healthcare costs and utilization.

Methods: This is a retrospective cohort study using QuintilesIMS health plan claims with independent variables from 2012 and outcomes from 2013. We included a population-based sample of 191,405 non-elderly adults with known sex, one or more opioid prescriptions, and continuous enrollment in 2012 and 2013. Three high-risk opioid use groups were identified in 2012 as (1) persons with 100+ morphine milligram equivalents per day for 90+ consecutive days (chronic users); (2) persons with 30+ days of concomitant opioid and benzodiazepine use (concomitant users); and (3) individuals diagnosed with an opioid use disorder. The length of time that a person had been characterized as a high-risk user was measured. Three healthcare costs (total, medical, and pharmacy costs) and four binary utilization indicators (the top 5% total cost users, the top 5% pharmacy cost users, any hospitalization, and any emergency department visit) derived from 2013 were outcomes. We applied a generalized linear model (GLM) with a log-link function and gamma distribution for costs while logistic regression was employed for utilization indicators. We also adopted propensity score weighting to control for the baseline differences between high-risk and non-high-risk opioid users.

Results: Of individuals with one or more opioid prescription, 1.45% were chronic users, 4.81% were concomitant users, and 0.94% were diagnosed as having an opioid use disorder. After adjustment and propensity score weighting, chronic users had statistically significant higher prospective total (40%), medical (3%), and pharmacy (172%) costs. The increases in total, medical, and pharmacy costs associated with concomitant users were 13%, 7%, and 41%, and 28%, 21% and 63% for users with a diagnosed opioid use disorder. Both total and pharmacy costs increased with the length of time characterized as high-risk users, with the increase being statistically significant. Only concomitant users were associated with a higher odds of hospitalization or emergency department use.

Conclusions: Individuals with high-risk prescription opioid use have significantly higher healthcare costs and utilization than their counterparts, especially those with chronic high-dose opioid use.

Keywords: Chronic high-dose opioid users, Concomitant users of opioid and benzodiazepine, Opioid shoppers, Healthcare costs, Resource utilization

---

* Correspondence: galexand@jhsph.edu
[2]Center for Drug Safety and Effectiveness, Johns Hopkins University, Baltimore, MD, USA
[4]Department of Epidemiology, Johns Hopkins Bloomberg School of Public Health, 615 N. Wolfe Street W6035, Baltimore, MD 21205, USA
Full list of author information is available at the end of the article

Background

Over the last two decades, adverse events from prescription opioids have soared in the United States [1–3]. In 2015, more Americans died of these products than ever before [4]; in addition, roughly 3.8 million people misused pain relievers every month and more than 2 million individuals are estimated to have an opioid use disorder every year, the majority of whom are not yet in treatment [5]. Given the morbidity and mortality from prescription opioids, several studies have investigated the direct and indirect societal costs of prescription opioid use disorders. For example, two widely cited studies, using claims data and publicly available secondary sources, estimated that the societal costs of prescription opioid use disorders skyrocketed from $8.6 billion in 2001 to $56 billion in 2007, while healthcare costs increased from $2.6 billion to $25 billion [6, 7]. Further, one review estimated that individuals with an opioid use disorder had annual healthcare costs that were $14,054–$20,546 greater than their counterparts among the privately insured, while commensurate increases among those with Medicaid ranged from $5870 to $15,183 per year [8]. More recent studies suggest similar additional expenses associated with opioid use disorders, ranging from $10,627 [9] to $20,760 [10] per year. This problem is not unique to the United States; for example, across the five largest European countries, the estimates of the incremental healthcare costs associated with prescription opioid abuse ranged from €900 to €2551 per person per year [11]. However, despite insights from prior studies, many analyses have adopted diagnosis codes rather than prescription drug utilization to identify high-risk opioid users [9, 10, 12–17], yet the vast majority of individuals with opioid use disorders are yet to be diagnosed. In addition, most studies have not explored the association between the extent of an individuals' high-risk use and their healthcare costs and resource utilization [9, 18–20]. Finally, in many analyses, comparisons between high-risk users and their counterparts have not been well controlled, increasing the likelihood of confounding [18, 19, 21].

In this study, we used longitudinal claims to characterize the healthcare costs and utilization among three groups of individuals with alternative measures of high-risk prescription opioid use. In addition to examining the overall associations, we were also interested in examining whether there was a dose–response relationship between the associations of interest.

Methods
Data
We used QuintilesIMS patient-level administrative claims, which are derived from participating health plans across the United States, including commercial plans and those contracting with Medicare and Medicaid; however, the fee-for-service portion of the Medicare or Medicaid data was not present in the QuintilesIMS data. We included enrollees from the largest multi-region commercial plan. Other than demographic and enrollment information, the database also included diagnosis, procedure, medication, and cost information from inpatient, outpatient, and Emergency Department (ED) settings. Patient information was de-identified to comply with the Health Insurance Portability and Accountability Act.

Study design and subjects
This is a 2-year retrospective cohort study (2012–2013). We used 2012 data to construct baseline covariates and three indicators of high-risk opioid users; for each type of high-risk opioid use, we also assigned an individual to a four-level indicator representing the magnitude of their opioid use. We used 2013 data to define our outcomes. Among 1,267,605 enrollees with continuous medical and pharmacy enrollment in 2012 and 2013, we restricted to 893,835 (70.51%) individuals between 18 and 64 years of age and with known sex; among them, 191,405 (21.41%) enrollees had at least one prescription opioid claim in 2012.

Identification of high-risk opioid users
High-risk group membership was identified using 2012 claims. First, we used files provided by the Centers for Disease Control and Prevention to define the prescription opioids and benzodiazepines of interest [22]. These files contained information on strength per unit and a morphine milligram equivalent (MME) conversion factor at the National Drug Code (NDC) level. The MME provides a standardized measure across quantities and strength. Next, we used the 2012 medical and pharmacy claims to define three patient groups at elevated risks of adverse events from prescription opioids. We defined 'chronic users' as those consuming more than 100 MMEs per day for more than 90 consecutive days [23, 24]. Chronic opioid use is related to higher medical utilization and a greater likelihood of overdose death [20, 21, 25]. We defined 'concomitant users' as patients filling more than 30-days of concomitant opioids and benzodiazepines [23, 24]. Benzodiazepines are associated with approximately one-third of overdose deaths involving prescription opioids [26] and the odds of dying by overdose is four-fold higher among veterans with current benzodiazepine prescriptions [27]. Finally, we defined 'opioid disorders' as patients with one or more diagnosis codes representing opioid use disorders (Appendix 1) [9, 12, 14–16, 28, 29].

We used two approaches to examine a dose–response association between high-risk opioid use and healthcare utilization. First, we categorized high-risk users into tertiles based on their magnitude of high-risk opioid use (level 1–3); we included non-high-risk opioid users as a reference group (level 0). For 'chronic users', we determined the number of days an individual was considered a chronic user to define the magnitude of high-risk opioid use; for 'concomitant users', we used the number of days with both drugs on hand; for those with opioid disorders, we adopted the number of months diagnosed with opioid use disorders. Second, we counted the number of high-risk groups each enrollee belonged to (0–3).

Outcome variables

Outcomes were derived from 2013 claims data. We calculated total, medical, and pharmacy costs (we also calculated pharmacy costs associated with prescription opioids only) and four binary measures of utilization (being among the top 5% total cost users, being among the top 5% pharmacy cost users, having any hospitalization, and having any ED visit) as our outcome variables. The annual costs were derived from claims and represents the sum of allowed amounts, reflecting what the insurance plan paid for services.

Control variables

We derived control variables from the Johns Hopkins Adjusted Clinical Group (ACG v11.0) Risk Adjustment System, using both medical and pharmacy claims as inputs. The ACG system is a widely used morbidity measure [30–37]; it has been validated against costs [33, 35, 36], utilization [32, 38], and death [39]. The ACG system assigns all ICD codes to one of 32 Aggregated Diagnostic Clusters (ADGs). Each ADG is a morbidity group consisting of clinically homogeneous diagnosis codes with a similar expected need for medical resources. Based on their ADGs, age, and sex, individuals are assigned to one of 93 discrete ACG categories. The ACG system also assigns each NDC code to one of 67 Rx-defined morbidity groups (RxMG) based on the combination of active ingredient and route of administration [30, 40]. The ACG system also calculates the number of chronic conditions/active ingredients using the diagnosis codes/NDC an individual encountered. In addition, the ACG system generates a risk score for concurrent total costs, including independent variables such as diagnosis-based overall disease burden, high-impact chronic conditions, diagnoses representing a high likelihood of hospitalization, and acute conditions.

Statistical analysis

We first described the characteristics of all enrollees, enrollees with any opioid use, and high-risk opioid users. Then, we constructed statistical models to evaluate the impact of being a high-risk user and the magnitude of high-risk opioid use on the prospective healthcare costs and utilization.

We used propensity score weighting to control for baseline differences in patient characteristics between high-risk and non-high-risk opioid users. Logistic regression was applied to derive a propensity score of becoming a high-risk user based on patient sex, four age categories (18–34, 35–44, 45–54, and 55–64), 32 diagnosis-based ADGs, 67 medication-based RxMGs, number of chronic conditions, number of active ingredients, and a concurrent risk score. An individual had three propensity score weights corresponding to each measure of high-risk use. We chose propensity score weighting because we could include all high-risk users, as might not occur with matching, and we wanted one interpretable overall effect, which might be impossible with stratification. We derived an average treatment effect of the treated weighting because we could estimate the average effect of treatment on the treated subjects, thus making comparisons between the actual outcomes of high-risk users and the expected outcomes under the counterfactual if they had not been high-risk users. This is especially useful when the study sample differs systematically from the overall population [41].

We examined the performance of our propensity score weighting based on comparisons of (1) high-risk users versus non-high-risk users with an opioid prescription and (2) high-risk users versus enrollees without an opioid prescription. We restricted our analyses to the first comparison because, after applying propensity score weighting, the average of the absolute standardized differences of all variables in the models reduced to less than 0.1; such differences were larger for the second comparison.

We used a generalized linear model (GLM) with a log-link function and gamma distribution to model costs, given the non-negative and positively skewed distribution of costs as well as a much higher proportion of people with very high costs [42–44]. We added $1 to all costs so that non-users could be included in the model. The log-link function provides an estimate of the proportional change in mean costs. We applied logistic regression for binary utilization indicators and included the same set of covariates from the propensity score model to control for residual confounding. We constructed both a crude and adjusted model with covariates and weights to explore the relationship between being high-risk opioid users and each outcome. For analyses of the dose–response association, we constructed a crude mode and an adjusted model with covariates since propensity scores were usually generated for binary outcomes.

As a sensitivity analysis, we also performed multivariate linear regression to test the robustness of our findings, since it is widely used to analyze costs, delivers intuitive results, and often performs similarly as other statistical models (such as a two-part log-normal model) with a sufficiently large sample size [8, 9, 33, 45]. These results yielded substantive similar findings and are reported in Appendix 2, but not discussed further herein.

Results
Characteristics of the eligible participants

Of 893,835 eligible enrollees, we identified 0.31% chronic users, 1.03% concomitant users, and 0.27% individuals with a diagnosis of an opioid disorder (Table 1). Of the 191,405 enrollees with any opioid use, the respective proportions of individuals with chronic use (2778/1.45%), concomitant use (9200/4.81%), and an opioid use disorder (1798/0.94%) were greater. The mean age of eligible enrollees was 42.4 years old, and about half (49.52%) were female; enrollees with any opioid prescription were slightly older (44.2 years old) and mostly female (55.14%). Individuals with opioid disorders were more likely to be younger and male than those in the other two high-risk groups.

Of the three high-risk groups examined, individuals with opioid use disorders had the lowest total ($25,000+) and pharmacy (~$4400) costs concurrently and prospectively; chronic users had the highest total (~$30,000) and pharmacy costs (~$11,000), but the lowest medical costs (~$20,000). Notably, more than one-third of chronic users' total costs were due to pharmacy costs, while pharmacy costs of those with opioid use disorders accounted for less than one-fifth of their total costs. In addition, the amount of pharmacy costs accounted for by prescription opioids varied across the three groups, with chronic users having the greatest proportion (more than 50%), compared to individuals with opioid use disorders (45%) and concomitant users (~20%).

Chronic users had lower rates of concurrent and prospective hospital (~15%) and ED (~28%) utilization, while those with opioid disorders had the highest rates of such utilization, although they declined over time. For example, among those with opioid disorders, the rates of hospitalization decreased from 29% concurrently to 18% prospectively, and the rates of ED visits decreased from 41% concurrently to 34% prospectively. Among the three high-risk groups, concomitant users had the highest morbidity across five ACG-based indicators, both concurrently and prospectively, while patients with opioid use disorders had the lowest morbidity prospectively.

The overlap across these three high-risk groups was low; the highest was 44.13% for chronic users being also concomitant users while the lowest was 5.04% for concomitant users being patients with opioid disorders. In the concurrent year, chronic users had 116 days being considered as chronic users, concomitant users had 150 days being concomitant users, and patients with opioid disorders had 3.7 months with a diagnosis of opioid disorders. On average, chronic users were included in 1.63 high-risk groups, concomitant users in 1.18, and patients with opioid disorders in 1.55.

Prospective healthcare costs associated with high-risk use

High-risk opioid use was associated with statistically significant increases in prospective total, medical, and pharmacy costs (Table 2). For example, after adjustment and weighting, chronic use was associated with greater prospective total (40%), medical (3%), and pharmacy (172%) costs. Similarly, corresponding increased costs were 13% (total costs), 7% (medical costs), and 41% (pharmacy costs) for concomitant users, and 28% (total costs), 21% (medical costs), and 63% (pharmacy costs) for patients with opioid use disorders.

Total and pharmacy costs, but not medical costs, increased as the magnitude of high-risk opioid use increased. After adjustment, each additional level in magnitude showed a statistically significant association with 19%/79% increases in total/pharmacy costs among chronic users, 4%/14% increases among concomitant users, and 19%/27% increases among patients with opioid use disorders. Costs were also greater among individuals with multiple high-risk group membership; each additional membership was statistically significantly associated with a 17% increase in total costs, a 6% increase in medical costs, and a 64% increase in pharmacy costs.

Prospective medical utilization associated with high-risk use

High-risk users were also associated with a statistically significantly greater likelihood of falling into the top fifth percentile of total and pharmacy spending, but only concomitant users had a statistically significantly higher likelihood of having any hospitalization and any emergency room visit (Table 3). For example, after accounting for covariates and weights, concomitant users were statistically significantly more likely to fall into the top 5% of total spending (odds ratio (OR) 1.18, 95% confidence interval (CI) 1.08–1.29) and pharmacy spending (OR 1.61, CIs 1.48–1.75), use

Table 1 Characteristics of three high-risk opioid groups, patients with any opioid and the whole study sample

	Chronic users	Concomitant users	Opioid disorders	Patients with any opioid use	All patients
Number of study subjects	2778	9200	1798	191,405	893,835
Age	47.22 (10.60)	49.47 (9.64)	38.59 (12.90)	44.16 (12.64)	42.43 (13.09)
Female	47.16%	65.76%	42.83%	55.14%	49.52%
Concurrent medical utilization in 2012					
Total cost	30,486 (57,670)	28,818 (61,406)	29,097 (50,380)	14,005 (34,238)	5456 (19,116)
Medical cost	19,275 (53,908)	22,195 (57,710)	23,662 (49,056)	11,888 (32,241)	4321 (17,632)
Pharmacy cost	11,211 (15,483)	6623 (15,638)	5435 (8119)	2117 (8120)	1135 (5357)
Opioid medication cost	6169 (11,315)	1393 (5560)	2494 (4158)	169 (1622)	36 (754)
1+ Hospitalization	15.95%	17.59%	29.14%	9.28%	2.98%
1+ Emergency visit	29.84%	33.55%	40.71%	27.76%	12.36%
Prospective medical utilization in 2013					
Total cost	31,045 (69,822)	27,040 (58,601)	26,061 (61,520)	11,176 (37,069)	5972 (23,001)
Medical cost	19,663 (65808)	20,008 (54,226)	20,758 (60,462)	8896 (34,402)	4739 (21,325)
Pharmacy cost	11,382 (17,539)	7033 (18,156)	5302 (7968)	2280 (10,617)	1233 (6530)
Opioid medication cost	6079 (13,170)	1459 (6506)	2416 (4606)	174 (1842)	40 (857)
1+ Hospitalization	14.25%	15.03%	17.96%	6.10%	3.03%
1+ Emergency visit	27.54%	31.07%	34.32%	18.61%	12.01%
Concurrent morbidity in 2012					
Count of ADGs	8.40 (4.34)	9.40 (4.22)	8.73 (4.36)	6.55 (3.78)	4.12 (3.49)
Count of RxMGs	8.85 (4.53)	10.31 (4.13)	7.77 (4.51)	5.98 (3.41)	3.00 (3.09)
Count of chronic conditions	4.00 (3.11)	4.43 (3.13)	4.11 (2.95)	2.26 (2.40)	1.31 (1.85)
Count of active ingredients	13.10 (8.16)	15.84 (8.09)	11.65 (8.37)	8.42 (5.79)	4.03 (4.64)
Concurrent risk score	4.67 (6.81)	4.95 (6.96)	5.16 (6.77)	2.49 (4.33)	1.14 (2.66)
Prospective morbidity in 2013					
Count of ADGs	8.25 (4.52)	9.13 (4.45)	7.73 (4.63)	5.86 (4.01)	4.18 (3.58)
Count of RxMGs	8.76 (4.64)	10.02 (4.41)	7.15 (4.65)	5.07 (3.92)	3.12 (3.19)
Count of chronic conditions	4.03 (3.26)	4.45 (3.26)	3.64 (3.11)	2.20 (2.48)	1.41 (1.96)
Count of active ingredients	12.75 (8.29)	15.17 (8.38)	10.42 (8.12)	7.13 (6.34)	4.18 (4.81)
Concurrent risk score	4.75 (7.42)	4.88 (7.10)	3.99 (6.22)	2.17 (4.33)	1.22 (2.95)
Overlap between three high-risk opioid groups in 2012					
Chronic users	–	13.33%	29.48%	1.45%	0.31%
Concomitant users	44.13%	–	25.80%	4.81%	1.03%
Opioid disorders	19.08%	5.04%	–	0.94%	0.27%
Magnitude of high-risk use in 2012	115.72 (85.23) / Days	150.72 (102.72) / Days	3.74 (3.29) / Months	–	–
Count of high-risk user membership in 2012					
Count of membership	1.63 (0.60)	1.18 (0.43)	1.55 (0.66)	0.07 (0.30)	0.02 (0.14)
0	–	–	–	93.87%	98.62%
1	43.05%	83.52%	54.39%	5.15%	1.17%
2	50.68%	14.59%	35.93%	0.89%	0.19%
3	6.26%	1.89%	9.68%	0.09%	0.02%

Table 2 Impact of being high-risk opioid users and its magnitude on prospective costs

	Total cost	Medical cost	Drug cost
Crude cost ratio – binary indicator			
Chronic users	2.85** (2.69–3.03)	2.25** (2.11–2.40)	5.30** (4.96–5.67)
Concomitant users	2.61** (2.52–2.69)	2.40** (2.32–2.49)	3.45** (3.32–3.58)
Opioid disorder	2.36** (2.19–2.54)	2.36** (2.18–2.56)	2.36** (2.17–2.56)
Adjusted cost ratio (with covariates and weighting) – binary indicator			
Chronic users	1.40** (1.39–1.42)	1.03* (1.02–1.04)	2.72** (2.69–2.75)
Concomitant users	1.13** (1.12–1.14)	1.07** (1.06–1.08)	1.41** (1.40–1.43)
Opioid disorder	1.28** (1.26–1.29)	1.21** (1.20–1.23)	1.63** (1.62–1.65)
Crude cost ratio (one level/count increase in magnitude/membership: 0–3)			
Magnitude of chronic users	1.62** (1.57–1.66)	1.44** (1.39–1.49)	2.17** (2.10–2.25)
Magnitude of concomitant users	1.54** (1.52–1.57)	1.48** (1.45–1.50)	1.76** (1.73–1.79)
Magnitude of opioid disorder	1.48** (1.43–1.54)	1.48** (1.42–1.54)	1.48** (1.42–1.54)
Count of high-risk group membership	2.18** (2.12–2.23)	2.02** (1.96–2.07)	2.81** (2.73–2.89)
Adjusted cost ratio (with covariates; one level/count increase in magnitude/membership: 0–3)			
Magnitude of chronic users	1.19** (1.16–1.23)	1.01 (0.98–1.04)	1.79** (1.74–1.84)
Magnitude of concomitant users	1.04** (1.03–1.06)	1.02 (1.00–1.03)	1.14** (1.13–1.16)
Magnitude of opioid disorder	1.19** (1.14–1.23)	1.20** (1.15–1.26)	1.27** (1.22–1.32)
Count of high-risk group membership	1.17** (1.14–1.20)	1.06** (1.03–1.10)	1.64** (1.59–1.68)

*$p < 0.05$; **$p < 0.01$

an inpatient service (OR 1.09, CIs 1.00–1.19), or visit the ED (OR 1.13, CI 1.06–1.21). Similar patterns were observed when examining the association between the magnitude of high-risk use and medical utilization; individuals with greater high-risk use or membership in various high-risk groups were statistically significantly more likely to fall into the top fifth percentile of total and pharmacy costs, but not necessarily have greater odds of any hospitalization or ED utilization.

Discussion

We used a large, commercially insured population to identify and characterize three groups of high-risk opioid users: 'chronic high-dose users', 'concomitant users' (of opioids and benzodiazepines), and individuals diagnosed with an opioid use disorder. All high-risk use was associated with much higher prospective pharmacy and total costs and, among the three groups examined, costs were greatest among chronic users (40% increase in total costs) and modestly lower among those with a diagnosed opioid use disorder (28%) or concomitant users (13%). In addition, high-risk use was associated with a greater likelihood of falling into the top fifth percentile of spending but not necessarily having higher resource use. Similar patterns were observed between a longer duration of such use and a greater likelihood of higher healthcare costs and resource utilization. These results are important given how commonly high-risk use occurs and the significant questions that remain regarding its impact on healthcare costs and utilization.

Most of the available studies identifying patients with opioid disorders rely on similar diagnosis codes. However, the definition of chronic users varies as do their denominators; for example, chronic users were defined as

Table 3 Impact of being high-risk opioid users and its magnitude on prospective medical utilization

	Top 5% total cost	Top 5% drug cost	Any hospitalization	Any emergency visit
Crude odds ratio (without covariates) – binary indicator				
Chronic users	4.07** (3.68–4.50)	13.58** (12.55–14.70)	2.61** (2.35–2.91)	1.68** (1.54–1.82)
Concomitant users	3.92** (3.69–4.16)	5.97** (5.65–6.31)	2.96** (2.78–3.14)	2.06** (1.96–2.15)
Opioid disorder	2.92** (2.54–3.35)	3.63** (3.19–4.13)	3.44** (3.04–3.88)	2.31** (2.09–2.55)
Adjusted odds ratio (with covariates and weighting) – binary indicator				
Chronic users	1.41** (1.20–1.66)	4.97** (4.31–5.74)	1.03 (0.87–1.20)	1.00 (0.89–1.14)
Concomitant users	1.18** (1.08–1.29)	1.61** (1.48–1.75)	1.09* (1.00–1.19)	1.13** (1.06–1.21)
Opioid disorder	1.20 (0.95–1.50)	1.65** (1.32–2.06)	0.94 (0.78–1.13)	1.03 (0.88–1.21)
Crude odds ratio (one level/count increase in magnitude/membership: 0–3)				
Magnitude of chronic users	1.79** (1.71–1.87)	3.07** (2.96–3.19)	1.47** (1.40–1.54)	1.24** (1.19–1.29)
Magnitude of concomitant users	1.76** (1.72–1.81)	2.15** (2.10–2.20)	1.57** (1.53–1.61)	1.36** (1.33–1.39)
Magnitude of opioid disorder	1.52** (1.43–1.62)	1.71** (1.61–1.81)	1.65** (1.56–1.74)	1.37** (1.31–1.44)
Count of high-risk group membership	2.62** (2.52–2.73)	4.14** (3.98–4.30)	2.20** (2.11–2.29)	1.69** (1.64–1.75)
Adjusted odds ratio (with covariates; one level/count increase in magnitude/membership: 0–3)				
Magnitude of chronic users	1.18** (1.11–1.25)	2.53** (2.41–2.67)	0.97 (0.92–1.03)	1.01 (0.97–1.06)
Magnitude of concomitant users	1.06** (1.03–1.10)	1.27** (1.23–1.31)	1.00 (0.97–1.04)	1.05** (1.03–1.08)
Magnitude of opioid disorder	1.12* (1.02–1.24)	1.27** (1.16–1.39)	1.11* (1.02–1.10)	0.99 (0.93–1.06)
Count of high-risk group membership	1.17** (1.10–1.25)	2.22** (2.09–2.35)	1.02 (0.96–1.08)	1.08** (1.03–1.13)

*$p < 0.05$; **$p < 0.01$

having 180+ days of supply among the insured with a medical or pharmacy claim [21], 100 MMEs or above per day in a year among enrollees with an opioid prescription [20], or at least 120 days of opioid prescription over any continuous 6 month period among enrollees with continuous enrollment [46]. Thus, the prevalence of patients diagnosed with opioid disorders in our study was on par with those from previous studies, ranging from 0.16% to 0.87% [9, 10, 16, 47], while that of chronic users was considerably different to those reported (0.65–2.8%) [20, 21, 46]; these differences must be taken into account when making comparisons across studies.

Out of 2378 eligible enrollees with a diagnosis of opioid disorders, 580 (24.39%) did not have any opioid prescription; thus, they were excluded from our analysis and the final sample size for patients with opioid disorders was reduced to 1798. This phenomenon has been reported by other researchers; indeed, in one study, approximately one-third of patients with an opioid abuse diagnosis did not have any opioid prescription [16], while in another study, 0.01% of the pharmacy-based non-opioid group still had a diagnosis of opioid abuse [21]. Among the 580 patients that did not have any opioid prescription, about two-fifths did not have their first diagnosis until July 2012 or later; therefore, these patients had enough time to obtain an opioid prescription prior to the first diagnosis, assuming that opioids would not be prescribed for patients with such diagnoses. It is likely that the illicit use of prescription opioid plays an important role in this finding, as approximately 3.8 million people misused pain relievers every month in 2015 [5].

Our findings extend previous analyses of the direct costs of prescription opioid use, although we used both prescription and medical claims to define our groups and adopted a more comprehensive set of covariates to decrease the potential for confounding. Based on our results, we estimated that the incremental total costs among patients with chronic use, concomitant use, and an opioid use disorder were $8870, $3111, and $5385, respectively. Our estimates are lower than prior estimates, which have generally ranged from $10,627 to $20,546 [9, 10, 16, 46]; such reductions may be in part due to better adjustment for potential confounders and our selection of a comparison group. For example, many prior studies have matched groups based on demographics only [10, 16, 17, 20], while even those matching on morbidity or baseline utilization [9] have only reported simple differences in average costs between high- and low-risk groups, leading to possible residual confounding [9, 10, 16, 20, 46]. In addition, others have used comparison groups including enrollees with an opioid claim [10, 17, 20], any medical claim [9], any medical or pharmacy claim [21], or just continuous enrollment [46]; however, these studies have not evaluated the comparability of their low- and high-risk groups. On the other hand, our estimate that individuals with an opioid use disorder had 28% greater total costs is similar to what was reported in another study with matching and outcome modelling [17].

Healthcare payers are an increasingly important stakeholder in the opioid epidemic, given the financial incentives to manage the resource use associated with the epidemic and the imperative to reduce injuries and deaths from these products. Health plans have access to patients' healthcare and prescription drug utilization, which allows for observation of events such as ED visits or hospitalizations associated with an opioid injury, as well as the quality and comprehensiveness of their primary care. Payers can engage to improve the care of high-risk patients, including minimizing early opioid exposure, using surveillance to identify high-risk prescribing and utilization, and providing greater assistance to those with opioid use disorders. For example, 'First-fill' education programs and early interventions to decrease patient's progression from acute to chronic use offer an important window of opportunity given the risks of long-term use associated with early fill patterns [48, 49]. Provider-targeted programs are also important since provider prescribing is associated with the patients' long-term use [50], and the remarkable variation in opioid prescribing across providers [51–53]. Warm handoffs [54] and early access to comprehensive medication assisted treatment after overdose [55] have also been promoted, given the high proportion of patients that resume prescription opioid use after an opioid-related adverse event [56] and the potential for patients to resume prescription opioid use during or following periods of buprenorphine receipt [57].

Our study had several limitations. First, we identified high-risk opioid use through claims data and thus could not identify the non-medical use of opioids diverted from friends or family. Our data also do not allow for us to examine heroin or illicit fentanyl use, and it is unclear to what degree we underestimate the true costs and resource use associated with the epidemic. Second, since we only had 2 years of data, we did not evaluate the long-term impact of high-risk opioid use. Third, we excluded Medicare and Medicaid enrollees and thus our results are not generalizable to all opioid users, but rather, reflect the experience of a group of commercially insured individuals; future work among the Medicare and Medicaid enrollees would provide important information. Fourth, studies have used different methods to define high-risk groups, yielding different estimates of their prevalence [9, 10, 16, 20, 21, 46, 47], making the direct comparison of estimates across studies difficult. Fifth, by requiring 2-year continuous enrollment, we excluded patients who died or lost job/insurance in 2013, which more likely concentrated on high-risk opioid users. Therefore, our results may underestimate the costs and utilization associated with high-risk opioid use. Sixth, even though we adopted propensity score weighting to control for baseline differences between groups, it is still possible that confounding exists, especially from those confounders not included in the propensity score model. Finally, we did not examine the experience of another high-risk opioid user group 'opioid shoppers', who obtain opioid prescriptions from multiple pharmacies and providers, since our data did not include a consistent means of identifying individual providers and pharmacies.

Conclusions

Three measures of high-risk prescription opioid use are associated with greater prospective costs. While our findings were modestly lower than previous estimates, the total cost of high-risk users was 4–6 times higher than that of all eligible enrollees and average pharmacy costs were as much as 4- to 11-fold higher. Given that opioid abuse-related injuries and deaths show no signs of abating, our findings underscore yet another dimension of the epidemic and the value of payer-driven interventions to reverse it.

Appendix 1
ICD-9-CM codes used to identify patients with 'opioid disorders'
Opioid-type dependence (304.0X).
  Combination of opioid abuse with any other (304.7X).
  Opioid abuse (305.5X).
  Poisoning by opiates and related narcotics, not heroin (965.0, 965.00, 965.02, 965.09)

Appendix 2

Table 4 Impact of being high-risk opioid group and its severity on prospective costs

	Total cost	Medical cost	Drug cost
Crude cost change – binary indicator			
Chronic users	20,161** (18,775–21,547)	10,925** (9637–12,213)	9236** (8841–9632)
Concomitant users	16,666** (15,893–17,439)	11673** (10,954–12,392)	4993** (4772–5214)
Opioid disorder	15,026** (13,306–16,746)	11,974** (10,377–13,571)	3051** (2559–3544)
Adjusted cost change (with covariates and weighting) – binary indicator			
Chronic users	6216** (5678–6754)	281 (−123 to 795)	5935** (5808–6063)
Concomitant users	637* (134–1140)	−1036** (−1518 to −553)	1673** (1546–1799)
Opioid disorder	1558** (1039–2076)	671** (161–1181)	887** (809–964)
Crude cost change (one level increase in severity) – severity level (0–3)			
Severity of chronic users	8845** (8205–9486)	4523** (3928–5119)	4322** (4139–4505)
Severity of concomitant users	7343** (6987–7700)	4959** (4628–5291)	2384** (2282–2486)
Severity of opioid disorder	6206** (5390–7022)	4880** (4123–5637)	1326** (1093–1560)
Adjusted cost change (with covariates: one level increase in severity) – severity level (0–3)			
Severity of chronic users	3337** (2695–3978)	263 (−344 to 869)	3074** (2887–3261)
Severity of concomitant users	1209** (840–1579)	315 (−34 to 664)	895** (787–1002)
Severity of opioid disorder	1136* (206–2067)	809 (−70 to 1688)	328* (56–599)

* $p < 0.05$; ** $p < 0.01$

Disclosures
Dr. Alexander is Chair of the FDA's Peripheral and Central Nervous System Advisory Committee, serves as a paid consultant and Chairs a QuintilesIMS Advisory Board, serves on the Advisory Board of MesaRx Innovations, and is a member of OptumRx's National P&T Committee. This arrangement has been reviewed and approved by Johns Hopkins University in accordance with its conflict of interest policies.
In addition, this study applies the ACG case-mix/risk adjustment methodology, developed at Johns Hopkins Bloomberg School of Public Health. Although ACGs are an important aspect of the paper, the goal of this paper is not to directly assess or evaluate the methodology. The Johns Hopkins University receives royalties for non-academic use of software based on the ACG methodology. Dr. Chang, Dr. Kharrazi, Dr. Bodycombe, and Dr. Weiner receive a portion of their salary support from this revenue.

Authors' contributions
HC designed the study, managed data, performed the analyses, and drafted the manuscript. HK, DB, and JPW secured data, provided critical comments, and revised the manuscript. GCA designed the study and drafted the manuscript. All authors read and approved the final manuscript.

Competing interests
Dr. Alexander serves as the Chair of the FDA's Peripheral and Central Nervous System Advisory Committee, serves as a paid consultant and Chairs a QuintilesIMS Advisory Board, serves on the Advisory Board of MesaRx Innovations, and is a member of OptumRx's National P&T Committee. This arrangement has been reviewed and approved by Johns Hopkins University in accordance with its conflict of interest policies. In addition, this study applies the ACG case-mix/risk adjustment methodology, developed at Johns Hopkins Bloomberg School of Public Health. Although ACGs are an important aspect of the paper, the goal of this paper is not to directly assess or evaluate the methodology. The Johns Hopkins University receives royalties for non-academic use of software based on the ACG methodology. Dr. Chang, Dr. Kharrazi, Dr. Bodycombe and Dr. Weiner receive a portion of their salary support from this revenue.

Author details
[1]Department of Health Policy & Management, Johns Hopkins Bloomberg School of Public Health, Baltimore, MD, USA. [2]Center for Drug Safety and Effectiveness, Johns Hopkins University, Baltimore, MD, USA. [3]Center for Population Health Information Technology, Johns Hopkins University, Baltimore, MD, USA. [4]Department of Epidemiology, Johns Hopkins Bloomberg School of Public Health, 615 N. Wolfe Street W6035, Baltimore, MD 21205, USA. [5]Division of General Internal Medicine, Department of Medicine, Johns Hopkins Medicine, Baltimore, MD, USA.

References

1. Alexander GC, Frattaroli S, Gielen AC, editors. The Prescription Opioid Epidemic: An Evidence-Based Approach. Baltimore: Johns Hopkins Bloomberg School of Public Health; 2015.
2. Dart RC, Surratt HL, Cicero TJ, Parrino MW, Severtson SG, Bucher-Bartelson B, Green JL. Trends in opioid analgesic abuse and mortality in the United States. N Engl J Med. 2015;372(3):241–8.
3. Kolodny A, Courtwright DT, Hwang CS, Kreiner P, Eadie JL, Clark TW, Alexander GC. The prescription opioid and heroin crisis: a public health approach to an epidemic of addiction. Annu Rev Public Health. 2015;36:559–74.
4. Rudd RA, Aleshire N, Zibbell JE, Gladden RM. Increases in Drug and Opioid Overdose Deaths - United States, 2000-2014. MMWR Morb Mortal Wkly Rep. 2016;64(50–51):1378–82.
5. Center for Behavioral Health Statistics and Quality. Key Substance Use and Mental Health Indicators in the United States: Results from the 2015 National Survey on Drug Use and Health. In: HHS Publication No. SMA 16–4984, NSDUH Series H-51. Rockville: Substance Abuse and Mental Health Services Administration; 2016.
6. Birnbaum HG, White AG, Reynolds JL, Greenberg PE, Zhang M, Vallow S, Schein JR, Katz NP. Estimated costs of prescription opioid analgesic abuse in the United States in 2001: a societal perspective. Clin J Pain. 2006;22(8):667–76.
7. Birnbaum HG, White AG, Schiller M, Waldman T, Cleveland JM, Roland CL. Societal costs of prescription opioid abuse, dependence, and misuse in the United States. Pain Med. 2011;12(4):657–67.
8. Meyer R, Patel AM, Rattana SK, Quock TP, Mody SH. Prescription opioid abuse: a literature review of the clinical and economic burden in the United States. Popul Health Manag. 2014;17(6):372–87.
9. Rice JB, Kirson NY, Shei A, Cummings AK, Bodnar K, Birnbaum HG, Ben-Joseph R. Estimating the costs of opioid abuse and dependence from an employer perspective: a retrospective analysis using administrative claims data. Appl Health Econ Health Policy. 2014;12(4):435–46.
10. Roland CL, Joshi AV, Mardekian J, Walden SC, Harnett J. Prevalence and cost of diagnosed opioid abuse in a privately insured population in the United States. J Opioid Manag. 2013;9(3):161–75.
11. Shei A, Hirst M, Kirson NY, Enloe CJ, Birnbaum HG, Dunlop WC. Estimating the health care burden of prescription opioid abuse in five European countries. Clinicoecon Outcomes Res. 2015;7:477–88.
12. White AG, Birnbaum HG, Mareva MN, Daher M, Vallow S, Schein J, Katz N. Direct costs of opioid abuse in an insured population in the United States. J Manag Care Pharm. 2005;11(6):469–79.
13. Yang Z, Wilsey B, Bohm M, Weyrich M, Roy K, Ritley D, Jones C, Melnikow J. Defining risk of prescription opioid overdose: pharmacy shopping and overlapping prescriptions among long-term opioid users in medicaid. J Pain. 2015;16(5):445–53.
14. White AG, Birnbaum HG, Schiller M, Tang J, Katz NP. Analytic models to identify patients at risk for prescription opioid abuse. Am J Manag Care. 2009;15(12):897–906.
15. Dufour R, Mardekian J, Pasquale MK, Schaaf D, Andrews GA, Patel NC. Understanding predcitors of opioid abuse: predictive model development and validation. Am J Pharm Benefits. 2014;6(5):208–16.
16. White AG, Birnbaum HG, Schiller M, Waldman T, Cleveland JM, Roland CL. Economic impact of opioid abuse, dependence, and misuse. Am J Pharm Benefits. 2011;3(4):e59–70.
17. Pasquale MK, Joshi AV, Dufour R, Schaaf D, Mardekian J, Andrews GA, Patel NC. Cost drivers of prescription opioid abuse in commercial and Medicare populations. Pain Pract. 2014;14(3):E116–25.
18. Cochran BN, Flentje A, Heck NC, Van Den Bos J, Perlman D, Torres J, Valuck R, Carter J. Factors predicting development of opioid use disorders among individuals who receive an initial opioid prescription: mathematical modeling using a database of commercially-insured individuals. Drug Alcohol Depend. 2014;138:202–8.
19. Braden JB, Russo J, Fan MY, Edlund MJ, Martin BC, DeVries A, Sullivan MD. Emergency department visits among recipients of chronic opioid therapy. Arch Intern Med. 2010;170(16):1425–32.
20. Gwira Baumblatt JA, Wiedeman C, Dunn JR, Schaffner W, Paulozzi LJ, Jones TF. High-risk use by patients prescribed opioids for pain and its role in overdose deaths. JAMA Intern Med. 2014;174(5):796–801.
21. Cicero TJ, Wong G, Tian Y, Lynskey M, Todorov A, Isenberg K. Co-morbidity and utilization of medical services by pain patients receiving opioid medications: data from an insurance claims database. Pain. 2009;144(1 2):20 7.
22. Analyzing Prescription Data and Morphine Milligram Equivalents [https://www.cdc.gov/drugoverdose/resources/data.html]. Accessed 02 May 2018.
23. Chang HY, Murimi IB, Jones CM, Alexander GC. Relationship between high-risk patients receiving prescription opioids and high-volume opioid prescribers. Addiction. 2018;113(4):677–86.
24. Chang HY, Murimi I, Faul M, Rutkow L, Alexander GC. Impact of Florida's prescription drug monitoring program and pill mill law on high-risk patients: A comparative interrupted time series analysis. Pharmacoepidemiol Drug Saf. 2018;27(4):422–9.
25. Gomes T, Mamdani MM, Dhalla IA, Paterson JM, Juurlink DN. Opioid dose and drug-related mortality in patients with nonmalignant pain. Arch Intern Med. 2011;171(7):686–91.
26. Jones CM, McAninch JK. Emergency department visits and overdose deaths from combined use of opioids and benzodiazepines. Am J Prev Med. 2015;49(4):493–501.
27. Park TW, Saitz R, Ganoczy D, Ilgen MA, Bohnert AS. Benzodiazepine prescribing patterns and deaths from drug overdose among US veterans receiving opioid analgesics: case-cohort study. BMJ. 2015;350:h2698.
28. McAdam-Marx C, Roland CL, Cleveland J, Oderda GM. Costs of opioid abuse and misuse determined from a Medicaid database. J Pain Palliat Care Pharmacother. 2010;24(1):5–18.
29. Rice JB, White AG, Birnbaum HG, Schiller M, Brown DA, Roland CL. A model to identify patients at risk for prescription opioid abuse, dependence, and misuse. Pain Med. 2012;13(9):1162–73.
30. Chang HY, Boyd CM, Leff B, Lemke KW, Bodycombe DP, Weiner JP. Identifying consistent high-cost users in a health plan: comparison of alternative prediction models. Med Care. 2016;54(9):852–9.
31. Chang HY, Clark JM, Weiner JP. Morbidity trajectories as predictors of utilization: multi-year disease patterns in Taiwan's national health insurance program. Med Care. 2011;49(10):918–23.
32. Chang HY, Lee WC, Weiner JP. Comparison of alternative risk adjustment measures for predictive modeling: high risk patient case finding using Taiwan's National Health Insurance claims. BMC Health Serv Res. 2010;10:343.
33. Chang HY, Weiner JP. An in-depth assessment of a diagnosis-based risk adjustment model based on national health insurance claims: the application of the Johns Hopkins Adjusted Clinical Group case-mix system in Taiwan. BMC Med. 2010;8:7.
34. Starfield B, Hankin J, Steinwachs D, Horn S, Benson P, Katz H, Gabriel A. Utilization and morbidity: random or tandem? Pediatrics. 1985;75(2):241–7.
35. Starfield B, Weiner J, Mumford L, Steinwachs D. Ambulatory care groups: a categorization of diagnoses for research and management. Health Serv Res. 1991;26(1):53–74.
36. Weiner JP, Starfield BH, Steinwachs DM, Mumford LM. Development and application of a population-oriented measure of ambulatory care case-mix. Med Care. 1991;29(5):452–72.
37. Chang HY, Richards TM, Shermock KM, Elder Dalpoas S, J Kan H, Alexander GC, Weiner JP, Kharrazi H. Evaluating the Impact of Prescription Fill Rates on Risk Stratification Model Performance. Med Care. 2017;55(12):1052–60.
38. Chang HY. The impact of morbidity trajectories on identifying high-cost cases: using Taiwan's National Health Insurance as an example. J Public Health. 2014;36(2):300–7.
39. Reid RJ, Roos NP, MacWilliam L, Frohlich N, Black C. Assessing population health care need using a claims-based ACG morbidity measure: a validation analysis in the Province of Manitoba. Health Serv Res. 2002;37(5):1345–64.
40. Forrest CB, Lemke KW, Bodycombe DP, Weiner JP. Medication, diagnostic, and cost information as predictors of high-risk patients in need of care management. Am J Manag Care. 2009;15(1):41–8.
41. Austin PC. An introduction to propensity score methods for reducing the effects of confounding in observational studies. Multivariate Behav Res. 2011;46(3):399–424.
42. Manning WG, Mullahy J. Estimating log models: to transform or not to transform? J Health Econ. 2001;20(4):461–94.
43. Leisegang R, Cleary S, Hislop M, Davidse A, Regensberg L, Little F, Maartens G. Early and late direct costs in a Southern African antiretroviral treatment programme: a retrospective cohort analysis. PLoS Med. 2009;6(12):e1000189.
44. Nguyen H, Ivers R, Jan S, Pham C. Analysis of out-of-pocket costs associated with hospitalised injuries in Vietnam. BMJ Global Health. 2017;2(1):e000082.

45. Shen Y, Ellis RP. How profitable is risk selection? A comparison of four risk adjustment models. Health Econ. 2002;11(2):165–74.
46. Leider HL, Dhaliwal J, Davis EJ, Kulakodlu M, Buikema AR. Healthcare costs and nonadherence among chronic opioid users. Am J Manag Care. 2011;17(1):32–40.
47. Ghate SR, Haroutiunian S, Winslow R, McAdam-Marx C. Cost and comorbidities associated with opioid abuse in managed care and Medicaid patients in the United Stated: a comparison of two recently published studies. J Pain Palliat Care Pharmacother. 2010;24(3):251–8.
48. Deyo RA, Hallvik SE, Hildebran C, Marino M, Dexter E, Irvine JM, O'Kane N, Van Otterloo J, Wright DA, Leichtling G, et al. Association between initial opioid prescribing patterns and subsequent long-term use among opioid-naive patients: a statewide retrospective cohort study. J Gen Intern Med. 2017;32(1):21–7.
49. Shah A, Hayes CJ, Martin BC. Characteristics of initial prescription episodes and likelihood of long-term opioid use – United States, 2006–2015. MMWR Morb Mortal Wkly Rep. 2017;66(10):265–9.
50. Barnett ML, Olenski AR, Jena AB. Opioid-prescribing patterns of emergency physicians and risk of long-term use. N Engl J Med. 2017;376(7):663–73.
51. Kim H, Hartung DM, Jacob RL, McCarty D, McConnell KJ. The concentration of opioid prescriptions by providers and among patients in the Oregon Medicaid Program. Psychiatr Serv. 2016;67(4):397–404.
52. Chang HY, Lyapustina T, Rutkow L, Daubresse M, Richey M, Faul M, Stuart EA, Alexander GC. Impact of prescription drug monitoring programs and pill mill laws on high-risk opioid prescribers: a comparative interrupted time series analysis. Drug Alcohol Depend. 2016;165:1–8.
53. Rutkow L, Chang HY, Daubresse M, Webster DW, Stuart EA, Alexander GC. Effect of Florida's Prescription Drug Monitoring Program and Pill Mill Laws on opioid prescribing and use. JAMA Intern Med. 2015;175(10):1642–9.
54. Rago G. Overdose to ER, a 'Warm Handoff' could save lives: USA Today; 2017. https://www.ydr.com/story/news/2017/03/29/overdose-er-warm-handoff-could-save-lives/99736074/. Accessed 02 May 2018.
55. Medication-Assisted Treatment Data. http://preventoverdoseri.org/medication-assisted-therapy/. Accessed 02 May 2018.
56. Larochelle MR, Liebschutz JM, Zhang F, Ross-Degnan D, Wharam JF. Opioid prescribing after nonfatal overdose and association with repeated overdose: a cohort study. Ann Intern Med. 2016;164(1):1–9.
57. Daubresse M, Saloner B, Pollack HA, Alexander GC. Non-buprenorphine opioid utilization among patients using buprenorphine. Addiction. 2017;112(6):1045–53.

Malaria elimination in remote communities requires integration of malaria control activities into general health care: an observational study and interrupted time series analysis in Myanmar

Alistair R. D. McLean[1,2], Hla Phyo Wai[1], Aung Myat Thu[1], Zay Soe Khant[1], Chanida Indrasuta[1], Elizabeth A. Ashley[2], Thar Tun Kyaw[3], Nicholas P. J. Day[4,5], Arjen Dondorp[4,5], Nicholas J. White[4,5] and Frank M. Smithuis[1,2,5]*

Abstract

Background: Community health workers (CHWs) can provide diagnosis and treatment of malaria in remote rural areas and are therefore key to the elimination of malaria. However, as incidence declines, uptake of their services could be compromised if they only treat malaria.

Methods: We conducted a retrospective analysis of 571,286 malaria rapid diagnostic tests conducted between 2011 and 2016 by 1335 CHWs supported by Medical Action Myanmar. We assessed rates of decline in *Plasmodium falciparum* and *Plasmodium vivax* incidence and rapid diagnostic test (RDT) positivity rates using negative binomial mixed effects models. We investigated whether broadening the CHW remit to provide a basic health care (BHC) package was associated with a change in malaria blood examination rates.

Results: Communities with CHWs providing malaria diagnosis and treatment experienced declines in *P. falciparum* and *P. vivax* malaria incidence of 70% (95% CI 66–73%) and 64% (59–68%) respectively each year of operation. RDT positivity rates declined similarly with declines of 70% (95% CI 66–73%) for *P. falciparum* and 65% (95% CI 61–69%) for *P. vivax* with each year of CHW operation. In four cohorts studied, adding a BHC package was associated with an immediate and sustained increase in blood examination rates (step-change rate ratios 2.3 (95% CI 2.0–2.6), 5.4 (95% CI 4.0–7.3), 1.7 (95% CI 1.4–2.1), and 1.1 (95% CI 1.0.1.3))).

Conclusions: CHWs have overseen dramatic declines in *P. falciparum* and *P. vivax* malaria in rural Myanmar. Expanding their remit to general health care has sustained community uptake of malaria services. In similar settings, expanding health services offered by CHWs beyond malaria testing and treatment can improve rural health care while ensuring continued progress towards the elimination of malaria.

Keywords: *P. falciparum*, *P. vivax*, Malaria, Community health workers, Vertical integration, Health systems strengthening, Myanmar, Sustainability, Elimination

* Correspondence: frank.m.smithuis@gmail.com
[1]Medical Action Myanmar, Yangon, Myanmar
[2]Myanmar Oxford Clinical Research Unit (MOCRU), Yangon, Myanmar
Full list of author information is available at the end of the article

Background

The global burden of malaria has fallen substantially since the beginning of the millennium (37% global decrease between 2000 and 2015), primarily due to improvements in access to diagnosis and treatment and increased coverage of insecticide-treated bednets [1]. Many of the estimated 216 million malaria cases and 445,000 deaths in 2016 occurred in remote areas of the tropics where health services are weak or non-existent [2]. Myanmar has the greatest burden of malaria in the Greater Mekong Subregion. Much of the burden of malaria is borne by remote and hard-to-reach communities [2]. The health care system in these communities has been weakened by decades of conflict and under-investment. The infrastructure is poor, and most villagers have no access to trained health staff and resort to informal health care providers (known by the colloquial term "quack" in Myanmar). These providers are generally untrained villagers who sell medicines unofficially. Over the past 6 years, investment in rural health care services has increased substantially [3], supported by both the national government and international donors, in particular from *The 3 Millennium Development Goal Fund* (a consortium of bilateral donors for Myanmar) and *The Global Fund to Fight AIDS, Tuberculosis and Malaria*. There has been particular support for malaria control (community health workers (CHWs) and long-lasting insecticide-treated net (LLIN) distribution) [4, 5]) for hard-to-reach communities. As a consequence, the national malaria incidence is estimated to have decreased by 49% since 2012: from 8.1 per 1000 to 4.2 per 1000 in 2015 [6].

Community-based malaria management using rapid diagnostic tests (RDTs) and good quality treatment, implemented by CHWs, can substantially improve malaria management in remote communities. CHWs can also distribute LLIN [7]. This approach has been successful in reducing malaria in many settings [8–11] although it has failed in other contexts where community uptake of services was not maintained [12–14]. Maintaining strong community uptake of CHW services is essential to sustain blood examination rates and good malaria control [12, 13, 15, 16] and to provide longitudinal surveillance data from case detection to estimate the true malaria incidence [17]. However, as malaria transmission and incidence falls, the proportion of febrile cases that are malaria, and receive antimalarial treatment, declines correspondingly. Community uptake of CHW programmes that offer only malaria testing and treatment is therefore likely to reduce. Patients attend a health worker because they have fever for which they want treatment. As the probability that a febrile patient has malaria and receives treatment declines, the perceived value of the malaria-only CHW programme declines too, and so the CHWs may become victims of their own success. In order to be appreciated and therefore used by their communities, CHW programmes need to provide relevant services of perceived value and benefit. To achieve this, 'malaria-only' CHWs can broaden their service to provide an integrated health care package to address common health problems.

Medical Action Myanmar (MAM), a medical aid organisation, has been supporting a network of CHWs in the most remote communities in Myanmar. These initially provided malaria control activities exclusively. However, as malaria decreased rapidly in these communities, CHWs were trained to offer an extended basic health care (BHC) package in addition to the malaria services. This was initiated in 2013 and 2014 in an effort to meet health needs and to ensure continued community participation with the CHW malaria programme. This extended BHC package incorporated treatment of malnutrition, diarrhoea, and respiratory tract infections, in line with the integrated community case management statement of the World Health Organization (WHO) and United Nations International Children's Fund (UNICEF) [18]. It also supported referral of severely ill patients and patients suspected to have tuberculosis to the nearest hospital.

All countries in the Greater Mekong Subregion have set national targets for malaria elimination in the near future. Despite interest in integrated CHW programmes, and their proven efficacy in reducing morbidity and mortality from acute respiratory infections [19–23] and diarrhoeal disease [19, 21, 23], there is relatively little information on their efficacy in malaria control and their effect on community uptake in the context of malaria elimination [24]. We conducted a retrospective analysis of 1335 MAM-supported CHWs operating in Myanmar between 2011 and 2016. We assessed the rates of decline in *Plasmodium falciparum* and *Plasmodium vivax* malaria incidence and RDT positivity with each year of CHW operation. In addition, we investigated the effects of the addition of a BHC package on the uptake of malaria services in four cohorts of CHWs which had provided malaria services only for at least 1 year.

Methods

Study area and population

Routine monitoring data were obtained from the network of CHWs in remote border areas of Myanmar, adjacent to Thailand, China, India and Bangladesh (Fig. 1). The terrain varies from forested hills to flat areas with many streams and rivers. Yearly rainfall is high (2500–5000 mm/year). During the rainy (malaria) season, many villages are inaccessible. Malaria transmission is heterogeneous ranging from low to high even over small geographic distances and occurs for most of the year with a peak of intensity during and after the rainy season.

In 2011, in cooperation with the Myanmar National Malaria Control Programme, MAM instituted a network of CHWs in remote communities in Mon State, South-East Myanmar, to provide community-based malaria

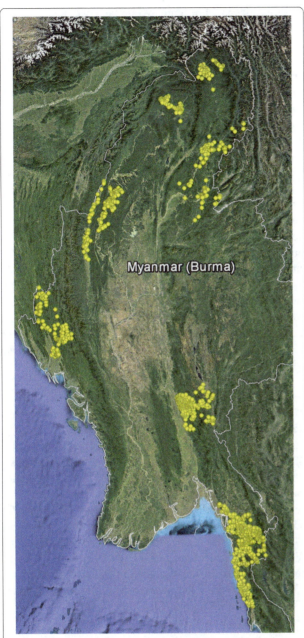

Fig. 1 Locations of community health workers within Myanmar supported by Medical Action Myanmar in 2016. Google Earth, US Dept of State Geographer 2018 Google, Image Landsat/Copernicus, Data SIO, NOAA, US Navy, NGA, GEBCO

management. Initially, 103 village volunteers were selected after consultation with village leaders and screening for literacy and education level. The volunteers were trained to perform malaria RDTs for all patients in their villages with complaints of fever and to provide treatment accordingly. *P. falciparum* malaria was treated with oral artemether-lumefantrine according to national guidelines. This was provided according to body weight in colour-coded blister packages. A single dose of primaquine (0.75mg/kg) was added on the first day of treatment to reduce transmissibility of the infection. *P. vivax* malaria was treated with 3 days of chloroquine (25 mg base/kg) plus primaquine, which was given initially once a day (0.25 mg base/kg) for 14 days without G6PD testing. After November 2015, this policy was changed to 15 mg, 30 mg, and 45 mg of primaquine for 5–9 year olds, 10–14 year olds, and 15 year olds respectively once weekly for 8 weeks to mitigate the risk of haemolysis in people who were G6PD deficient. The CHW recorded the test results and treatment provided, together with basic patient information details on standard forms, and these reports were provided to the regional Vector Borne Disease Control office each month. CHWs agreed to be available in their village every day for a minimum of 1 h to provide diagnosis and treatment, usually early morning or late afternoon when villagers returned from their fields. The CHWs received a fixed monthly incentive ($\approx$\$4 USD) and a small incentive ($\approx$\$0.4 USD) for every patient tested (Additional file 1). All activities were supported by health education and community engagement discussions to inform the community and to seek their feedback.

During 2013 and 2014, it became clear that the incidence of malaria had decreased markedly since the introduction of malaria-focused CHWs and that other important unaddressed health needs had become relatively more common and pressing. A BHC package was therefore added to the CHW malaria services which comprised four components:

1) Management of selected common diseases, including respiratory tract infections, diarrhoea, and skin infections
2) Detection of acute malnutrition with mid-upper-arm-circumference measurement and treatment with ready-to-use therapeutic food (plumpy'nut™)
3) Active case finding of patients suspected to have tuberculosis and referral to the nearest government hospital
4) Referral of complicated and severely ill patients with life threatening or disabling diseases to the nearest government hospital

Over the next 2 years, the network of CHWs trained expanded and, by the end of 2016, had grown to 1326. The CHWs received training in line with the curricula of the National Malaria Control Programme and National TB Programme (further training details in Additional file 1).

Statistical analysis

To assess temporal changes in incidence, RDT positivity rates and monthly blood examination rates, negative binomial mixed effects regression models were constructed with random intercepts and slopes. Seasonal variations in outcomes were accounted for by the inclusion of harmonic functions of time as a covariate. As a sensitivity analysis, we fitted alternate models with (1) adjustment for seasonality with a categorical month indicator, (2) no adjustment for seasonality, and (3) adjustment with a first-order autoregressive variance structure (Additional file 2). Plots of residuals were inspected for signs of autocorrelation. When modelling incidence and RDT positivity rates, the outcome was RDT-positive results (per month, per CHW) and the primary exposure was years of CHW operation. The exposure variable for the incidence model was the population served by a CHW, and the exposure variable for the RDT positivity rate model was the number of RDTs performed.

When modelling monthly blood examination rates, the population each CHW served was incorporated as the exposure variable and the outcome variable was total RDTs performed. To assess the impact of the introduction of BHC package services on CHW blood examination rate, we adopted standard methods for interrupted time series analysis [25]. We identified cohorts of CHWs from the same state/region where at least ten CHWs had been providing malaria-only services for more than 12 months and where these CHWs received BHC package training over 2 months. The announcement and introduction of BHC services was expected to affect consultation rates immediately, so we made the a priori decision to construct a slope and level change model, estimating the immediate change and change in time trend at time of BHC implementation. A likelihood ratio test comparing a level change model (BHC main effect only) to the slope and level change model provided a p value for the change in slope at BHC implementation. Statistical analyses were performed using Stata 14.2 (StataCorp, College Station, TX) and R software (version 3.4.4, The R Foundation for Statistical Computing, Vienna, Austria).

Results
CHW recruitment and population coverage
In 2011, a group of 103 CHWs were recruited, trained, and supplied to diagnose and treat malaria in remote communities in Mon State, Myanmar, covering a population of 163,171. This network of CHWs was expanded subsequently, and over the next 5 years, 1335 CHWs were trained and supplied. Of these, 1326 (98%) were still operational in 2016 in the following states and divisions: Mon, Kayah, Kayin, and Thanintharyi in the East; Kachin and Sagaing in the North; and Chin and Rakhine in the West, covering an estimated population of 728,057 (Fig. 1). This is approximately 1.3% of the Myanmar population.

Over this period, 571,286 RDTs were performed by the CHWs and 10,604 *P. falciparum* infections and 10,657 *P. vivax* infections were detected and treated. The median (interquartile range) overall blood examination rate (i.e. percentage of the total population who had blood tested) across all CHWs was 4.2% (1.9–7.6%) per month. The populations serviced by individual CHWs were generally small (median 309 (IQR 170–597)). Median monthly blood examination rates were higher in CHWs serving smaller populations: 7.5% (IQR 4.3–12.6%) for CHWs with a catchment population less than 250, and 4.2% (IQR 2.4–6.3%) for those with a catchment population of 250–500 compared with 1.6% (IQR 0.8%–2.9%) for those with a catchment population greater than 500.

P. falciparum and *P. vivax* incidence and RDT positivity rates
There was considerable heterogeneity in the initial incidence and positivity rates of *P. falciparum* and *P. vivax* in newly opened CHW posts (Table 1, Additional files 3 and 4). Across the study villages, the incidence and RDT positivity rates of both *P. falciparum* and *P. vivax* malaria declined markedly after institution of the CHWs (Fig. 2). For each year of CHW operation, there was a 70% (95% CI 66–73%) decrease in *P. falciparum* incidence (Fig. 2a) and a 64% (95% CI 59–68%) decrease in *P. vivax* incidence (Fig. 2b). Similar declines in RDT positivity rates were observed; each year of CHW operation was associated with a 70% (95% CI 66–73%) decrease in the *P. falciparum* (Fig. 2c) and a 65% (95% CI 61–69%) decrease in the *P. vivax* RDT positivity rates (Fig. 2d). Similar declines in

Table 1 Malaria in the first year of community health worker operation in eight regions of Myanmar

Region	Programme started	*P. falciparum*		*P. vivax*	
		Positivity rate[a]	Incidence[b]	Positivity rate[a]	Incidence[b]
Chin	May 2016[c]	22.6	14.7	4.3	2.8
Kachin	April 2014	0.6	0.1	0.8	0.2
Kayah	August 2014	1.3	0.3	3.9	0.8
Kayin	March 2012	11.7	5.3	16.9	7.7
Mon	September 2011	2.8	0.4	5.1	0.7
Rakhine	November 2016[c]	1.0	0.1	0	0
Sagaing	March 2016[c]	1.3	0.2	0.4	0.1
Tanintharyi	March 2014	0.1	0.04	0.2	0.1

[a]Per 100 rapid diagnostic tests. [b]Per 1000 person months. [c]Summary data covers months from start date until December 2016

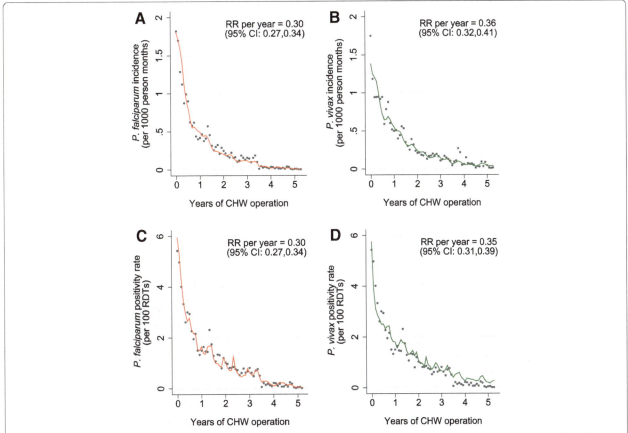

Fig. 2 Malaria incidence and RDT positivity rates by years of CHW operation. Grey dots denote observed aggregated data, and the line indicates the prediction from a mixed effects negative binomial regression model for **a** *P. falciparum* incidence (per 1000 person months), **b** *P. vivax* incidence (per 1000 person months), **c** *P. falciparum* RDT positivity rate (%), and **d** *P. vivax* RDT positivity rate (%). Models were constructed from activities of 1335 CHWs and 571,286 RDT results. CHW: community health worker, RR: rate ratio, 95% CI: 95% confidence interval as calculated from the model

incidence and RDT positivity rates were obtained from three sensitivity analyses, which (1) accounted for seasonality with a monthly indicator, (2) did not adjust for seasonality, and (3) accounted for seasonality with a first-order autoregressive variance structure (Additional file 2). In sensitivity analysis 3, estimates of the decline in *P. falciparum* incidence, *P. vivax* incidence, and *P. vivax* RDT positivity rates were of slightly smaller magnitude (64%, 60%, and 62% declines respectively) than estimates obtained in the primary analysis.

Blood examination rates before and after the introduction of a basic health care package

Training of CHWs to provide the BHC package in addition to the malaria activities began in April 2013 with 43 CHWs. By the end of 2016, 1040 CHWs were providing a BHC package. In 2016, CHWs provided 284,658 BHC consultations, including diagnosis of 14,509 cases of pneumonia and identification and referral to the nearest hospital of 6278 patients with suspected tuberculosis and 859 patients for other severe disease causes.

The monthly blood examination rates of the four cohorts of CHWs that introduced the BHC package after providing malaria-only services for at least a year were investigated. These cohorts comprised 154 CHWs who were all based in Eastern Myanmar (three cohorts in Mon state and one cohort in Kayin state, Table 2). The RDT positivity rate before BHC package introduction was highest in the Kayin cohort (18.1% and 11.4% respectively, in the 2 years preceding BHC), while the cohorts from Mon State had lower RDT positivity rates (7.4% and 6.2%; 9.4% and 5.4%; and 1.8% and 0.9% in the 2 years preceding the introduction of the BHC package).

In the pre-introduction period when the CHWs provided malaria services only, cohorts 1, 2, and 4 were experiencing significant declines in blood examination rates ($p < 0.0001$ for all) while in cohort 3 the decline was small and was not significant ($p = 0.91$; Fig. 3, Table 3). The introduction of the BHC package was associated with an immediate step-change increase in the blood examination rate in all four cohorts, (rate ratios post-BHC relative to pre-BHC: 2.3, 5.4, 1.7, and 1.1 respectively, $p < 0.0001$ for cohorts 1 to 3 and $p = 0.16$ for

Table 2 Characteristics of the cohorts included in interrupted time series analysis

	Cohort 1	Cohort 2	Cohort 3	Cohort 4
Number of CHWs	44	18	19	73
Total monthly reports	2759	1039	1214	3252
Total RDTs performed	60,461	13,904	33,585	64,909
State	Mon	Mon	Mon	Kayin
Townships	Kyaikmaraw, Ye	Ye	Kyaikmaraw, Mudon, Paung	Kyainseikgyi
Date first CHW operational	September 2011	September 2011	September 2011	March 2012
Dates BHC package introduced	May–June 2013	August–September 2013	March 2014	May 2014
Total population covered	47,831	6415	31,724	54,595
Median (IQR) community population	850 (387–1459)	388 (259–430)	1285 (905–2644)	548 (281–870)
MBER (year prior to BHC)	1.2%	1.7%	1.5%	3.4%
RDT (+) rate (1–2 years prior to BHC)	7.4%	9.4%	1.8%	18.1%
RDT (+) rate (year prior to BHC)	6.2%	5.4%	0.9%	11.4%
RDT (+) rate (year post-BHC)	1.4%	0.8%	0.3%	6.0%

CHW community health worker, *RDT* rapid diagnostic test for malaria, *BHC* basic health care, *MBER* monthly blood examination rate, *IQR* interquartile range

cohort 4, Fig. 3, Table 3). The three cohorts (1, 2, and 4) that experienced significant blood examination rate declines prior to BHC implementation experienced significant positive changes in slope after BHC implementation (likelihood ratio test for interaction $p < 0.0001$, $p < 0.0001$, and $p = 0.01$ respectively), while in cohort 3 blood examination rates were stable over time prior to BHC implementation and did not deteriorate with time after the step-change increase. We repeated the interrupted time series analysis of blood examination rates in three sensitivity analyses, which (1) accounted for seasonality with a monthly indicator, (2) did not adjust for seasonality, and (3) accounted for seasonality with a first-order autoregressive variance structure (Additional file 2). Results were broadly similar across these sensitivity analyses with the exception of the estimate of the step change in cohort 4 (rate ratio = 1.1 in the primary analysis and in sensitivity analysis 1; rate ratio = 1.5 in sensitivity analysis 2 and sensitivity analysis 3). Across the entire programme, CHWs offering a malaria-only service had an average blood examination rate of 1.63 per 100 persons per month (158,425 RDTs over 9.72×10^6 person months). CHWs offering a BHC package had an average blood examination rate of 3.20 per 100 persons per month (412,861 RDTs over 1.29×10^7 person months).

Discussion

Malaria elimination is now firmly on the agenda in much of the tropical world [26], and many countries, particularly in Southeast Asia, have set ambitious timelines for achieving it. In Myanmar, as in many low- and middle-income countries, CHWs are key to the delivery of malaria diagnosis and treatment in remote areas. This retrospective analysis clearly demonstrates the substantial public health benefit, in terms of reduced malaria incidence, of instituting trained CHWs in remote malaria-affected villages. The two-thirds annual reduction in incidence in these communities compares with an estimated decrease of 20% per year for the overall Myanmar yearly malaria incidence between 2012 and 2015 [6]. Thus, with relatively little training, but reliable supplies and careful monitoring, these community members provided a popular and highly effective public health service. The most likely explanation for the CHWs' success in reducing malaria is that provision of community-based early diagnosis and effective quality-assured treatment, coupled with LLIN distribution, significantly reduced malaria transmission.

The continued function of CHWs is essential to drive malaria to elimination, and to ensure continued monitoring of any imported malaria cases once local transmission has ceased. But having achieved large reductions in malaria, the CHW who treats only malaria becomes increasingly inactive and irrelevant as fewer and fewer patients with acute febrile illness are diagnosed with malaria and receive specific treatment. From the febrile patient's perspective, it matters little what the cause of their fever is, as long as it is treated effectively, so the incentive to seek treatment from the "malaria only" CHW declines as malaria incidence declines. Malaria-only community health workers recognise that when malaria declines, febrile patients are less likely to consult them, and wish to be able to provide help to patients with non-malaria fever [27]. Patients return to untrained informal health care providers, who provide inappropriate medicines and interventions. This was our concern when the numbers of patients seeking malaria RDTs in remote Myanmar villages declined.

To improve access to health care and to remedy the declining consultation rate, the remit of the CHWs was broadened to include other common febrile illnesses and

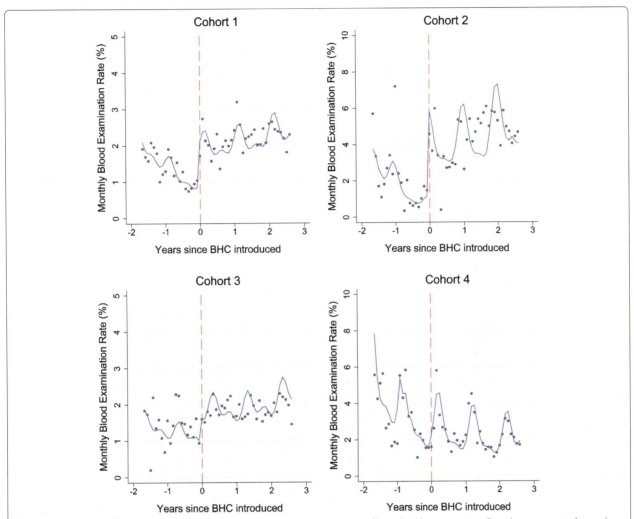

Fig. 3 Monthly blood examination rates in four cohorts of CHWs pre/post addition of basic health care services. Grey dots represent observed aggregated data, and the blue line indicates the prediction from a mixed effects negative binomial regression model. Vertical red line denotes the time when the basic health care package was introduced. Graphs are displayed for time points where data were available from all cohorts for consistency. BHC: basic health care. For model coefficients, see Table 3

referral of severely ill patients to the nearest hospital. This initiative was welcomed by the communities as non-malaria febrile illnesses now received a specific treatment as well, and for malaria control activities, it had the major advantage of sustaining quality. In this retrospective assessment, there was a decrease in health seeking behaviour and malaria RDT testing after malaria transmission had gone down, but this trend reversed after broadening the health care package of the CHWs. A limitation of this study was that it was observational, not experimental. However, the consistency and magnitude of the estimates observed, across four separate cohorts, suggest that the improvements in malaria RDT testing rates are real, accurate, and representative of what

Table 3 Interrupted time series analysis: monthly blood examination rates pre/post-basic health care package introduction

Cohort	Pre-BHC trend (per year) Rate Ratio (95% CI); p value	Step change at BHC introduction Rate ratio (95% CI); p value	Post-BHC trend (per year) Rate ratio (95% CI); p value	p value for change in trend[a]
1	0.60 (0.52,0.69); < 0.0001	2.28 (1.97,2.64); < 0.0001	1.08 (1.01,1.16); 0.03	< 0.0001
2	0.40 (0.31,0.53); < 0.0001	5.38 (3.96,7.32); < 0.0001	1.01 (0.87,1.18); 0.86	< 0.0001
3	0.99 (0.83,1.17); 0.91	1.71 (1.41,2.08); < 0.0001	1.03 (0.88,1.22); 0.71	0.51
4	0.76 (0.66,0.86); < 0.0001	1.10 (0.96,1.26); 0.16	0.89 (0.82,0.96); 0.002	0.01

BHC basic health care, *CI* confidence interval
[a] Change in trend from pre-BHC to post-BHC

could be expected in future implementations of integrated care. Of note, we observed different magnitudes of effect across different cohorts, suggesting that the context of a given community will be an important factor in service uptake. Cohort 4 had the smallest magnitude step-increase in blood examination rate, though in sensitivity analyses this estimate was higher when seasonality was not accounted for, or was accounted for using first-order autoregression (Additional file 2). Cohort 4 also had the highest malaria RDT positivity rate prior to BHC package introduction; a small step-increase was consistent with an expectation that this intervention will be most effective in communities that feel malaria is no longer a primary concern. Interrupted time series analyses are well suited to the evaluation of intervention effects in real-world settings [28], and as it seems unlikely that the incidence of febrile illnesses changed coincidentally with the change in CHW practice, a causal relationship is likely.

Most health professionals recognise that CHWs can have an important positive effect on malaria diagnosis and treatment in the community and that the success of community case management can be replicated for other common diseases. WHO and UNICEF outlined their support for integrated community case management in 2012 [18], noting that appropriately trained, supervised, and supported CHWs can identify and correctly treat most childhood respiratory tract infections and diarrhoea [29]. It has been estimated that community management of childhood pneumonia could reduce mortality from pneumonia in children less than 5 years old by 70% [22]. Oral rehydration salts and zinc reduce the mortality of diarrhoeal disease in community settings; community promotion of oral rehydration salts was estimated to reduce the number of deaths due to diarrhoea by 69% (95% CI 51–80%) [30], and zinc supplementation is estimated to decrease diarrhoea mortality by 23% (95% CI 15–31%) [31]. The approach of integrating disease-specific programmes with other health services (the "diagonal approach") is likely to be appropriate for other narrow disease-specific programmes, which can also see their sustainability threatened by their own success, and is critical for effective health systems strengthening [32, 33].

During the period of this study, financial incentive schemes for CHWs in Myanmar varied across different organisations; the value of incentives offered by MAM was neither the highest nor the lowest, among organisations supporting Myanmar CHWs [34]. There are concerns that per test incentives that are too high can have a negative influence on CHW diagnostic practices. Conversely, when incentives are too low or absent, the CHW may stop testing altogether and retention may become difficult. More research is needed to identify the correct balance of monthly incentive and test incentive in low-income areas. Ultimately, frequent monitoring and supervision are essential under any incentive scheme to maintain high standards of care and to check for aberrant practices.

Some policy makers worry that CHWs are not capable of providing the correct diagnosis for patients with non-malaria fevers. In several countries, CHWs are allowed to prescribe antimalarials but not antibiotics. Health professionals fear that CHWs may become the new generation of informal health care providers, over-prescribing unnecessary antibiotics without proper diagnosis. Instead, they suggest that it is better to refer patients with non-malaria febrile illnesses to the nearest government health service. However, in remote areas with poor infrastructure, numerous barriers of geographical access, availability, affordability, and acceptability hamper access to government health services [35, 36], and such a strategy is simply not feasible. Even when trusted CHWs refer patients to the nearest hospital, many will not go [37, 38]. Smaller villages are generally more remote and face more barriers to health service access so typically have a higher uptake of CHW services. It is in these villages that integration of community-based health services is most important. Integrated CHWs can be carefully regulated, which could diminish irrational antibiotic use, prevent antimicrobial resistance, and substantially reduce morbidity and mortality in a cost-effective manner.

This retrospective analysis includes over half a million malaria RDT results from a large number of communities (1335) over 5 years. The downward trends of incidence for both *P. falciparum* and *P. vivax* malaria after the introduction of community-based malaria management are substantial and convincing. By contrast, the analysis of the impact of the introduction of a BHC package was performed only in a relatively small number of cohorts (four) including 154 communities. This was unavoidable as the number of CHWs with enough data before and after introduction of the BHC package was limited, but the results are likely to be relevant to other remote communities.

Conclusions

In summary, this study demonstrates the clear benefits of the integration of basic health care into CHW services to sustain uptake of malaria services. Malaria has decreased significantly over the past years, and a further decline of morbidity and mortality is expected. As malaria approaches elimination, National Malaria Control Programmes must plan for likely reductions in funding and ensure that the capabilities for vector control and malaria diagnosis and treatment are maintained. A diagonal approach to health systems strengthening is needed to ensure effective, sustainable, and cost-effective health services in remote communities. A CHW for malaria-only is not sustainable and must become the CHW for an integrated package of common health problems. This will benefit the community and will ensure that malaria is eliminated and then stays eliminated.

Additional files

Additional file 1: Community Health Workers Training, Monitoring and Incentives: Additional details of the training, monitoring and incentive structure of Medical Action Myanmar community health workers.

Additional file 2: Sensitivity analyses. Sensitivity analyses of models of malaria incidence and RDT positivity rates by years of CHW operation and of the interrupted times series analysis of basic health care package introduction.

Additional file 3: Malaria incidence and RDT positivity rates by calendar year for Kachin, Kayah, Mon, Rakhine, Sagaing, Tanintharyi. (A) *P. falciparum* incidence (per 1000 person months); (B) *P. vivax* incidence (per 1000 person months); (C) *P. falciparum* RDT positivity rate (%); (D) *P. vivax* RDT positivity rate (%). RDTs = Rapid Diagnostic Tests. Chin and Kayin are presented separately in Additional file 3 for legibility.

Additional file 4: Malaria incidence and RDT positivity rates by calendar year for Chin and Kayin. (A) *P. falciparum* incidence (per 1000 person months); (B) *P. vivax* incidence (per 1000 person months); (C) *P. falciparum* RDT positivity rate (%); (D) *P. vivax* RDT positivity rate (%). RDTs = Rapid Diagnostic Tests. Other state/regions are presented separately in Additional file 2 for legibility.

Abbreviations

BHC: Basic health care; CHW: Community health worker; CI: Confidence interval; IQR: Interquartile range; MAM: Medical Action Myanmar; RDT: Rapid diagnostic test; UNICEF: United Nations International Children's Fund; WHO: World Health Organization

Acknowledgements

We thank all MAM field staff and community health workers in remote communities who were essential for the success of the programme, the National Malaria Control Programme, the Karen Department of Health and Welfare, Community and Health Development Network and staff from United Nations Office for Project Services in Myanmar, the 3 Millennium Development Goal Fund, and The Global Fund to Fight AIDS, Tuberculosis and Malaria. We thank Julie Simpson for her valuable feedback and comments. MOCRU is part of the Mahidol Oxford Research Unit, supported by the Wellcome Trust of Great Britain.

Funding

Funding was received from The Global Fund to Fight AIDS, Tuberculosis and Malaria, the 3 Millennium Development Goal Fund, Planet Wheeler Foundation, Kadoorie Charitable Foundation, DAK Foundation, and The Wellcome Trust. The funding bodies played no role in the design of the study; collection, analysis, and interpretation of the data; writing the manuscript; or the decision to publish.

Authors' contributions

AM, EA, ND, AD, NW, and FS contributed to the conceptualization. HPW, AMT, ZSK, TTK, and FS contributed to the investigation. AM, NW, and FS contributed to the formal analysis. AM, NW, and FS contributed to the writing of the original draft preparation. AM, HPW, AMT, ZSK, CI, EA, TTK, ND, AD, NW, and FS contributed to the writing and review and editing of the manuscript. All authors read and approved the final manuscript.

Competing interests

The authors declare that they have no competing interests.

Author details

[1]Medical Action Myanmar, Yangon, Myanmar. [2]Myanmar Oxford Clinical Research Unit (MOCRU), Yangon, Myanmar. [3]Department of Public Health, Ministry of Health and Sports, Nay Pyi Taw, Myanmar. [4]Mahidol-Oxford Tropical Medicine Research Unit (MORU), Faculty of Tropical Medicine, Mahidol University, Bangkok, Thailand. [5]Centre for Tropical Medicine and Global Health, Nuffield Department of Clinical Medicine, University of Oxford, Oxford, UK.

References

1. Cibulskis RE, Alonso P, Aponte J, Aregawi M, Barrette A, Bergeron L, Fergus CA, Knox T, Lynch M, Patouillard E, et al. Malaria: global progress 2000 - 2015 and future challenges. Infect Dis Poverty. 2016;5(1):61.
2. World Health Organization. World malaria report 2017. Geneva: World Health Orgnaization; 2017.
3. Mu TT, Sein AA, Kyi TT, Min M, Aung NM, Anstey NM, Kyaw MP, Soe C, Kyi MM, Hanson J. Malaria incidence in Myanmar 2005-2014: steady but fragile progress towards elimination. Malar J. 2016;15(1):503.
4. Nyunt MH, Aye KM, Kyaw KT, Han SS, Aye TT, Wai KT, Kyaw MP. Challenges encountered by local health volunteers in early diagnosis and prompt treatment of malaria in Myanmar artemisinin resistance containment zones. Malar J. 2016;15:308.
5. Lwin MM, Sudhinaraset M, San AK, Aung T. Improving malaria knowledge and practices in rural Myanmar through a village health worker intervention: a cross-sectional study. Malar J. 2014;13:5.
6. Department of Public Health MoHaS, The Republic of the Union of Myanamar: National strategic plan 2016-2020 for intensifying malaria control and accelerating progress towards malaria elimination. 2017. http://www.searo.who.int/myanmar/documents/malarianationalstrategicplan2016-2020.pdf?ua=1. Accessed 20 Jul 2018.
7. Lin K, Aung S, Lwin S, Min H, Aye NN, Webber R. Promotion of insecticide-treated mosquito nets in Myanmar. Southeast Asian J Trop Med Public Health. 2000;31(3):444–7.
8. Lemma H, Byass P, Desta A, Bosman A, Costanzo G, Toma L, Fottrell E, Marrast AC, Ambachew Y, Getachew A, et al. Deploying artemether-lumefantrine with rapid testing in Ethiopian communities: impact on malaria morbidity, mortality and healthcare resources. Trop Med Int Health. 2010;15(2):241–50.
9. Delacollette C, Van der Stuyft P, Molima K: Using community health workers for malaria control: experience in Zaire. Bull World Health Organ 1996, 74(4):423–430.
10. Carrara VI, Sirilak S, Thonglairuam J, Rojanawatsirivet C, Proux S, Gilbos V, Brockman A, Ashley EA, McGready R, Krudsood S, et al. Deployment of early diagnosis and mefloquine-artesunate treatment of falciparum malaria in Thailand: the Tak Malaria Initiative. PLoS Med. 2006;3(6):e183.
11. Brenner JL, Kabakyenga J, Kyomuhangi T, Wotton KA, Pim C, Ntaro M, Bagenda FN, Gad NR, Godel J, Kayizzi J, et al. Can volunteer community health workers decrease child morbidity and mortality in southwestern Uganda? An impact evaluation. PLoS One. 2011;6(12):e27997.
12. Hamainza B, Moonga H, Sikaala CH, Kamuliwo M, Bennett A, Eisele TP, Miller J, Seyoum A, Killeen GF. Monitoring, characterization and control of chronic, symptomatic malaria infections in rural Zambia through monthly household visits by paid community health workers. Malar J. 2014;13:128.
13. Ohnmar, Tun M, San S, Than W, Chongsuvivatwong V. Effects of malaria volunteer training on coverage and timeliness of diagnosis: a cluster randomized controlled trial in Myanmar. Malar J. 2012;11:309.
14. Ali F, Mucache D, Scuccato R. Avaliação do Programa dos APEs. Maputo, Moçambique: Ministério da Saúde e Cooperação Suíça; 1994.
15. Hansen KS, Ndyomugyenyi R, Magnussen P, Lal S, Clarke SE. Cost-effectiveness analysis of malaria rapid diagnostic tests for appropriate treatment of malaria at the community level in Uganda. Health Policy Plan. 2017;32(5):676–89.
16. Collins D, Jarrah Z, Gilmartin C, Saya U. The costs of integrated community case management (iCCM) programs: a multi-country analysis. J Glob Health. 2014;4(2):020407.
17. World Health Organization. World malaria report 2015. Geneva: World Health Orgnaization; 2015.

18. Young M, Wolfheim C, Marsh DR, Hammamy D. World Health Organization/ United Nations Children's Fund joint statement on integrated community case management: an equity-focused strategy to improve access to essential treatment services for children. Am J Trop Med Hygiene. 2012;87(5 Suppl):6–10.
19. Ghimire M, Pradhan YV, Maskey MK. Community-based interventions for diarrhoeal diseases and acute respiratory infections in Nepal. Bull World Health Organ. 2010;88(3):216–21.
20. Yeboah-Antwi K, Pilingana P, Macleod WB, Semrau K, Siazeele K, Kalesha P, Hamainza B, Seidenberg P, Mazimba A, Sabin L, et al. Community case management of fever due to malaria and pneumonia in children under five in Zambia: a cluster randomized controlled trial. PLoS Med. 2010;7(9):e1000340.
21. Boschi-Pinto C, Dilip TR, Costello A. Association between community management of pneumonia and diarrhoea in high-burden countries and the decline in under-five mortality rates: an ecological analysis. BMJ Open. 2017;7(2):e012639.
22. Theodoratou E, Al-Jilaihawi S, Woodward F, Ferguson J, Jhass A, Balliet M, Kolcic I, Sadruddin S, Duke T, Rudan I, et al. The effect of case management on childhood pneumonia mortality in developing countries. Int J Epidemiol. 2010;39(Suppl 1):i155–71.
23. Das JK, Lassi ZS, Salam RA, Bhutta ZA. Effect of community based interventions on childhood diarrhea and pneumonia: uptake of treatment modalities and impact on mortality. BMC Public Health. 2013;13(Suppl 3):S29.
24. Smith Paintain L, Willey B, Kedenge S, Sharkey A, Kim J, Buj V, Webster J, Schellenberg D, Ngongo N. Community health workers and stand-alone or integrated case management of malaria: a systematic literature review. Am J Trop Med Hygiene. 2014;91(3):461–70.
25. Wagner AK, Soumerai SB, Zhang F, Ross-Degnan D. Segmented regression analysis of interrupted time series studies in medication use research. J Clin Pharm Ther. 2002;27(4):299–309.
26. Rabinovich RN, Drakeley C, Djimde AA, Hall BF, Hay SI, Hemingway J, Kaslow DC, Noor A, Okumu F, Steketee R, et al. malERA: an updated research agenda for malaria elimination and eradication. PLoS Med. 2017;14(11):e1002456.
27. Ngor P, White L, Chalk J, Lubell Y, Favede C, Cheah P, Nguon C, Ly P, Maude R, Sovannaroth S, et al. Smartphones for community health in rural Cambodia: a feasibility study [version 1; referees: 2 approved with reservations]. Wellcome Open Res. 2018;3:69.
28. Kontopantelis E, Doran T, Springate DA, Buchan I, Reeves D. Regression based quasi-experimental approach when randomisation is not an option: interrupted time series analysis. BMJ. 2015;350:h2750.
29. Rowe SY, Kelly JM, Olewe MA, Kleinbaum DG, McGowan JE Jr, McFarland DA, Rochat R, Deming MS. Effect of multiple interventions on community health workers' adherence to clinical guidelines in Siaya district, Kenya. Trans R Soc Trop Med Hyg. 2007;101(2):188–202.
30. Munos MK, Walker CL, Black RE. The effect of oral rehydration solution and recommended home fluids on diarrhoea mortality. Int J Epidemiol. 2010; 39(Suppl 1):i75–87.
31. Walker CL, Black RE. Zinc for the treatment of diarrhoea: effect on diarrhoea morbidity, mortality and incidence of future episodes. Int J Epidemiol. 2010; 39(Suppl 1):i63–9.
32. Ooms G, Van Damme W, Baker BK, Zeitz P, Schrecker T: The 'diagonal' approach to Global Fund financing: a cure for the broader malaise of health systems? Glob Health 2008, 4:6.
33. Marchal B, Cavalli A, Kegels G. Global health actors claim to support health system strengthening: is this reality or rhetoric? PLoS Med. 2009;6(4):e1000059.
34. Kyaw SS, Drake T, Thi A, Kyaw MP, Hlaing T, Smithuis FM, White LJ, Lubell Y. Malaria community health workers in Myanmar: a cost analysis. Malar J. 2016;15:41.
35. Jacobs B, Ir P, Bigdeli M, Annear PL, Van Damme W: Addressing access barriers to health services: an analytical framework for selecting appropriate interventions in low-income Asian countries. Health Policy Plan 2012, 27(4):288–300.
36. Sudhinaraset M, Briegleb C, Aung M, Khin HS, Aung T. Motivation and challenges for use of malaria rapid diagnostic tests among informal providers in Myanmar: a qualitative study. Malar J. 2015;14:61.
37. English L, Miller JS, Mbusa R, Matte M, Kenney J, Bwambale S, Ntaro M, Patel P, Mulogo E, Stone GS. Monitoring iCCM referral systems: Bugoye Integrated Community Case Management Initiative (BIMI) in Uganda. Malar J. 2016;15:247.
38. Simba DO, Warsame M, Kimbute O, Kakoko D, Petzold M, Tomson G, Premji Z, Gomes M. Factors influencing adherence to referral advice following pre-referral treatment with artesunate suppositories in children in rural Tanzania. Trop Med Int Health. 2009;14(7):775–83.

Quantifying the impact of social groups and vaccination on inequalities in infectious diseases using a mathematical model

James D. Munday[1,2*], Albert Jan van Hoek[1,2,3], W. John Edmunds[1,2] and Katherine E. Atkins[1,2,4]

Abstract

Background: Social and cultural disparities in infectious disease burden are caused by systematic differences between communities. Some differences have a direct and proportional impact on disease burden, such as health-seeking behaviour and severity of infection. Other differences—such as contact rates and susceptibility—affect the risk of transmission, where the impact on disease burden is indirect and remains unclear. Furthermore, the concomitant impact of vaccination on such inequalities is not well understood.

Methods: To quantify the role of differences in transmission on inequalities and the subsequent impact of vaccination, we developed a novel mathematical framework that integrates a mechanistic model of disease transmission with a demographic model of social structure, calibrated to epidemiologic and empirical social contact data.

Results: Our model suggests realistic differences in two key factors contributing to the rates of transmission—contact rate and susceptibility—between two social groups can lead to twice the risk of infection in the high-risk population group relative to the low-risk population group. The more isolated the high-risk group, the greater this disease inequality. Vaccination amplified this inequality further: equal vaccine uptake across the two population groups led to up to seven times the risk of infection in the high-risk group. To mitigate these inequalities, the high-risk population group would require disproportionately high vaccination uptake.

Conclusion: Our results suggest that differences in contact rate and susceptibility can play an important role in explaining observed inequalities in infectious diseases. Importantly, we demonstrate that, contrary to social policy intentions, promoting an equal vaccine uptake across population groups may magnify inequalities in infectious disease risk.

Keywords: Inequality, Mathematical modelling, Influenza, Rubella, Social groups, Vaccination

---

* Correspondence: James.Munday@lshtm.ac.uk
[1]Centre for Mathematical Modelling of Infectious Diseases, London School of Hygiene & Tropical Medicine, London, UK
[2]Department of Infectious Disease Epidemiology, Faculty of Epidemiology and Population Health, London School of Hygiene & Tropical Medicine, London, UK
Full list of author information is available at the end of the article

Background

Reductions in global infectious disease burden have uncovered inequalities in infectious disease health outcomes [1–7]. These inequalities often reflect a disproportionately high incidence observed amongst the most deprived and vulnerable in society [4, 8–10]. Implementing equitable public health care relies on prioritising effective interventions that control the drivers of these inequalities [11].

There may be many contributing factors to inequalities in reported infectious disease health outcomes. Some of these factors have a direct and proportional impact on the relative reported disease burden between social groups, for example, the severity of disease experienced [12, 13], the propensity to seek health care [14] and the reporting rate of disease [15]. In contrast, other factors affect the transmission of infection and may result in non-linear changes in the relative disease burden between social groups. This latter group of factors include differences in social contact, both within and between social groups, and differences in the susceptibility to infection and infectiousness.

Although indistinguishable when their effects are measured using reported disease burden, these drivers have different implications for delivering equitable public health interventions. For example, in the 2009 H1N1 pandemic influenza A (pH1N1) disparities in health outcomes between social groups were identified globally. In particular, British Pakistanis had a 3.4 times increased risk of mortality relative to the White British population [16]; many ethnic minority groups (Black, South Asian and Southeast Asian) had a higher risk (odds ratio (OR) of 1.33–4.5) of exposure than white Canadians in Ontario [17]; Pacific populations were twice as likely to be exposed to infection than the rest of the New Zealand population [18]. Although these examples would likely present as increased clinical burden in particular sub-groups, the drivers of these differences are difficult to determine. Even though the results from New Zealand indicate differences in transmission rate between sub-groups, the seroprevalence data do not provide enough information to identify the specific driver responsible.

Vaccination is an important intervention in infectious disease control because it reduces disease burden in those vaccinated as well as reducing onward transmission to unvaccinated people. The strength of this indirect protection non-linearly depends on the transmission rate [19]. Therefore, if inequalities are caused by differences in transmission between social groups, vaccination may benefit some groups more than others. The impact of vaccination on inequality in infectious disease outcome is therefore unclear.

To address this gap in our knowledge, we developed a novel mathematical model of the transmission of two vaccine-preventable infections circulating in a population with two social groups characterised by different transmission properties. To quantify the effect of differences in transmission on disease inequality between the social groups, we parameterised the model using realistic estimates of susceptibility and contact structure informed by empirical social mixing data. Using our model, we investigated how the overall impact of vaccination is distributed between two social sub-groups, as well as the effect on inequality in disease incidence.

In addition, we determined the optimal vaccine allocation needed to eliminate inequality.

Methods

We developed a novel mathematical model to evaluate whether differences in contact rate and the susceptibility to infection between two social groups can explain disease inequality across a population. We used this model to quantify how a vaccination programme affects these inequalities. Our mathematical model combined a dynamic epidemiological model of disease transmission with an age-structured population model of two distinct social groups (Fig. 1).

Population model

To simulate the demographics of a high-income country, we modelled a stable age distribution with birth rate equal to death rate, a life expectancy of 80 years and mortality only occurring after 70 years of age at a constant rate. The population model was stratified into n_{age} = 15 age groups (0–4, 5–9, …, 65–69, 70+ years) with continuous ageing between age groups. The age-structured population model was further stratified into two social groups of equal size, with the same proportion of male and female and an identical age structure. Throughout the paper, the social groups with high and low transmission are labelled group H and group L, respectively.

Epidemiological model

Our dynamic transmission model tracked the proportion of the population as susceptible (S), infected but not infectious (E), infectious (I) and permanently immune to infection (R) (Fig. 1a).

The transmission between and within the two social groups was captured by three mechanisms. The first two control the underlying differences between the two social groups that are potential drivers of inequality: (1) a difference in contact intensity between the two groups, expressed as the relative rate at which members of group L interact with members of their own group, compared to the rate at which members within group H interact with one another ('contact intensity', $0 < \chi < 1$), and (2) a difference in susceptibility to infection, expressed as the relative susceptibility for members of group L compared to members of group H ('susceptibility', $0 < \eta < 1$). The

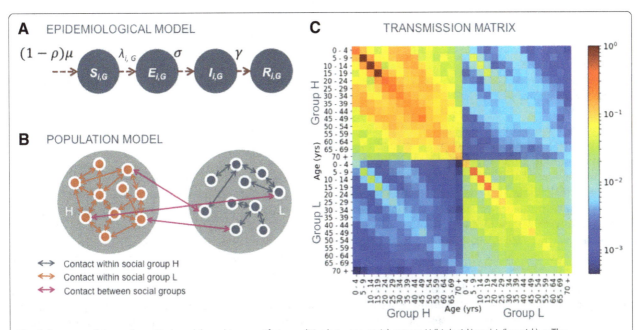

Fig. 1 Summary of the mathematical model used to quantify inequalities between social groups H (high risk) and L (low risk). **a** The epidemiological model, where $S_{i,G}$, $E_{i,G}$, $I_{i,G}$, $R_{i,G}$ and $\lambda_{i,G}$ are the proportion susceptible, infected but not infectious, infectious, recovered and force of infection in age group i and social group G (either group H or group L), ρ is the proportion vaccinated, σ is the rate at which infected individuals become infectious and γ is the rate of recovery from infection. Population also moves out of these groups into other age groups and are removed when they die (not shown in this schematic). **b** A schematic of the population model with higher contact rate in group H than group L; the groups also differ in susceptibility (not shown). **c** An example transmission matrix, showing the relative transmission rate between age and social groups with all social mixing and susceptibility assumptions included with parameterisation $\chi = 0.6$, $\eta = 0.6$, $\xi = 0.05$ (rates normalised such that the highest transmission group 10–14 years old in group H has a rate of 1. The same age group has a rate of 0.36 within group L (low susceptibility and reduced contact rate, χ and η), 0.05 from group L to group H (between-group contact rate, ξ) and 0.03 from group H to group L (between-group contact rate and reduced susceptibility, ξ and η)

third mechanism determines the integration of the two social groups: (3) the relative rate at which individuals from one social group contact members of the opposite social group ('integration', $0 < \xi < 1$). For example, $\xi = 0.15$ corresponds to contact between group H and group L at 15% of the rate of contact within group H. The rate of contact between the groups remained symmetrical; i.e. the rate of contact from group H to group L was the same as the rate of contact from group L to group H. The force of infection, λ, for the susceptible population in age group i and social group H or L is therefore dependent on the social group-specific susceptibility, the age- and social group-specific contact rate and the reproductive number, R_0, of the disease (Fig. 1c) and can be expressed as:

$$\lambda_{i,H} = \sum_{j=1}^{15} r\beta_{ij}\left(I_{j,H} + \xi I_{j,L}\right) \quad (1)$$

$$\lambda_{i,L} = \sum_{j=1}^{15} r\eta\beta_{ij}\left(\xi I_{j,H} + \chi I_{j,L}\right) \quad (2)$$

where β_{ij} is the age-specific transmission rate from age group j to age group i, and $I_{j,H}$ and $I_{j,L}$ are the proportion infectious in age group j and social groups H and L, respectively.

To keep R_0 constant when the relative contact rate (χ), susceptibility (η) and integration (ξ) of the social groups were changed, we scaled the force of infection using a linear operator, r. This approach allows parameters of interest (relative contact rate (χ), susceptibility (η), integration (ξ) and R_0) to be varied independently from each other (Additional file 1). All modelling and analysis was performed using Python 2.7.12 [20].

Parameterisation

Disease scenarios

We parameterised our model for two vaccine-preventable diseases: seasonal influenza and rubella. We quantified the incidence in the total population for both diseases. For influenza, we also quantified the incidence in those aged 60 years and over, who are at risk for severe complications following infection. For rubella, we quantified the incidence in women of childbearing age (WCA) (15–45 years), who serve as a proxy for children born with congenital rubella syndrome after their mothers become infected during pregnancy. The reproduction number, incubation period and infectious period for both diseases were parameterised from the literature (Table 1). The contact rate between age groups was parameterised with empirical social mixing data collected in the UK arm of the POLYMOD contact survey [21].

Inequality mechanisms

Integration We informed the parameterisation of ξ, the rate of contact between social groups, relative to the rate of contact within group H, using social contact data from the UK arm of the POLYMOD study [21]. We assumed that all household contacts were within their own social group, with a further 70–90% of non-household contacts also within their own social group. The relative rate of contact between social groups, ξ, was estimated as 0.05–0.25 (Additional file 1).

Relative contact rate The feasible range for the contact intensity parameter, χ, the relative rate contact within group L compared to group H, was also informed by the POLYMOD contact data. For each of the 15 age groups we sorted the participants into quintiles by their household size. We then recombined the age groups, quintile by quintile, to recover five equally sized groups. For each participant, we calculated the total number of contacts from within each person's own social group (using the same assumption as above that all household contacts and 70–90% of non-household contacts were with members of their own social group). The contact intensity parameter χ was then estimated by evaluating the ratio of the total number of within-group contacts for individuals in every unique pair of quintiles. We estimated the range of ratios as 0.65–0.95 (Additional file 1).

Relative susceptibility Given the disease-specific consideration regarding previous exposure to obtain a parameter for the relative susceptibility (ξ), we investigated the same range of 65–95% susceptibility in group L compared to group H.

Primary analysis: quantifying inequalities

The inequality in the population was expressed by the relative risk of infection in the high mixing group (group H) relative to the low mixing group (group L). We calculated this relative risk across the overall population and for the disease-specific risk groups. For influenza, we calculated the cumulative relative risk over the course of a single outbreak. For rubella, we measured the relative annual infection risk at endemic equilibrium to ensure that both rate of transmission and age-specific prior exposure to infection were accounted for in our calculation.

Vaccination

For both diseases, we assumed that a proportion of individuals become immunised after vaccination—an 'effective coverage'. Consistent with disease-specific immunity profiles, we assumed no waning of vaccine protection over the period of evaluation (lifetime for rubella or one influenza season). Effective coverage for influenza vaccination was identical across all age groups from the beginning of the season; for rubella, vaccine was administered at birth.

Table 1 Model parameter values used in base case and sensitivity analyses

	Symbol	Primary analysis	Sobol range[b]
Population parameters			
Difference in transmission (either):[a]			
Within-group mixing ('contact')	χ	0.65–0.95	0.65–1.54
Relative susceptibility of group L to group H ('susceptibility')	η	0.65–0.95	0.65–1.54
Quantity of out-group mixing relative to within-group mixing of group H ('integration')	ξ	0.05–0.25	0.05–0.25
Relative vaccine uptake in group H to group L	V_H/V_L	1.0	0.70–1.43
Epidemiological parameters			
Basic reproduction number [48, 49]	R_0		
Influenza		1.8	1.5–4.0
Rubella		6.5	5.0–8.0
Pre-infectious period (days) [50]	σ		
Influenza		2.6	2.6
Rubella		14.0	14.0
Infectious period (days) [50]	γ		
Influenza		4.0	4.0
Rubella		11.0	11.0

[a]One parameter value set to 1.0 whilst the other adjusted over the 'primary analysis range'
[b]Ranges were set so the mid value is the 'base case', which was 1.0 (no difference) for factors which vary for group L relative to group H

To allow comparison of results between the two diseases with different R_0 values, we express the effective vaccine coverage as a fraction of the critical vaccination threshold (CVT), $1 - 1/R_0$, i.e. the minimum proportion of the population required to be vaccinated to interrupt transmission. We evaluated the relative risks of infection with no vaccination and with vaccination at 80% of the CVT. Unless otherwise stated, the effective coverage was assumed to be identical between social groups.

Identifying the drivers of inequality
To evaluate the relative importance of the model parameters as drivers for inequality, we used a variance-based global sensitivity analysis, the total Sobol' sensitivity index (S_T) [22, 23], which calculates the proportion of the variance in the relative risk attributable to each parameter and combinations thereof.

Results
Underlying epidemiology
We ran simulations with no vaccination and no epidemiological differences between group H and group L (i.e. setting $\chi, \eta, \xi = 1$). We found that the influenza epidemic lasted approximately 21 weeks with a cumulative attack rate of 62% across all age groups and 40% amongst those older than 60 years. For rubella at endemic equilibrium 99.4% of the population were infected before death (95% before the age of 30 years), and the mean age of infection was 8 years. The annual incidence amongst WCA was 66 per 100,000 (Fig. 2).

Pre-vaccination inequalities
Influenza
Without vaccination, introducing a relative contact rate of 0.65–0.95 within group L compared to group H led to a change in cumulative attack rate in both social groups, and hence a change in the relative risk of infection between the two groups (Fig. 2). In particular, across base case values of susceptibility and integration, group H experienced a relative risk of infection 1.04–1.44 compared to group L (Fig. 3a). This relative risk increased to 1.06–1.62 (an increase of 1–12%) amongst the elderly in group H. Less integration between the two groups exacerbated this inequality; when contact between groups was decreased by 67% compared to the base case scenario ($\xi = 0.05$), the relative risk for group H increased to 1.06–1.84 (Fig. 4a).

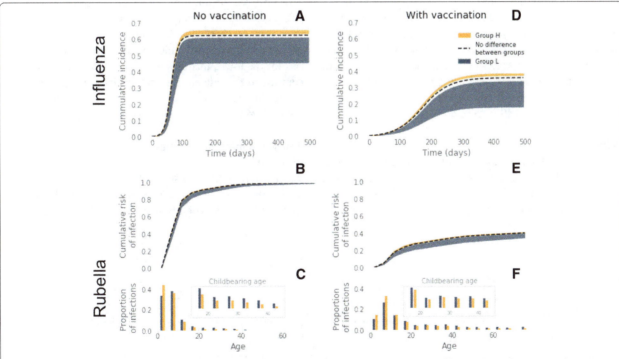

Fig. 2 Epidemiology predicted by the mathematical model for seasonal influenza and rubella with no differences between two population groups (*black dashed line*) and with differences in susceptibility and contact rate for group H (*orange region*) and group L (*navy region*) across feasible range of contact rate within social groups ($\chi = 0.65 - 0.95$) and base case values of integration ($\xi = 0.15$) and susceptibility (Table 1). **a** Cumulative incidence of influenza over a single outbreak with no vaccination. **b** Proportion of population infected with rubella by age at endemic equilibrium with no vaccination. **c** Proportion of all infections acquired in each 5-year age group, with no vaccination. **d** Cumulative incidence of influenza with 37% vaccine uptake (80% of the critical vaccination threshold (CVT)). **e** Proportion of population infected with rubella by age with 67% vaccine uptake (80% of the CVT). **f** Proportion of all infections acquired in each 5-year age group, with 67% vaccine uptake (80% of the CVT)

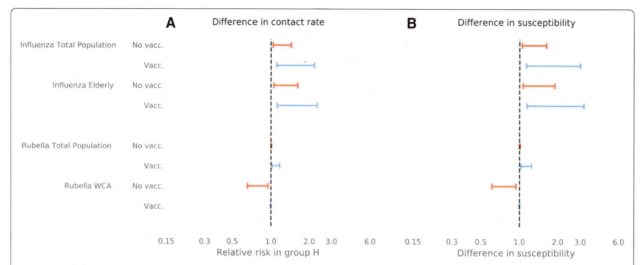

Fig. 3 Risk of infection in group H relative to group L in the total population and in risk groups, elderly and women of childbearing age (*WCA*). Relative risks shown with no vaccination and vaccination at 80% of critical vaccination threshold (37% for influenza and 67% for rubella). Forest plots show ranges of relative risk for fixed integration of $\xi = 0.15$ and a range of **a** ratio of in-contact rate in social groups ($\chi = 0.65$–0.95) and **b** ratio of susceptibility in social groups ($\eta = 0.65$–0.95)

Reducing the susceptibility in group L by a factor of 0.65–0.95 relative to group H, whilst maintaining base case values of within-group contact and between group integration, led to 1.05–1.63 times more infections in group H than group L over the course of the outbreak (Fig. 3b). Again, the relative risk amongst the elderly in group H was higher than that of the social group as a whole, with a relative risk of 1.05–1.63 under base case assumptions of integration. Relative risk of infection in group H increased when the social groups were less integrated relative to the base case scenario to 1.08–2.04 ($\xi = 0.05$) and up to 2.49 in the elderly.

Rubella

Unlike our influenza model results, differences in contact rate and susceptibility between the social groups did not result in an inequality in the risk of rubella infection in the whole population (Fig. 3). However, a more intense contact rate in group H or a lower susceptibility in group L led to a lower age of infection in group H relative to group L (Fig. 2). This difference in the age of infection resulted in a relative risk of infection for WCA in group H of 0.64–0.95 across feasible ranges of both within-group contact rates and susceptibility. In contrast to the influenza risk group, therefore, our model suggests there is an elevated risk for the low-transmission social group (Fig. 3). Again, in contrast to the influenza model results, varying the level of integration between social groups only marginally affected the relative risk of infection across WCA (Fig. 4b).

Post-vaccination inequalities
Influenza

Vaccination with a 37% uptake (80% of the CVT) reduced the cumulative attack rate of seasonal influenza from 62% to 30% when transmission in the social groups

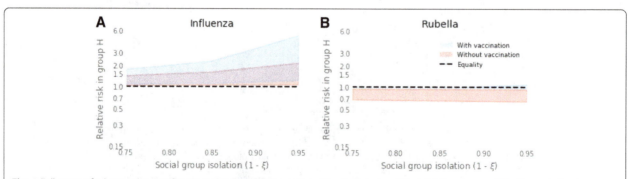

Fig. 4 Full range of relative risk in **a** influenza in the elderly (60+ years) and **b** rubella in women of childbearing age (15–45 years), due to differences in contact rate ($\chi = 0.6$–0.9) as isolation between sub-groups varies ($\xi = 0.05$–0.15). *Red shaded region* shows range of relative risk with no vaccination, *blue shaded region* shows relative risk with vaccination at 80% of the critical vaccination threshold (37% coverage for influenza, 67% coverage for rubella)

was identical (Fig. 2d). However, with differences in contact rate and susceptibility between the two social groups, introducing vaccination increased the inequality between the social groups (Fig. 3). For example the relative risk of 1.04–1.84 before vaccination increased to 1.11–2.18 after vaccination with differences in contact rate, and for differences in susceptibility relative risk increased from 1.05–2.04 before vaccination to 1.13–3.00 after vaccination (with base case integration, $\xi = 0.15$).

Consistent with the results without vaccination, relative risk of infection for group H increased when the two social groups were less integrated (Fig. 4a). When the inequality was driven by feasible changes in either within-group contact rate or susceptibility to infection, the relative risk across the whole of group H reached 4.83 and 6.99, respectively, when integration was at its lowest value ($\xi = 0.05$). Therefore, vaccination increased the inequality of disease risk in the social group most at risk of infection by 5–241% (Table 2).

Although the percentage increase in relative risk after vaccination was less amongst the elderly in group H (5–203%), the relative risk remained higher than in the total population, with a maximum relative risk of 5.19 and 7.52 for differences in contact rate and susceptibility, respectively (Fig. 4a).

The marked increase in inequality in risk of influenza infection as a result of vaccination corresponds to the social group H benefiting substantially less from the vaccination programme than group L.

Sensitivity analysis shows robustness of these results to variation in the relative size and community structure of group L and group H (Additional file 1: Figure S15).

Table 2 Percentage increase in risk of infection in group H relative to group L due to vaccination

Driver of inequality	Infection	Population group	Increase in relative risk
Difference in contact rate	Influenza	All	4–162%
		Elderly	3–137%
	Rubella	All	2–39%
		WCA	4–72%
Difference in susceptibility	Influenza	All	5–241%
		Elderly	5–203%
	Rubella	All	2–49%
		WCA	5–86%

Percentage increases in relative risk of infection for the total population (all), women of childbearing age (WCA) and elderly. Results calculated when either the relative within-group contact rate of the two social groups is varied ('contact' parameter) or when the relative susceptibility of group L to group H is varied ('susceptibility' parameter) (Table 1). Integration between the social groups is set at its base case value

Rubella
An effective vaccination uptake of 67% (80% of the CVT) greatly reduced lifetime risk of rubella in both social groups, with less than 40% of the unvaccinated population experiencing infection over their lifetime (Fig. 2d). With differences in contact rate between the social groups, vaccination caused an inequality to emerge. Specifically, the relative risk of infection in group H relative to group L increased from 1.01–1.02 to 1.02–1.42, across a feasible range of within-group mixing patterns (Fig. 3a). The same result was found as a consequence of susceptibility differences (Fig. 3b).

Furthermore, vaccination reduced the difference in the age of infection between the two social groups (Fig. 2). The combination of changes in relative risk of infection before death and in age at infection caused a switch in the group most at risk for infection in WCA. Before vaccination the highest relative risk was amongst women in group L, whereas with vaccination the WCA in group H tended to have a higher risk, with relative risk ranging from 0.99 to 1.16.

Sensitivity analysis shows robustness of these results to variation in the relative size and community structure of group L and group H (Additional file 1: Figure S16).

Vaccinating to prevent inequality
By increasing the vaccine uptake in group H relative to group L, the inequalities driven by vaccination, differences in contact rate and differences in susceptibility can be mitigated. To achieve equality in risk of infection for influenza across the entire population, group H had to receive 52–70% of the total number of vaccine doses across the feasible ranges of population parameters (Fig. 5a). In contrast, small changes in vaccine dose allocation were required to curb inequality in rubella (50.3–52.3%) (Fig. 5b). The level of integration between the two social groups did not affect the vaccine uptake required in each group to eliminate inequality (results not shown).

Ranking drivers of inequalities
Pre-vaccination era
Without vaccination the magnitude of the inequality (i.e. relative risk of infection for the high-transmission group) in influenza was most sensitive to the relative susceptibility of the social groups ($S_T = 0.55$) and their relative contact rate ($S_T = 0.48$) (Fig. 6a). The same was true for rubella (for relative susceptibility $S_T = 0.58$; for relative within-group contact rate $S_T = 0.46$). By comparison, sensitivity to integration between the two groups was relatively small, however greater for influenza than rubella ($S_T = 0.03$ vs. 0.004, respectively) (Fig. 6b).

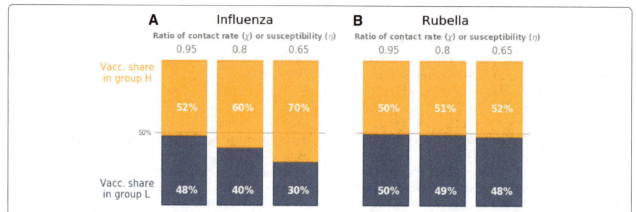

Fig. 5 Optimal vaccine allocation between social groups required to control disease inequalities in **a** influenza and **b** rubella. Results shown for ratio of contact rate in social groups ($\chi = 0.65$–0.95) and ratio of susceptibility in social groups ($\eta = 0.65$–0.95). The total vaccination coverage is 80% of the critical vaccination threshold (37% vaccine uptake for influenza, 67% vaccine uptake for rubella)

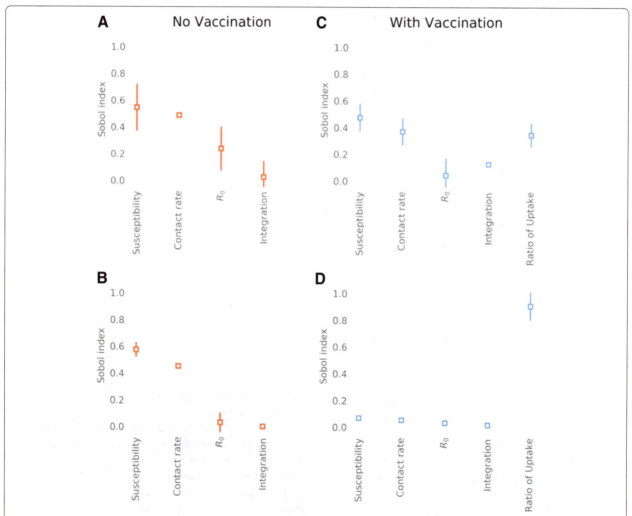

Fig. 6 Total Sobol' indices, S_T, for contact (χ), susceptibility (η), integration (ξ), infectivity (R_0) and difference in vaccination coverage (V_H/V_L) relative risks for rubella and influenza. **a** Influenza in the elderly (60+ years) with no vaccination. **b** Rubella in women of childbearing age (15–45 years) with no vaccination. **c** Influenza in the elderly with vaccination coverage at 37% (80% of the critical vaccination threshold). **d** Rubella in women of childbearing age (15–45 years) with vaccination coverage at 67% (80% of the critical vaccination threshold). Error bars show 95% confidence interval

Vaccination era
Additional variance introduced by differences in vaccine uptake between social groups caused a reduction in the relative sensitivity of inequalities to all other parameters, with the exception of integration. Nonetheless, for influenza, inequality in the disease risk between the two social groups remained most sensitive to relative susceptibility and contact rate ($S_T = 0.48$; $S_T = 0.37$). In contrast, inequalities were relatively insensitive to relative vaccine uptake ($S_T = 0.35$) (Fig. 6c). Sensitivity to the integration between social groups also increased relative to no vaccination ($S_T = 0.13$). For rubella, relative vaccine uptake between the two social groups had the greatest influence on inequality ($S_T = 0.91$), diminishing the relative sensitivity of inequality to relative susceptibility and contact rate of the social groups such that they were negligible (Fig. 6d).

Discussion

Differences in incidence of infectious diseases between social groups have been observed; however, the factors that drive these inequalities are not well quantified. Moreover, the impact of vaccination on these inequalities is unclear. We developed a novel mathematical model to simulate influenza and rubella in two connected social groups and assessed the role of differences in two key factors—contact rate and susceptibility—on inequalities as well as the impact of vaccination. Our model suggested that these factors could be responsible for substantial differences in disease epidemiology between social groups. Therefore, these factors may play a significant role in driving observed inequalities in infectious disease outcomes. Furthermore, the results suggest that the impact of these factors on inequalities depends on the characteristics of the pathogen, as we show that the same differences in transmission are likely to cause greater inequality in influenza than rubella. Vaccination can exacerbate the inequalities even when the uptake is equal between the groups.

These observations have four important implications for public health and immunisation strategies. First, inequality in health is an area of high importance amongst public health authorities [5, 24]. As such, there is an appetite for policy that avoids and reduces inequalities in infectious disease outcome [25, 26]. To this end, effort is spent attempting to provide equal distribution of vaccination across social groups in the population [27]. However, our results indicate that equal vaccination uptake could, paradoxically, increase inequalities into high-transmission groups, if the vaccine coverage is not high enough to eliminate disease. This result indicates that equal vaccination is not an appropriate measure of equitable intervention, and inequality in disease burden must be evaluated directly.

Second, groups who have social characteristics that place them at a higher risk of infection and who also have a reduced vaccination uptake may be vulnerable to amplified inequalities. For example, during pH1N1 in 2009, Black and Hispanic populations had a lower uptake of influenza vaccination than the White population in the USA [28]. In addition, countries with self-financed or partially self-paid vaccination programmes may discourage more materially deprived groups from vaccinating; studies [29, 30] in Poland and South Korea have identified that lower uptake of vaccination correlates with low socio-economic status. This leaves the possibility that low uptake may correlate with factors contributing to transmission.

Third, the factors that most influence inequality depend on the underlying disease dynamics; therefore, intervention efforts must be disease- and population-specific. For example, our results indicate that differences in vaccine uptake are more important in creating inequalities in rubella than differences in factors associated with transmission rate. This is reflected in the small (0.3–2.3%) change from equal vaccine uptake required to mitigate differences in contact rate or susceptibility (Fig. 4). However, inequalities in influenza are more sensitive to differences in transmission-related factors than differences in vaccine uptake. This contrast was evidenced when low vaccine uptake in more affluent social groups created 'a reversal of health inequalities' with higher prevalence in more affluent areas during a measles outbreak in London, UK in 2001–2002 [31]. In contrast, the same geographical region saw a higher attack rate of pH1N1 in more deprived areas [9] only 7 years later. This finding suggests that, notwithstanding the potential to increase existing inequalities, for diseases like rubella, equal vaccine uptake may be the most practicable target for minimising post-vaccination inequalities in disease burden. However, the same approach may not be optimal for influenza.

Finally, we identified that inequalities resulting from differences in transmission are highly sensitive to the level of integration of sub-groups. The importance of integration between social groups becomes more pronounced for diseases with sub-optimal vaccine uptake. This result suggests that inequalities driven by differences in transmission rate or a difference in vaccine uptake may be more likely to occur in highly segregated populations. Our finding could explain inequalities in incidence of infectious disease in urban centres, where there is geographical clustering of social and ethnic groups. For example, central Birmingham, UK, which was heavily affected by pH1N1 in 2009, is an area where up to 80% of the population is South Asian, an ethnic group associated with higher risk of transmission [8]. This phenomenon may also contribute to increased risk of outbreaks of measles, often observed in isolated communities with low vaccination coverage [32, 33]. Our findings reinforce the notion that communities that are more isolated should be of particular focus when considering public health strategies for infectious disease. Further, our results highlight the importance of understanding the role of transmission-related factors in inequality in populations where social and ethnic groups are becoming more segregated, as inequalities could be set to increase [34].

Our influenza model predicts a relative risk of infection in an unvaccinated population of up to 2.05, within feasible values of social group mixing and susceptibility. This is broadly consistent with data from the pH1N1 epidemic in 2009. For example, a case-control study from Ontario, Canada shows that East/Southeast Asian, South Asian and Black ethnicities had a significantly increased risk of acquiring pH1N1 relative to White Canadians (OR 1.33–4.50) [17]. Similarly, in New Zealand a seroprevalence study showed that Pacific Island populations were twice as likely to be infected during the 2009 pandemic than those of European ethnic identity [18]. Whilst there are many examples of observed inequalities in influenza [8, 9, 35–39], studies of inequalities associated with rubella and other endemic childhood infections are often focused on disparities in vaccine uptake rather than disease outcome [40].

Whilst much attention has been given to investigating the impact of transmission heterogeneity on the overall effectiveness of control strategies [41, 42], we build on this work by considering the role of heterogeneity in influencing inequalities in infectious disease outcomes, rather than the overall disease burden. Transmission models have previously been developed to evaluate the impact of social structure on observed inequalities in reported incidence of pandemic and seasonal influenza [43, 44]. By using socio-economic census data, these studies can replicate some of the location-specific inequalities between pre-defined social groups. However, because it is difficult to disentangle the drivers of inequality underlying these socio-economic groups, the models do not provide a fully generalisable framework in which to evaluate inequality. To overcome this issue, we developed a 'bottom up' approach, in which potential transmission-related drivers of inequality are isolated and evaluated. By parameterising our model with empirical social mixing data, we can explicitly capture the contact patterns between age and social groups and the effect of vaccination. Our generalised framework therefore allows us to disentangle the relative impact of different drivers of inequality and the impact of vaccination on this inequality.

To enable a mechanistic understanding of the drivers of inequality, we made some simplifying assumptions. We assumed that the two social groups in our model have identical age structures and birth rates. It has been shown that differences in age structure and other demographic differences such as birth rate can also result in changes in transmission which lead to inequalities in incidence [43, 44] and the effectiveness of vaccination [45]. To remain consistent with this assumption, we corrected for age distribution when we calculated the range of differences in contact rate between the groups. Furthermore, we assumed gender non-specific contact patterns. In some settings gender differences may exist, particularly in rates of contact between adults and infants [46, 47]. Whilst this gender difference may also differ between social groups, a recent survey suggests that contact rates between mothers and children are broadly consistent across ethnic and socio-economic groups [47]. Our approach is general and aims to establish the relative impact of various drivers of inequality. As such, our results should not be considered as indicative of the magnitude of specific inequalities, but rather as the potential for difference in transmission to explain inequalities and the qualitative nature of the inequalities that may arise from such drivers. We hope the results can be used to target additional analyses at specific scenarios where differences in transmission may arise, for example, where differences in household size distribution or high levels of segregation between social groups prevail.

Conclusion

Differences in contact behaviour and susceptibility to infection could cause substantial inequality in infectious disease-related health outcomes, particularly those related to influenza outbreaks or infections with similar epidemiology. Such inequalities have a highly non-linear relationship with vaccination, which is sensitive to the underlying epidemiology of the infection, ultimately resulting in an increase in inequality after sub-optimal vaccination, even when uptake is equal across the entire population. As such, we advocate measurement of health outcomes rather than vaccination coverage when quantifying the equality of protection across multiple social groups. Moreover, targeted vaccination in known risk groups may reduce overall inequalities in the case of influenza outbreaks. However, due to the high sensitivity of rubella inequalities to differences in vaccination coverage, this is not a recommended course of action in this case or for similar infections.

Abbreviations
CVT: Critical vaccination threshold; pH1N1: Pandemic influenza A H1N1 (2009); WCA: Women of childbearing age

Acknowledgements
JM thanks Sebastian Funk, Petra Klepac and Mark Jit for discussions and comments on the original manuscript. The authors also thank Jan Medlock for providing the Python script used to convert contact survey data to symmetrical contact matrices.

Funding
JM, AJvH and KEA received funding from the National Institute for Health Research Health Protection Research Unit (NIHR HPRU) in immunisation at the London School of Hygiene & Tropical Medicine in partnership with Public Health England. The views expressed are those of the authors and not necessarily those of the UK National Health Service, the UK NIHR, the UK Medical Research Council, the UK Department of Health or Public Health England.

Authors' contributions
JM, AJvH, WJE and KEA conceived and designed the study. JM analysed the contact survey data, implemented the model and conducted the sensitivity analyses. JM, AJvH and KEA analysed and interpreted the model outputs. JM, AJvH, WJE and KEA wrote and revised the manuscript. All authors read and approved the final manuscript.

Competing interests
The authors declare that they have no competing interests.

Author details
[1]Centre for Mathematical Modelling of Infectious Diseases, London School of Hygiene & Tropical Medicine, London, UK. [2]Department of Infectious Disease Epidemiology, Faculty of Epidemiology and Population Health, London School of Hygiene & Tropical Medicine, London, UK. [3]National Institute for Public Health and the Environment (RIVM), Bilthoven, The Netherlands. [4]Centre for Global Health, Usher Institute of Population Health Sciences and Informatics, Edinburgh Medical School, The University of Edinburgh, Edinburgh, UK.

References
1. Millett ERC, Quint JK, Smeeth L, Daniel RM, Thomas SL. Incidence of community-acquired lower respiratory tract infections and pneumonia among older adults in the United Kingdom: a population-based study. PLoS One. 2013;8:e75131.
2. Blain AP, Thomas MF, Shirley MDF, Simmister C, Elemraid MA, Gorton R, et al. Spatial variation in the risk of hospitalization with childhood pneumonia and empyema in the north of England. Epidemiol Infect. 2014;142:388–98.
3. Myles PR, McKeever TM, Pogson Z, Smith CJP, Hubbard RB. The incidence of pneumonia using data from a computerized general practice database. Epidemiol Infect. 2009;137:709–16.
4. Chapman KE, Wilson D, Gorton R. Invasive pneumococcal disease and socioeconomic deprivation: a population study from the north east of England. J Public Health (Oxf). 2013;35:558–69.
5. Semenza JC, Suk JE, Tsolova S. Social determinants of infectious diseases: a public health priority. Eur Commun Dis Bull. 2010;15:2–4.
6. Semenza JC, Giesecke J. Intervening to reduce inequalities in infections in Europe. Am J Public Heal. 2008;98:787–92.
7. Semenza JC. Strategies to intervene on social determinants of infectious diseases. Eur Commun Dis Bull. 2010;15:32–9.
8. Inglis NJ, Bagnall H, Janmohamed K, Suleman S, Awofisayo A, De Souza V, et al. Measuring the effect of influenza A(H1N1)pdm09: the epidemiological experience in the West Midlands, England during the "containment" phase. Epidemiol Infect. 2014;142:428–37.
9. Balasegaram S, Ogilvie F, Glasswell A, Anderson C, Cleary V, Turbitt D, et al. Patterns of early transmission of pandemic influenza in London — link with deprivation. Influenza Other Respir Viruses. 2012;6:e35–41.
10. Jordan R, Verlander N, Olowokure B, Hawker JI. Age, sex, material deprivation and respiratory mortality. Respir Med. 2006;100:1282–5.
11. Kawachi I, Subramanian SV, Almeida-Filho N. A glossary for health inequalities. J Epidemiol Community Health. 2002;56:647–52.
12. Levy NS, Quyen Nguyen T, Westheimer E, Layton M. Disparities in the severity of influenza illness: a descriptive study of hospitalized and nonhospitalized novel H1N1 influenza-positive patients in New York City: 2009-2010 influenza season. J Public Heal Manag Pract. 2013;19:16–24.
13. Mayoral JM, Alonso J, Garín O, Herrador Z, Astray J, Baricot M, et al. Social factors related to the clinical severity of influenza cases in Spain during the A (H1N1) 2009 virus pandemic. BMC Public Health. 2013;13:118.
14. Haroon SMM, Barbosa GP, Saunders PJ. The determinants of health-seeking behaviour during the A/H1N1 influenza pandemic: an ecological study. J Public Health (Oxf). 2011;33:503–10.
15. Nyland GA, McKenzie BC, Myles PR, Semple MG, Lim WS, Openshaw PJM, et al. Effect of ethnicity on care pathway and outcomes in patients hospitalized with influenza A(H1N1)pdm09 in the UK. Epidemiol Infect. 2015;143:1129–38.
16. Zhao H, Harris RJ, Ellis J, Pebody RG. Ethnicity, deprivation and mortality due to 2009 pandemic influenza A(H1N1) in England during the 2009/2010 pandemic and the first post-pandemic season. Epidemiol Infect. 2015;143:3375–83.
17. Navaranjan D, Rosella LC, Kwong JC, Campitelli M, Crowcroft N. Ethnic disparities in acquiring 2009 pandemic H1N1 influenza: a case–control study. BMC Public Health. 2014;14:214.
18. Wilson N, Barnard LT, Summers JA, Shanks GD, Baker MG. Differential mortality rates by ethnicity in 3 influenza pandemics over a century. Emerg Infect Dis: New Zealand; 2012.
19. Fine P, Eames K, Heymann DL. "Herd immunity": a rough guide. Clin Infect Dis. 2011;52:911–6.
20. Python Software Foundation. Python language reference, version 2.7. Python Software Foundation. 2013. https://www.python.org.
21. Mossong J, Hens N, Jit M, Beutels P, Auranen K, Mikolajczyk R, et al. Social contacts and mixing patterns relevant to the spread of infectious diseases. PLoS Med. 2008;5:e74.
22. Sobol IM. Global sensitivity indices for nonlinear mathematical models and their Monte Carlo estimates. Math Comput Simul. 2001;55:271–80.
23. Herman J, Usher W. SALib: An open-source Python library for Sensitivity Analysis. J Open Source Softw. 2017;2:97.
24. Commission on Social Determinants of Health (CSDH). Closing the gap in a generation. Geneva: World Health Organization; 2008.
25. Hutchins SS, Truman BI, Merlin TL, Redd SC. Protecting vulnerable populations from pandemic influenza in the United States: a strategic imperative. Am J Public Health. 2009;99(Suppl2):S243–8.
26. Blumenshine P, Reingold A, Egerter S, Mockenhaupt R, Braveman P, Marks J. Pandemic influenza planning in the United States from a health disparities perspective. Emerg Infect Dis. 2008;14:709–15.
27. Peng Y, Xu Y, Zhu M, Yu H, Nie S, Yan W. Chinese urban-rural disparity in pandemic (H1N1) 2009 vaccination coverage rate and associated determinants: a cross-sectional telephone survey. Public Health. 2013;127:930–7.
28. Uscher-Pines L, Maurer J, Harris KM. Racial and ethnic disparities in uptake and location of vaccination for 2009-H1N1 and seasonal influenza. Am J Public Health. 2011;101:1252–5.
29. Ganczak M, Dmytrzyk-Daniłów G, Karakiewicz B, Korzeń M, Szych Z. Determinants influencing self-paid vaccination coverage, in 0–5 years old Polish children. Vaccine. 2013;31:5687–92.
30. Lee K-C, Han K, Kim JY, Nam GE, Han B-D, Shin K-E, et al. Socioeconomic status and other related factors of seasonal influenza vaccination in the South Korean adult population based on a nationwide cross-sectional study. PLoS One. 2015;10:e0117305.
31. Atkinson P, Cullinan C, Jones J, Fraser G, Maguire H. Large outbreak of measles in London: reversal of health inequalities. Arch Dis Child. 2005;90:424–5.
32. Baugh V, Figueroa J, Bosanquet J, Kemsley P, Addiman S, Turbitt D. Ongoing measles outbreak in orthodox Jewish community, London, UK. Emerg Infect Dis. 2013;19:1707–9.
33. Gastañaduy PA, Budd J, Fisher N, Redd SB, Fletcher J, Miller J, et al. A measles outbreak in an underimmunized Amish community in Ohio. N Engl J Med. 2016;375:1343–54.

34. Casey L. The Casey review: a review into opportunity and integration. London: Ministry of Housing, Communities & Local Government; 2016.
35. Rutter PD, Mytton OT, Mak M, Donaldson LJ. Socio-economic disparities in mortality due to pandemic influenza in England. Int J Public Health. 2012; 57:745–50.
36. Dee DL, Bensyl DM, Gindler J, Truman BI, Allen BG, D'Mello T, et al. Racial and ethnic disparities in hospitalizations and deaths associated with 2009 pandemic influenza A (H1N1) virus infections in the United States. Ann Epidemiol. 2011;21:623–30.
37. Quinn SC, Kumar S. Health inequalities and infectious disease epidemics: a challenge for global health security. Biosecur Bioterror. 2014;12:263–73.
38. Kumar S, Quinn SC, Kim KH, Daniel LH, Freimuth VS. The impact of workplace policies and other social factors on self-reported influenza-like illness incidence during the 2009 H1N1 pandemic. Am J Public Health. 2012;102:134–40.
39. Yousey-Hindes KM, Hadler JL. Neighborhood socioeconomic status and influenza hospitalizations among children: New Haven County, Connecticut, 2003-2010. Am J Public Health. 2011;101:1785–9.
40. Doherty E, Walsh B, O'Neill C. Decomposing socioeconomic inequality in child vaccination: results from Ireland. Vaccine. 2014;32:3438–44.
41. Garnett GP, Anderson RM. Sexually transmitted diseases and sexual behavior: insights from mathematical models. J Infect Dis. 1996;174:S150–61.
42. Woolhouse ME, Dye C, Etard JF, Smith T, Charlwood JD, Garnett GP, et al. Heterogeneities in the transmission of infectious agents: implications for the design of control programs. Proc Natl Acad Sci U S A. 1997;94:338–42.
43. Kumar S, Piper K, Galloway DD, Hadler JL, Grefenstette JJ. Is population structure sufficient to generate area-level inequalities in influenza rates? An examination using agent-based models. BMC Public Health. 2015;15:947.
44. Hyder A, Leung B. Social deprivation and burden of influenza: testing hypotheses and gaining insights from a simulation model for the spread of influenza. Epidemics. 2015;11:71–9.
45. Metcalf CJE, Lessler J, Klepac P, Cutts F, Grenfell DBT. Impact of birth rate, seasonality and transmission rate on minimum levels of coverage needed for rubella vaccination. Epidemiol Infect. 2012;140:2290–301.
46. Van Hoek AJ, Andrews N, Campbell H, Amirthalingam G, Edmunds WJ, Miller E. The social life of infants in the context of infectious disease transmission; social contacts and mixing patterns of the very young. PLoS One. 2013;8:e76180.
47. Campbell PT, Mcvernon J, Shrestha N, Nathan PM, Geard N. Who's holding the baby? A prospective diary study of the contact patterns of mothers with an infant. BMC Infect Dis. 2017;17:634.
48. Edmunds WJ, Van De Heijden OG, Eerola M, Gay NJ. Modelling rubella in Europe. Epidemiol Infect. 2000;125:617–34.
49. Baguelin M, Flasche S, Camacho A, Demiris N, Miller E, Edmunds WJ. Assessing optimal target populations for influenza vaccination programmes: an evidence synthesis and modelling study. PLoS Med. 2013;10:e1001527.
50. Heymann DL. Control of communicable disease manual. 20th ed. Washington, DC: American Public Health Association; 2014.

Vaccination with chemically attenuated *Plasmodium falciparum* asexual blood-stage parasites induces parasite-specific cellular immune responses in malaria-naïve volunteers: a pilot study

Danielle I. Stanisic[1*], James Fink[2], Johanna Mayer[2], Sarah Coghill[2], Letitia Gore[2], Xue Q. Liu[1], Ibrahim El-Deeb[1], Ingrid B. Rodriguez[1], Jessica Powell[1], Nicole M. Willemsen[1], Sai Lata De[1], Mei-Fong Ho[1], Stephen L. Hoffman[3], John Gerrard[2] and Michael F. Good[1*]

Abstract

Background: The continuing morbidity and mortality associated with infection with malaria parasites highlights the urgent need for a vaccine. The efficacy of sub-unit vaccines tested in clinical trials in malaria-endemic areas has thus far been disappointing, sparking renewed interest in the whole parasite vaccine approach. We previously showed that a chemically attenuated whole parasite asexual blood-stage vaccine induced CD4$^+$ T cell-dependent protection against challenge with homologous and heterologous parasites in rodent models of malaria.

Methods: In this current study, we evaluated the immunogenicity and safety of chemically attenuated asexual blood-stage *Plasmodium falciparum* (Pf) parasites in eight malaria-naïve human volunteers. Study participants received a single dose of 3×10^7 Pf pRBC that had been treated in vitro with the cyclopropylpyrroloindole analogue, tafuramycin-A.

Results: We demonstrate that Pf asexual blood-stage parasites that are completely attenuated are immunogenic, safe and well tolerated in malaria-naïve volunteers. Following vaccination with a single dose, species and strain transcending *Plasmodium*-specific T cell responses were induced in recipients. This included induction of *Plasmodium*-specific lymphoproliferative responses, T cells secreting the parasiticidal cytokines, IFN-γ and TNF, and CD3$^+$CD45RO$^+$ memory T cells. Pf-specific IgG was not detected.

Conclusions: This is the first clinical study evaluating a whole parasite blood-stage malaria vaccine. Following administration of a single dose of completely attenuated Pf asexual blood-stage parasites, *Plasmodium*-specific T cell responses were induced while Pf-specific antibodies were not detected. These results support further evaluation of this chemically attenuated vaccine in humans.

Keywords: Malaria, *Plasmodium falciparum*, Vaccines, Chemically attenuated malaria parasites, T cell responses

---

* Correspondence: d.stanisic@griffith.edu.au; Michael.Good@griffith.edu.au
[1]Institute for Glycomics, Griffith University, Parklands Drive, Southport, Queensland, Australia
Full list of author information is available at the end of the article

Background

Plasmodium spp. parasites cause more than 200 million clinical cases of malaria and 438,000 deaths per year, with the majority of deaths occurring in children < 5 years of age [1]. An effective vaccine capable of inducing long-lasting immunity is not currently available. Disappointing results following the testing of sub-unit vaccines in clinical trials [2–5] have highlighted some of the limitations of sub-unit vaccines that need to be addressed, including antigenic polymorphism in critical epitopes.

The limited protection induced by sub-unit vaccine candidates has resulted in renewed interest in the whole organism vaccine approach. The fundamental rationale for a whole parasite vaccine is that by maximising the number of antigens presented to the immune system, including those that are conserved between different parasite strains, the impact of antigenic polymorphism will be diminished. There has been considerable progress with injectable whole parasite *Plasmodium falciparum* sporozoite (PfSPZ) vaccines [6–11]. The administration of whole blood-stage parasites in the context of controlled human malaria infection (CHMI) in human volunteers is not new [12]; deliberate malaria infection was used as a treatment for neurosyphilis (malariotherapy) in the early 1900s (reviewed in [13, 14]). CHMI with whole blood-stage parasites is also used for the in vivo assessment of malaria vaccine and drug candidate efficacy (reviewed in [12]). However, there have been no published clinical studies of whole parasite blood-stage malaria vaccines [15].

Cyclopropylpyrroloindole analogues, such as centanamycin (CM) and tafuramycin-A (TF-A) have been used to successfully attenuate both sporozoite and asexual blood-stage malaria parasites [16–20]. These compounds bind covalently to poly-A regions of DNA [21]. Studies in mice involving vaccination with chemically attenuated sporozoites demonstrated induction of protective immunity [16, 17]. To adapt this for a blood-stage vaccine approach, we vaccinated mice with a single dose of ring-stage *Plasmodium chabaudi* AS parasitised red blood cells (pRBC) that had been treated in vitro with CM or the related compound, TF-A, and demonstrated long-lasting protection from homologous and heterologous blood-stage challenge [18]. Similar protection was observed when mice were vaccinated with chemically attenuated *Plasmodium yoelii* 17X, although three doses of vaccine provided superior protection compared to one dose [19]. Although an adjuvant was not required for induction of protective immune responses, vaccine efficacy was ablated if the red cell membrane was disrupted [18]. These data suggested that the red cell membranes were required to target the attenuated parasites to dendritic cells in the spleen and liver, which was observed post-vaccination. Protective immunity was dependent on $CD4^+$ T cells present at the time of challenge, and a strong IFN-γ response was induced by the vaccine [18, 19]. Parasite-specific antibodies were induced only in the *P. yoelii* 17X model and contributed to protection. Vaccination also led to a significant $CD8^+$ T cell response, although depletion of these cells did not ablate vaccine-induced immunity. In previous pre-clinical studies involving other types of whole parasite blood-stage vaccines, it was shown that cellular immunity or IFN-γ played critical roles in protection [22–24]. The importance of IFN-γ in immunity to human malaria has also been demonstrated in individuals in malaria-endemic areas [25–28] and in a controlled human experimental infection study [29].

To facilitate transition of the chemically attenuated vaccine approach into humans, pre-clinical in vitro and in vivo studies with *P. falciparum* (Pf) were undertaken. Treatment of parasites with 2 μM CM resulted in complete parasite attenuation in vitro [18]. In vivo studies in *Aotus* monkeys showed that following inoculation of TF-A-treated parasites, they persisted at sub-patent levels for up to 8 days (as determined by qPCR) [30]. Pf-specific T cell responses, but not Pf-specific IgG, were induced. Collectively, these data supported the evaluation of this vaccine approach in clinical studies.

We previously manufactured clinical-grade cultured Pf asexual blood-stage cell banks [31] and demonstrated their infectivity in vivo in malaria-naïve volunteers [32]. In this present study, we used the Pf 7G8 cell bank to investigate the immunogenicity, safety and tolerability of chemically attenuated parasites in malaria-naïve individuals.

Methods

Aims and study participants

The main aims of the study were to (i) characterise the safety and tolerability of TF-A-treated Pf blood-stage parasites in humans and to (ii) characterise the immunogenicity of TF-A-treated Pf blood-stage parasites in humans. Griffith University was the study sponsor, and the study was conducted in the Clinical Trial Unit at Griffith University, Southport, Queensland, Australia, from July 2014 to August 2015. Study participants were healthy male, malaria-naïve individuals, aged 18–60 years ($n = 8$) (Additional file 1: Table S1). Volunteers were excluded if they had a history of malaria infection or travelled to/lived (> 2 weeks) in a malaria-endemic country during the previous 12 months. Other key eligibility criteria can be found in the listing on the Australian New Zealand Clinical Trials registry (www.anzctr.org.au); the identifier is ACTRN12614000228684.

Study participants received a single vaccination of 3×10^7 pRBC treated with 50 nM of TF-A (group A; $n = 3$) or 200 nM of TF-A (group B; $n = 5$) on study day 0. Follow-up visits were scheduled every 2 days (from study day 2 to day 26) following vaccination. At these visits, blood samples were collected to assess parasite levels in the blood of participants and to evaluate the immunogenicity of the vaccine in established assays. If the numbers of parasites in the blood increased exponentially and levels reached 11,500 pRBC/ml (as measured by quantitative PCR [qPCR]) or clinical symptoms of malaria developed, rescue treatment with a standard course of the anti-malarial artemether-lumefantrine (A/L) (Riamet) was commenced immediately. If rescue treatment with A/L was not initiated, 4 weeks following administration of the vaccine (day 28), participants were given a standard course of A/L.

For safety assessments at every visit, participants were evaluated by a medical investigator. This included a physical exam, measurement of vital signs (e.g. temperature, heart rate, blood pressure and respiratory rate) and recording of solicited and unsolicited adverse events. Blood was also collected for safety purposes at designated scheduled visits (days 0, 8, 16, 28, 90) for group B. For group A, this was undertaken at days 0, 8, the day of initiation of anti-malarial treatment for each participant (days 10–13), days 28 and 90. Sullivan Nicolaides Pathology tested samples collected prior to immunisation, on day 28 and day 90 for the presence of alloantibodies. Indirect anti-globulin testing was undertaken using column agglutination technology. An independent Safety Review Team, including an independent medical expert, was appointed to oversee the study and monitor its progress.

Culture of Pf for the production of chemically treated parasites

The culturing of Pf 7G8 for the production of chemically treated parasites was undertaken at Griffith University. All processes were carried out in compliance with Annex 13, Pharmaceutical Inspection Co-operation Scheme (PIC/S) Guide, in a monitored environment suitable for production of sterile biologics in accordance with approved protocols. For group A (P1, P2, P3) and three participants in group B (P4, P5, P6), cultures were initiated using seed vials from the clinical-grade Pf 7G8 cell bank [31] and were expanded using leukocyte-depleted group O RhD negative erythrocytes (Key Biologics, LLC, Memphis, TN, USA) as previously described for the production of the clinical-grade cell banks [31]. For two participants in group B (P7 and P8), the Pf 7G8 cell bank was expanded in erythrocytes derived from the blood of the study participant. Parasite cultures were checked regularly, at which time, thin blood films were made from collected samples, stained with Diff Quik (Bacto Laboratories) and read to ascertain the parasitemia. As required, the parasites were sub-cultured using freshly washed human erythrocytes. This culturing process was continued with the number of tissue culture dishes/flasks increasing until the malaria parasite was at ring-stage, and it was calculated that there were sufficient parasite numbers to manufacture the chemically treated pRBC.

Chemical treatment of Pf 7G8 with tafuramycin-A

The 2 mM TF-A stock solution was prepared according to published methods [18], and aliquots were stored at −80 °C. Fresh working stocks of 20 μM were made from this as required, and serial dilutions were performed in Roswell Park Memorial Institute (RPMI)-1640 (Gibco, Invitrogen Corporation, CA) to obtain the appropriate concentration of TF-A for the chemical treatment of pRBCs. Pf 7G8 cultures were centrifuged at $433g$ for 10 min, and the supernatant removed. The cell pellets were combined in a single tube, and a thin blood smear was prepared to determine parasitemia. The parasitemia of cultures for preparation of chemically treated pRBC was 3–5%. For each vented flask required, 500 μl of packed cells (pRBCs and uninfected red blood cells [uRBCs]) was added to 9 ml of pre-warmed RPMI-1640 medium. One millilitre of the appropriate TF-A solution was added to obtain a final concentration of either 50 nM (group A) or 200 nM of TF-A (group B). This cell suspension was incubated for 40 min in a 37 °C incubator with 5% O_2, 5% CO_2, and 90% N_2, and the flasks were gently agitated every 10 min. The packed cells were transferred to 50 ml conical tubes and washed with RPMI-1640 at $433g$ for 5 min, and the supernatant discarded. The pellet was resuspended in RPMI-1640 and incubated at 37 °C for a further 20 min. The pRBC were washed twice more with RPMI-1640 and a final wash in 0.9% saline for injection. Finally, the pellet was re-suspended in saline for injection and a cell count was performed to calculate the volume required for the immunising dose. This was re-suspended in saline for injection to give a final volume of 2 ml/dose.

Preparation and administration of the chemically treated Pf vaccine

The vaccine was dispensed into as many 2 ml syringes as required for administration to the study participants who were inoculated by intravenous injection. Study participants received an inoculum containing either 3×10^7 Pf 7G8 pRBC treated with 50 nM of TF-A (group A) or 3×10^7 Pf 7G8 pRBC treated with 200 nM of TF-A (group B). The number of parasites present in each batch of vaccine was verified retrospectively by undertaking qPCR on surplus material.

Evaluation of the chemically treated Pf vaccine

During preparation of each batch of chemically attenuated inocula, additional inocula were prepared in parallel for testing as described below.

Sterility testing of the chemically treated Pf vaccine

Sterility testing of in-process samples and inocula for the assessment of biocontamination with aerobic and anaerobic microorganisms was undertaken by Biotest Laboratories Pty Ltd. (Underwood, Australia) using the direct inoculation technique into tryptone soya broth and thioglycollate medium. Test parameters and acceptance criteria were defined according to the British Pharmacopoeia 2014, Appendix XVI A. Following a 14-day incubation period, there was no evidence of growth of aerobic or anaerobic microorganisms.

Measurement of residual tafuramycin-A in chemically treated vaccine

A bioanalytical method to determine the residual TF-A in a vaccine dose was developed and qualified by the Centre for Integrated Preclinical Drug Development (CIPDD), Herston, Australia). The range of detection of the assay was 5–200 ng/ml. A vaccine dose from each batch was frozen on dry ice and sent to CIPDD for analysis. During the manufacturing process, the majority of the TF-A is washed away; any residual compound is considered a by-product of manufacture and an impurity in the final product. In all batches produced, the amount of residual TF-A present was well below the limit described in the "European Union (EU) Guidelines on the limits of Genotoxic Impurities" of 1.5 µg/person/day (group A: $x = 86.04$ ng/vaccine dose; range: 14.4–206.8 ng/vaccine dose; and group B: $x = 114$ ng/vaccine dose; range: 82.4–136.8 ng/vaccine dose).

Growth of parasites, as assessed by tritiated hypoxanthine uptake

The viability of the parasites following chemical attenuation was assessed using the $[^3H]$-hypoxanthine growth inhibition assay. Chemically attenuated ring-stage parasites (2% haematocrit) were added to 96-well flat-bottomed plates (100 µl per well) in quadruplicate. Unattenuated ring-stage parasites and unparasitised red blood cells (uRBC) at 2% haematocrit were used as positive and background controls respectively. Plates were placed in a 37 °C incubator with 5% O_2, 5% CO_2, and 90% N_2. The assay duration was 48 h with $[^3H]$-hypoxanthine (0.2 µCi/well) added from the start of the experiment. Following incubation, plates were frozen, then subsequently thawed and harvested onto glass fibre mats (Perkin Elmer, Australia) using a Filtermate cell harvester (Perkin Elmer). Radioactivity was measured using a Microbeta^2 counter (Perkin Elmer). The remainder of the packed cells from the vaccine were placed in culture, and after 1 week, 2 weeks and 3 weeks of culture, cells were harvested and evaluated according to incorporation of $[^3H]$-hypoxanthine. Twice a week, fresh uRBC were added into the cultures and the medium changed. No growth was observed, as measured by lack of $[^3H]$-hypoxanthine incorporation, compared to unattenuated Pf 7G8 control samples that were cultured in parallel.

PCR

Sample preparation, DNA extraction and parasitemia, as measured by qPCR, were undertaken as previously described [33] with the following modifications. The standard curve was prepared from a lyophilized World Health Organisation (WHO) Pf international standard (NIBSC code: 04/176) [34] that was reconstituted in 500 µl of nuclease-free water and diluted in a 1:1 solution with 1 X phosphate buffered saline (PBS) (Gibco). DNA was isolated from 500 µl of this solution at a concentration of 5×10^8 IU/ml. Blood samples from study participants and standards were tested in triplicate. Established modified calculations [35] were used to equate international units (IU)/ml to parasites/ml, with 1 IU/ml equivalent to 0.5 parasites/ml. The number of parasites/ml was calculated using the CFX96 Touch Real Time Detection System software (BioRad, Australia).

Collection and processing of samples from study participants

Whole blood was collected from study participants in sodium heparin tubes and centrifuged at 433g for 10 min. Plasma was removed and stored at −80 °C until it was required for analysis. The cell pellet was diluted 1:1 in RPMI-1640, and peripheral blood mononuclear cells (PBMCs) were isolated by density centrifugation with Ficoll-Paque (Amersham). PBMCs were washed, resuspended at 1×10^7 cells/ml in 90% heat inactivated foetal bovine serum (FBS)/10% dimethyl sulfoxide and frozen to −80 °C at 1 °C/min in freezing containers for 24 h (Nalgene), before transfer to liquid N_2 for storage.

Enzyme-linked immunosorbent assay (ELISA)

NUNC Maxi-sorp immunoplates (Thermoscientific, Australia) were coated with 5 µg/ml of crude Pf 7G8 antigen in bicarbonate coating buffer, pH 9.6 and incubated overnight at 4 °C. After washing with 0.05% Tween20/PBS, plates were blocked with 10% skim milk buffer/0.05% Tween 20/PBS and incubated at 37 °C for 2 h. Following washing, plasma (diluted 1:50 in 5% skim milk buffer/0.05% Tween 20/PBS) was added to the plates and they were incubated at 37 °C for 1 h. The plates were washed again, and a goat anti-human IgG horseradish peroxidase conjugate (Abcam, Australia) or a goat anti-human IgM Fc5µ horseradish peroxidase conjugate (Merck Millipore) was added at 1:10,000 (IgG) or 1:2,500 (IgM) in 5% skim milk buffer/0.05% Tween 20/PBS and plates were incubated at 37 °C for 1 h. Following further washing, tetramethylbenzadine (TMB) substrate solution (Becton Dickinson, Australia) was added and plates were incubated at room temperature for 10–15 min. Absorbance was measured at 650 nM on an xMark micro-plate reader (Bio-rad, Australia). Positive control serum was obtained from residents of malaria-endemic areas. Negative control serum was obtained from unexposed Brisbane residents.

PBMC stimulation assays
Upon thawing, cells were washed thrice in complete medium (RPMI-1640 containing 10% heat inactivated human serum, 2 nM L-glutamine, 100 U/ml of penicillin and 100 mg/ml of streptomycin sulphate), re-suspended in complete medium, counted using trypan blue (Sigma) and aliquoted into U-bottom 96-well plates.

For T cell proliferation assays, 2×10^5 cells in 100 μl was added per well. Subsequently, 100 μl of purified fresh pRBCs at trophozoite/schizont stage (Pf 7G8, Pf NF54 or *Plasmodium knowlesi* A1H1.1) or uRBCs (6×10^5 cells/well), 1% phytohaemagglutinin (PHA; Gibco) or media only was added, and PBMCs were cultured for 7 days at 37 °C, 5% CO_2. Each treatment was tested in triplicate.

For intracellular cytokine staining, 5×10^5 cells in 100 μl were added per well. Subsequently, 100 μl of purified fresh Pf 7G8 pRBCs or uRBCs (1×10^6 cells/well), 1% PHA or media only was added, and PBMCs were cultured for 36 h at 37 °C, 5% CO_2. Each treatment was tested in triplicate. Sorbitol-synchronised, *Mycoplasma*-negative, live, late-stage trophozoite/schizont stage pRBCs used in the above in vitro assays were purified by magnetic separation over CS columns (Miltenyi Biotec) on a VarioMACs magnet (Miltenyi Biotec) for these assays.

Measurement of PBMC proliferation
For assessing proliferation of PBMCs via the incorporation of radioisotope, the unlabelled cells were pulsed with 1 μCi of $^3[H]$-thymidine/well (Perkin Elmer, Australia) for the final 18 h and plates were stored at − 80 °C. Following thawing, cells were harvested onto glass fibre mats (Perkin Elmer, Australia) using a Filtermate cell harvester (Perkin Elmer) and radioactivity was measured using a β-scintillation microplate counter (Perkin Elmer). The uptake of $^3[H]$-thymidine was measured as corrected counts per minute (CCPM), and results were expressed as deltaCPM, which is defined as the $^3[H]$-thymidine (CPM) in the presence of stimulus, subtracting the average $^3[H]$-thymidine (CPM) incorporated in the presence of the appropriate control stimulus (e.g. unparasitised red blood cells).

Detection of cytokines by cytometric bead array
After 6 days of culture, prior to the addition of radioisotope, cell culture supernatants were removed and frozen at − 80 °C. Cytokines were measured in the thawed culture supernatants using a Th1/Th2/Th17 cytometric bead array (CBA) kit (BD Biosciences) according to the manufacturer's instructions. Samples were analysed on a CyAn ADP flow-cytometer, and data analysis was performed using BD FCAPArray software. To determine agonist-specific cytokine induction, background levels from uRBC alone were subtracted. Selected plasma samples were also analysed with Th1/Th2/Th17 CBA kits according to the manufacturer's instructions.

Identification of cellular sources of cytokines by flow cytometry
For the final 4 h of incubation, Golgi-Plug (BD Biosciences) was added. Plates were removed from the incubator and centrifuged at 433g for 5 min. To enable dead cell exclusion, the LIVE/DEAD Aqua Fixable Dead Cell Stain (Thermofisher Scientific) was added to the cells according to manufacturer's instructions and incubated in the dark at room temperature for 30 min. Following washing, antibodies for staining of cell surface markers (γδ TCR PE-CF594, clone B1; CD3 PerCp, clone SK7; CD4 450, clone RPA-T4; CD8 PECy7, clone RPA-T8; CD45RO APC-H7, clone UCHL1; all from BD Biosciences) were diluted in FACs buffer (1% bovine serum albumin [BSA]/PBS), added to cells and incubated for 20 min in the dark on ice. Following washing with FACs buffer, cells were fixed in 40% v/v formalin at room temperature for 15 min. Cells were fixed and permeabilised using the BD Fix/Perm Kit (BD Biosciences) according to the manufacturer's instructions. Intracellular staining with cytokine-specific antibodies (IFN-γ APC, clone B27; TNF FITC, clone 6401.1111; IL-2 PE, clone MQ1-17H12; all from BD Biosciences) and the appropriate isotype controls was performed on ice for 30 min. Following washing, cells were resuspended in FACs buffer for analysis of the Cyan ADP flow cytometer (Beckman Coulter, Australia). Data analysis was performed using FlowJo V10 (FlowJo, LLC).

Statistics
All data were analysed and graphed using GraphPad PRISM 6. One-way ANOVA was performed on datasets followed by Dunnett's multiple comparisons test. For the antibody and T cell proliferative data, analyses were conducted at an individual level, using assay replicates and comparing responsiveness at day 0 with subsequent time points. For all other immunological analyses, data was combined for all individuals within a group at each time point, and comparisons were conducted between day 0 and subsequent time points.

Results

Parasite growth in volunteers post-inoculation
We initially established the minimal dose of TF-A necessary to completely attenuate Pf 7G8 and prevent growth of the parasite in vitro. We observed that a dose of 50 nM was sufficient as demonstrated by the lack of parasite growth measured by $^3[H]$ hypoxanthine

incorporation (Additional file 1: Figure S1). We then produced vaccine doses for administration to volunteers. The biological properties of the vaccine, including assessment of residual TF-A are described in the "Methods" section.

We treated three study participants in group A (P1 → P3), with a single vaccine dose containing 3×10^7 pRBC treated with 50 nM TF-A. The dose of 3×10^7 pRBC was chosen based on the lowest dose of a *P. chabaudi*-attenuated vaccine shown to be efficacious in mice (10^4) [18], with a correction for approximate weight differences. Surprisingly, all three participants developed a sub-patent Pf infection (Fig. 1a) necessitating initiation of anti-malarial treatment with A/L on days 10–13 (according to symptoms and the parasitemia threshold as defined in the study protocol [11,500 parasites per millilitre]). As a TF-A concentration of 50 nM was insufficient to completely attenuate the parasite, a higher dose was used to prepare the vaccine for the next study group (group B), which received a single vaccine dose of 3×10^7 pRBC treated with 200 nM TF-A. Apart from a sub-patent parasitemia detected by qPCR on day 2 only, all five participants (P4 → P8) remained parasite-negative until day 28, when drug treatment with A/L was initiated in accordance with the study protocol (Fig. 1b).

Adverse events and lab abnormalities

A number of adverse events (AEs) and abnormal laboratory values considered probably or possibly related to the vaccine were recorded for participants in group A (Additional file 1: Tables S2 and S3). The majority of these were typical of symptoms or blood abnormalities observed during Pf infection (malaria) and resolved following completion of anti-malarial drug treatment.

There were no AEs attributable to the vaccine recorded for the participants in group B.

Induction of alloantibodies

Blood group O RhD negative blood was used to manufacture the chemically attenuated pRBC inoculum for P1 → P6. However, we observed that P6 seroconverted to the minor Rh antigen "c" by day 28. While his Rh phenotype was "CDe", and the phenotype of the donor red blood cells was "ce", this was an unexpected finding as it had not been observed in any of > 380 volunteers previously given controlled human blood-stage malaria infections (J McCarthy, pers. comm. and DI Stanisic, unpublished data). As a result of this finding, the inocula for the last two volunteers in group B (P7 and P8) were manufactured using their own blood.

Induction of parasite-specific antibody responses

Plasma samples from study participants were tested for Pf 7G8-specific IgM and IgG by ELISA. In all participants in group A, the group that developed Pf infection, parasite-specific IgM was induced, with significantly higher levels present on day 28 compared to day 0 ($p < 0.01$ for P1 and P3; $p < 0.001$ for P2) (Fig. 2a). Levels of parasite-specific IgM in group B (Fig. 2b), the group that did not develop Pf infection, and IgG in groups A (Additional file 1: Figure S2A) and B (Additional file 1: Figure S2B) were not significantly elevated compared to day 0 during the course of the study ($p > 0.05$).

Induction of parasite-specific cellular responses

To assess cellular responses, parasite-specific lymphoproliferation (as measured by ^{3}[H]-thymidine incorporation)

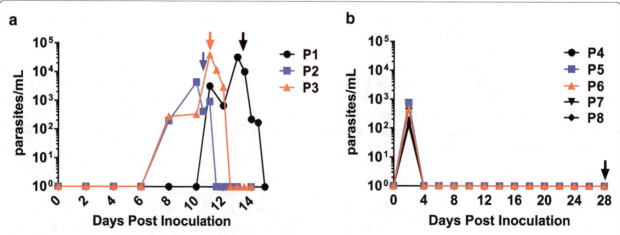

Fig. 1 The course of parasitemia in study participants inoculated with chemically treated *P. falciparum* 7G8. Parasite levels in study participants, as determined by qPCR, following inoculation with **a** 3×10^7 *P. falciparum* pRBC treated with 50 nM tafuramycin-A (TF-A) or **b** 3×10^7 *P. falciparum* pRBC treated with 200 nM TF-A. Arrows indicate initiation of drug treatment with artemether-lumefantrine

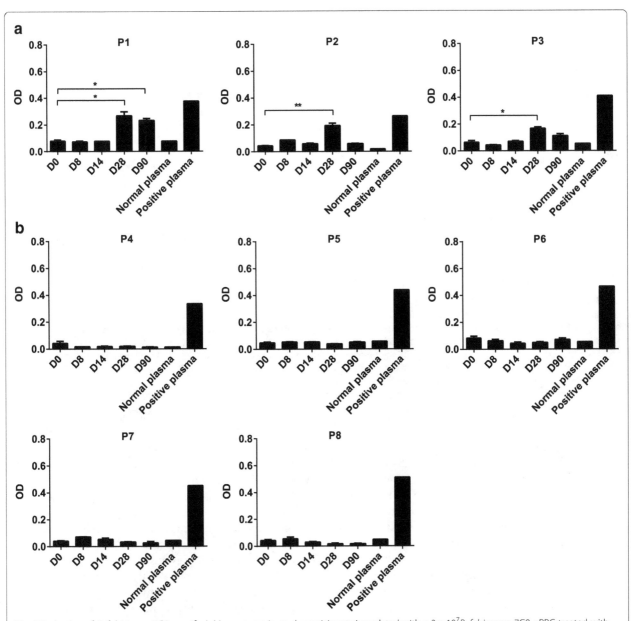

Fig. 2 Induction of *P. falciparum* 7G8-specific IgM responses in study participants inoculated with **a** 3×10^7 *P. falciparum* 7G8 pRBC treated with 50 nM TF-A or **b** 3×10^7 *P. falciparum* 7G8 pRBC treated with 200 nM TF-A. ELISAs were performed to detect IgM specific for crude *P. falciparum* 7G8 antigen using plasma collected at different time points following vaccination. Results are expressed as optical density (OD) at 650 nm. Samples were run in duplicate. Data represents mean ± SEM. An individual's data was analysed using a one-way ANOVA followed by Dunnett's multiple comparisons test; *$p < 0.01$, **$p < 0.001$

was assessed to homologous (7G8) and heterologous (PfNF54 and *P. knowlesi*) pRBC. In group A, responses to homologous parasites (7G8) did not increase significantly compared to day 0 ($p > 0.05$) (Fig. 3a). There was a decrease in responses between days 8–13, which was associated with the development of infection and the administration of anti-malarial treatment (Fig. 1). Proliferative responses to the heterologous parasites did not increase at any time point for P1 ($p > 0.05$) (Fig. 3a). For P2 and P3, significantly increased responses compared to day 0 were seen to PfNF54 and *P. knowlesi* at various time points ($p < 0.05$) (Fig. 3a).

In group B, proliferative responses to homologous parasites (Fig. 3b) were significantly increased at one or more time points compared to day 0 for all five individuals ($p < 0.04$ for all); for 3/5 individuals, this was observed at three or more time points. Additionally, for 3/5 individuals, this was observed at D90. For heterologous parasites, significantly increased responses were seen to PfNF54 at one of more time points in all participants

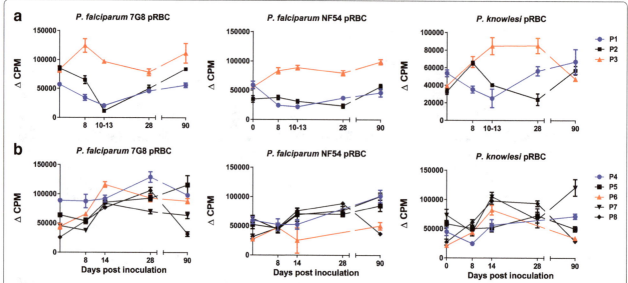

Fig. 3 Lymphoproliferative responses to homologous (*P. falciparum* 7G8) and heterologous (*P. falciparum* NF54 and *P. knowlesi*) pRBC in study participants inoculated with a single dose of **a** 3×10^7 *P. falciparum* 7G8 pRBC treated with 50 nM (group A) or **b** 200 nM (group B) TF-A. Peripheral blood mononuclear cells (PBMCs) were isolated from blood samples collected at different time points post-inoculation and cryopreserved. Following thawing, PBMCs were incubated with parasitised red blood cells (pRBC) or unparasitised red blood cells (uRBC) for 7 days; the last 18 h with ^{3}[H] thymidine. Proliferation of PBMCs was estimated by ^{3}[H] thymidine incorporation. Data represents mean ± SEM for each time point (tested in triplicate). CPM: counts per minutes. Delta CPM indicates that responses to pRBC were corrected against responses to uRBC. The day 28 samples for P4 and P6 were not available for testing against *P. falciparum* NF54 and *P. knowlesi*

($p \leq 0.02$ for all) and to *P. knowlesi* in 4/5 study participants (P4, P6, P7 and P8) ($p < 0.05$ for all) (Fig. 3b).

Cytokines present in the supernatants of the PBMC cultures in the 7-day assay following incubation with *P. falciparum* 7G8 pRBC were measured. Similar to the lymphoproliferative responses, for group A, the production of IFN-γ, TNF and IL-6 generally decreased compared to day 0 between days 8–13; in most instances, this returned to baseline levels by D90 (Fig. 4a and Additional file 1: Figure S3A). IL-4 and IL-10 levels increased in all individuals in parallel with the decrease in inflammatory cytokines. When combining data for all individuals in group A at each time point, there was a significant increase in IL-10 production at day 14 ($p = 0.018$) compared to day 0. Production of IL-2 and IL-17A was not consistent between individuals (Additional file 1: Figure S3A). In group B, an increase in IFN-γ, TNF and IL-10 production compared to day 0 was observed for all individuals (Fig. 4b). When combining data for all individuals in group B at each time point, for IFN-γ, this increase was significant at days 14 and 28 ($p < 0.02$ for both), and for IL-10, it was significant at day 14 ($p = 0.043$). Production of IL-2, IL-4, IL-6 and IL-17A varied over time and between individuals (Fig. 4b and Additional file 1: Figure S3B).

We were interested in the endurance of the altered immune response following vaccination. Four of the five individuals in group B demonstrated persisting altered immune responses, compared to day 0, to *P. falciparum* 7G8 pRBC resulting in production of the parasiticidal cytokine, IFN-γ, at day 90 and two of these individuals also had persisting TNF responses (Fig. 4b). The one individual (P4) whose response did not persist to day 90 was responsive until day 28.

Due to the appearance of clinical symptoms in participants in group A, we evaluated plasma levels of key inflammatory and anti-inflammatory cytokines in these individuals and compared these levels with those in plasma from participants in a previous study where we had evaluated the infectivity of the Pf 7G8 cell bank [32]. Similar parasitemias were observed in those study participants [32], who were asymptomatic at the time of initiation of A/L treatment and in whom it was initiated according to the same criteria for reaching the parasitemia threshold. Overall, higher levels of IL-6 and IL-10 were observed in individuals in the current study compared with the previous infectivity study (Additional file 1: Figure S4).

The intracellular production of IFN-γ, TNF and IL-2 in response to homologous pRBC in short-term in vitro assays was also examined in CD3$^+$ T cells. Initially, we examined CD3$^+$ T cells to identify monofunctional and polyfunctional T cells secreting the parasiticidal cytokines, IFN-γ and TNF. T cells secreting these cytokines individually or in combination were induced in both groups following inoculation (Fig. 5 and Additional file 1: Figure S5). In group B, T cells secreting IFN-γ alone or in combination with TNF were the most frequently detected (Fig. 5). When combining data for all individuals

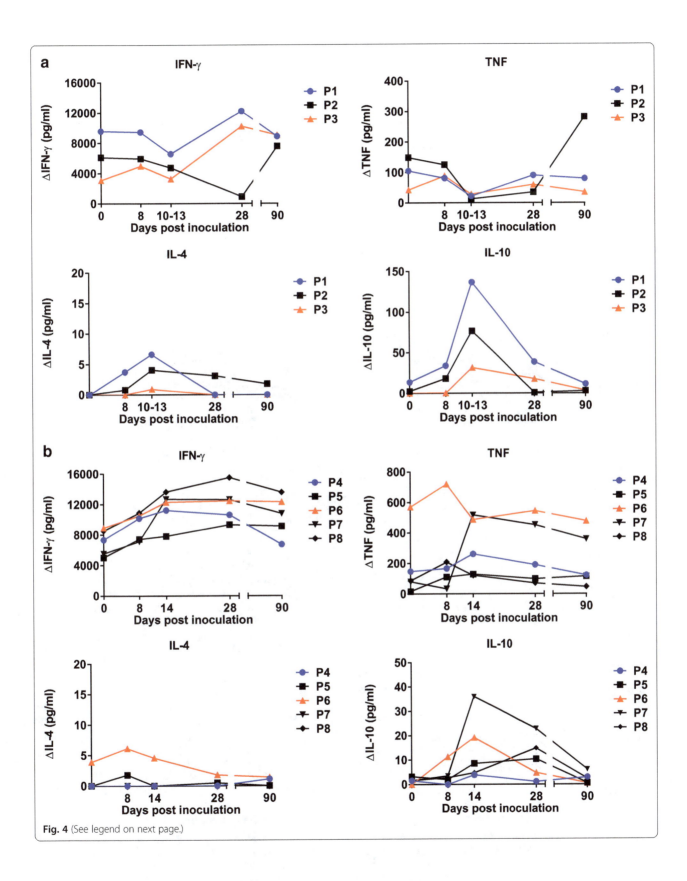

Fig. 4 (See legend on next page.)

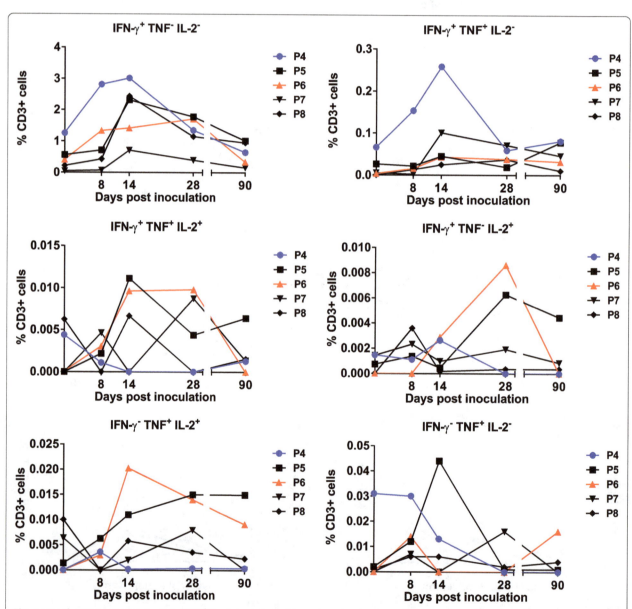

(See figure on previous page.)
Fig. 4 Cytokine responses to *P. falciparum* 7G8 in study participants inoculated with a single dose of **a** 3×10^7 *P. falciparum* 7G8 pRBC treated with 50 nM (group A) or **b** 200 nM (group B) TF-A. Peripheral blood mononuclear cells (PBMCs) were isolated from blood samples collected at different time points post-inoculation and cryopreserved. Following thawing, PBMCs were incubated with parasitised red blood cells (pRBC) or unparasitised red blood cells (uRBC) for 7 days. Eighteen hours before the end of the culture period, culture supernatants were collected, pooled ($n = 3$) and used in cytokine bead arrays to quantify the level of cytokines produced in response to *P. falciparum* 7G8 pRBCs by flow cytometric analysis. Delta cytokine indicates that responses to pRBC were corrected against responses to uRBC

Fig. 5 Monofunctional and polyfunctional CD3$^+$ T cells in study participants inoculated with a single dose of 3×10^7 *P. falciparum* 7G8 pRBC treated with 200 nM TF-A (group B). Peripheral blood mononuclear cells (PBMCs) were isolated from blood samples collected at different time points post-inoculation and cryopreserved. Following thawing, PBMCs were incubated with parasitised red blood cells (pRBC) or unparasitised red blood cells (uRBC) for 36 h. Cells from triplicate wells were collected and pooled prior to staining with antibodies for flow cytometric analysis to evaluate the proportion of CD3$^+$ T cells producing intracellular IFN-γ, TNF and IL-2. Responses to pRBC were corrected against responses to uRBC

in group B at each time point, there was a significant increase in cells secreting IFN-γ alone (i.e. IFN-γ⁺TNF⁻IL-2⁻) when comparing day 14 with day 0 ($p < 0.02$). Triple cytokine-secreting cells (IFN-γ, TNF and IL-2) were also detected, albeit at lower frequencies.

Intracellular production of the three cytokines in response to homologous pRBC was then examined individually in naïve ($CD3^+CD45RO^-$) and memory ($CD3^+CD45RO^+$) T cell populations. In both groups, all three cytokines were produced by both cell types with the cellular source and cytokine profile varying between individuals (Fig. 6 and Additional file 1: Figure S6). Importantly, memory T cells ($CD3^+CD45RO^+$) producing the three cytokines were induced following inoculation in all individuals in group B following inoculation (Fig. 6). When combining data for all individuals in group B at each time point, $CD3^+CD45RO^+$ cells secreting IFN-γ were significantly increased at day 14 compared with day 0 ($p = 0.04$).

Intracellular cytokine production was also examined according to $CD3^+$ T cell subset: helper T cells ($CD3^+CD4^+CD8^-$); cytotoxic T cells ($CD3^+CD4^-CD8^+$); and γδ T cell ($CD3^+γδ^+$) populations. There was heterogeneity in the cellular source and cytokine profile in individuals across both groups A and B (Fig. 7 and Additional file 1: Figure S7). Generally, in group B, with the exception of TNF production in $CD8^+$ T cells, IFN-γ and TNF production by the different T cell subsets increased following inoculation and peaked on day 14 (Fig. 7). In this group, γδ T cells were the T cell subset with the highest proportion of cells producing IFN-γ, TNF or IL-2. When combining data for all individuals in group B at each time point, and comparing responses to day 0, $CD8^+$ T cells producing IFN-γ were significantly increased at day 14 ($p = 0.007$) and $CD4^+$ T cells and γδ T cells secreting TNF were also significantly increased at day 14 ($p = 0.040$ and 0.036 respectively).

Discussion

Here, for the first time, we describe the preparation and administration to humans of chemically treated Pf pRBC and show that a single dose of attenuated Pf pRBC is able to induce strain and species-transcending cellular immune responses in malaria-naïve individuals. Pf-specific antibody responses were not detected. The dose-ranging component of this study indicates that doses of > 50 nM TF-A must be used in vitro to effectively attenuate *P. falciparum* and prevent the development of the clinical manifestations of Pf infection in vivo.

Lymphoproliferative responses were examined, and as previously shown, all individuals had pre-existing responses to pRBC at baseline [36], despite no previous exposure to Pf. This responsiveness could be due to cross-reactivity between parasite antigens and environmental organisms [36]. Critically, the responses to homologous pRBC increased following inoculation in individuals who received completely attenuated chemically treated Pf 7G8 (group B), and they persisted in a proportion of individuals for up to 90 days (the duration of the study). Proliferative responses to heterologous parasites were also observed in more than half of these individuals. It is possible that administration of additional doses of attenuated parasites will augment the breadth, magnitude and persistence of this response. Cytokine production in response to homologous parasites was also examined, and increased production of IFN-γ and TNF (as measured in culture supernatants) was observed following inoculation. Both IFN-γ and TNF are strongly implicated in protection against Pf infection [25–28, 37], and the latter also in pathology [38–40]. Increased levels of IL-10 were also observed; it is a regulatory cytokine thought to play a crucial role in *Plasmodium* spp. infection, due to its ability to regulate both innate and adaptive inflammatory responses, e.g. production of TNF (reviewed in [41]).

By using intracellular cytokine staining, we further examined production of IFN-γ, TNF and IL-2 by $CD3^+$ T cells. In group B, T cells secreting IFN-γ alone or in combination with TNF were the most frequently detected; however, a significant increase following vaccination was only seen at day 14 for $CD3^+$ T cells secreting IFN-γ alone. Previous studies on malaria and other infectious diseases have demonstrated a correlation between the presence of antigen-specific polyfunctional T cells and protective immunity induced following vaccination (e.g. [42–44]). Although the prevalence of these cells was low and the increases in these populations following vaccination were not significant, administration of additional vaccine doses may increase their prevalence and longevity. Future studies examining the protective efficacy of a chemically attenuated whole blood-stage parasite vaccine should examine the role of these polyfunctional T cells in protection. Importantly, we also observed the induction of cytokine-secreting memory T cells ($CD3^+CD45RO^+$) following inoculation. It would be of interest in future studies to undertake additional phenotyping to examine the pluripotency of this memory T cell population. Analysis of the $CD3^+$ T cell subsets following inoculation showed that there was a significant increase at day 14 in $CD4^+$ and γδ T cells producing TNF and in $CD8^+$ T cells producing IFN-γ.

Pf-specific IgM was detected only in individuals who developed an active malaria infection (group A). The lack of antibody production in group B may be a function of antigen dose, as they were exposed to a lower dose of parasites. It is possible that with administration of further doses of the completely attenuated parasites, an antibody response may be induced.

In a previous clinical study investigating the protective efficacy of multiple low-dose Pf infections

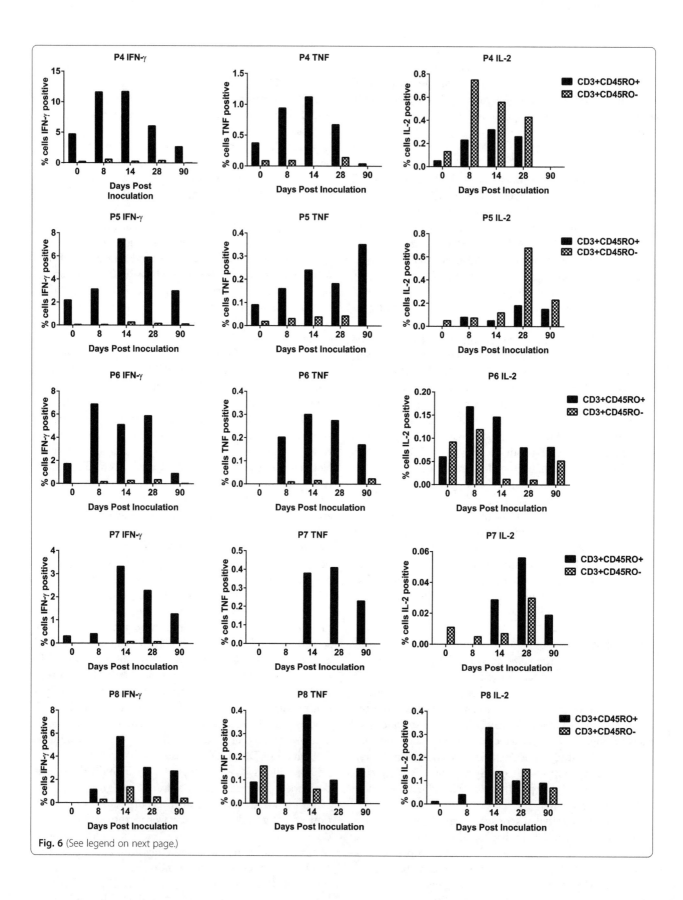

Fig. 6 (See legend on next page.)

(See figure on previous page.)
Fig. 6 Cytokine production in naïve and memory T lymphocytes in study participants inoculated with a single dose of 3×10^7 *P. falciparum* 7G8 pRBC treated with 200 nM TF-A (group B). Peripheral blood mononuclear cells (PBMCs) were isolated from blood samples collected at different time points post-inoculation and cryopreserved. Following thawing, PBMCs were incubated with parasitised red blood cells (pRBC) or unparasitised red blood cells (uRBC) for 36 h. Cells from triplicate wells were collected and pooled prior to staining with antibodies for flow cytometric analysis to evaluate the proportion of naïve T cells ($CD3^+CD45RO^-$) and memory T cells ($CD3^+CD45RO^+$) producing intracellular IFN-γ, TNF and IL-2. Responses to pRBC were corrected against responses to uRBC

attenuated in vivo with atovaquone/proguanil, we observed protection against homologous challenge in three out of four volunteers [29]. However, we could not exclude that protection was due in part to residual drug [45]. Pf-specific cellular immune responses were induced in the absence of Pf-specific antibody in that study, similarly to what we observed in the current study. However, the requirement for delayed anti-malarial drug administration is problematic for the feasibility of this in vivo treatment approach as a vaccine strategy. Our current approach of in vitro treatment of pRBC prior to administration offers a viable alternative.

Induction of parasite-specific cellular immune responses, in the absence of antibodies, was observed in previous rodent studies evaluating the protective efficacy of chemically attenuated *P. chabaudi* pRBC [18]. This is similar to what we observed in the current study, and it differs from the *P. yoelii* 17X rodent studies, where parasite-specific antibodies were also induced in addition to the cellular immune responses [19]. A further study involving administration of chemically treated Pf FVO

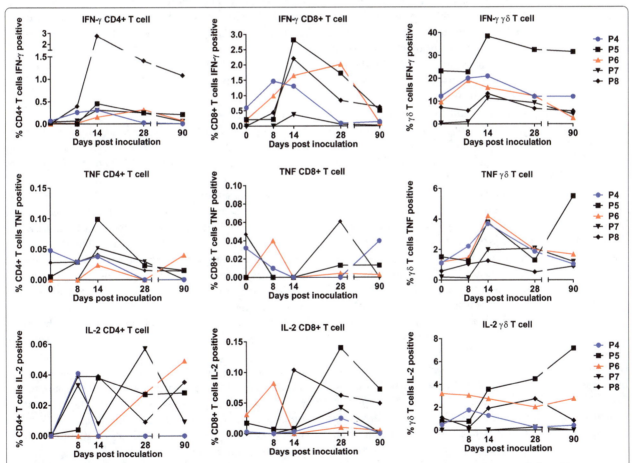

Fig. 7 Cytokine production in $CD3^+$ lymphocyte sub-populations in study participants inoculated with a single dose of 3×10^7 *P. falciparum* 7G8 pRBC treated with 200 nM TF-A (group B). Peripheral blood mononuclear cells (PBMCs) were isolated from blood samples collected at different time points post-inoculation and cryopreserved. Following thawing, PBMCs were incubated with parasitised red blood cells (pRBC) or unparasitised red blood cells (uRBC) for 36 h. Cells from triplicate wells were collected and pooled prior to staining with antibodies for flow cytometric analysis to evaluate intracellular IFN-γ, TNF and IL-2 production in helper T cells ($CD3^+CD4^+CD8^-$), cytotoxic T cells ($CD3^+CD4^-CD8^+$) and γδ T cells ($CD3^+$ γδ$^+$). Responses to pRBC were corrected against responses to uRBC

parasites to non-splenectomised *Aotus* monkeys demonstrated induction of Pf-specific cellular responses in the absence of IgG [30]. Following a single dose of chemically treated parasites, the vaccinated monkeys received a homologous blood-stage challenge with all developing parasitemia and requiring anti-malarial drug treatment. This suggests that more than one vaccine dose may be required for clinical protection.

Rodent studies investigating chemically attenuated *Plasmodium* spp. suggest that persistence of low levels of parasite antigen may be important for inducing an antibody-independent protective immune response [20]. Although persisting parasites could not be detected in this current study beyond day 2 post-inoculation, it is possible that they were persisting at levels below the limit of detection of the qPCR.

The development and clinical evaluation of this whole parasite asexual blood-stage vaccine approach presented a number of general and specific issues for consideration. The use of human red blood cells in the manufacturing process and the final vaccine product entailed specific regulatory and safety considerations, specifically the possibility of contamination with infectious adventitious agents and allo-immunisation. To address the first issue, we used transfusion-compatible blood products, with collection and screening undertaken according to current regulatory guidelines, and used a defined malaria parasite cell bank grown at Good Manufacturing Practices (GMP) standard that had also been rigorously screened according to regulatory guidelines [31]. Furthermore, the manufacturing process complied with current, local GMP requirements. The second issue, the possibility of allo-immunisation (the induction of antibodies against red blood cell antigens), was addressed by the use of blood from a group O RhD negative donor to manufacture the inoculum for group A and the first three participants in group B (P4-P6). In one study participant, P6, seroconversion to the minor Rh antigen "c" was observed following inoculation. As the Rh phenotype of the donor red blood cells that were used to manufacture the inoculum for the first three participants in group B were "ce" while P6's phenotype was "CDe", it is likely that the induction of "c" antibodies may have been due to injection with the chemically treated pRBC. Seroconversion was not observed in P1–P5 despite incompatibility with the donor red blood cells at the minor Rh antigens. Although it is not feasible to match donor blood with recipients at all of the minor Rh antigens, following this observation, the inocula for P7 and P8 were manufactured individually using their own red blood cells. In this current study, the inocula were prepared from cultures with a 5% parasitemia; thus, the total number of red blood cells being injected was 20-fold higher than the number of pRBC. To progress this vaccine strategy and to address the possible induction of alloantibodies, we believe it is critical to reduce the number of red blood cells in the inocula, which could be achieved by purifying the pRBC away from the uninfected red blood cells. This current study involved the administration of only a single dose of Pf pRBC; the impact of multiple doses of Pf pRBC on the induction of alloantibodies is being examined in ongoing studies.

TF-A is a compound with genotoxic potential, and while the majority is washed away during the manufacturing process, its use required the measurement of residual TF-A in an inoculum dose for each manufactured batch. According to the "EU Guidelines on the limits of Genotoxic Impurities" (which has been adopted by our local regulatory body, the Therapeutic Goods Administration), a value of 1.5 μg/day of genotoxic impurity is considered to be associated with acceptable risk. Notably, the US FDA stipulates a much higher threshold of 120 μg/day, and this is for up to 14 days of continuous administration. The amount of residual TF-A in our inoculum batches was considerably lower than both of these thresholds (group A: $x = 86.04$ ng/vaccine dose; group B: $x = 114$ ng/vaccine dose). Purification of pRBC away from uRBC would result in an even further reduction in the amount of residual TF-A.

Conclusions

This study represents the first clinical evaluation of chemically attenuated whole blood-stage parasites in malaria-naïve human volunteers. When the Pf parasites were completely attenuated, the inoculum was safe and well tolerated, although future studies may need to focus on the purification of pRBC (e.g. magnet purification of trophozoite-stage pRBC) for the inoculum to address the possibility of induction of alloantibodies. The induction of strain and species-transcending parasite-specific cellular immune responses following inoculation provides support for the whole blood-stage parasite approach as a means of increasing the breadth of the resulting immune response. While homologous and heterologous protection has been demonstrated in rodent models of malaria [18, 19], it is not known whether these cross-reactive immune responses will be protective in humans. These data support further clinical development of chemically attenuated whole blood-stage parasites as a vaccine strategy. Future studies will focus on a multi-dose immunisation regimen and will address whether lower doses of attenuated parasites are immunogenic.

Additional file

Additional file 1: Table S1. Demographics of study participants. **Table S2.** Adverse events reported in study participants in group A. **Table S3.** Abnormal laboratory values reported in study participants in group A.

Figure S1. In vitro growth of *P. falciparum* 7G8 following treatment with different doses of tafuramycin-A. **Figure S2.** Induction of *P. falciparum* 7G8 IgG responses in study participants inoculated with a single dose of (A) 3×10^7 *P. falciparum* 7G8 pRBC treated with 50 nM of TF-A or (B) 3×10^7 *P. falciparum* 7G8 pRBC treated with 200 nM of TF-A. **Figure S3.** Cytokine responses to *P. falciparum* 7G8 in study participants inoculated with a single dose of (A) 3×10^7 *P. falciparum* 7G8 pRBC treated with 50 nM (group A) or (B) 200 nM (group B) TF-A. **Figure S4.** Serum cytokine responses in study participants inoculated with a single dose of (A) 3×10^7 *P. falciparum* 7G8 pRBC treated with 50 nM TF-A (group A) or (B) 1,800 *P. falciparum* 7G8 pRBC (infectivity study) untreated. **Figure S5.** Monofunctional and polyfunctional CD3[+] T cells in study participants inoculated with a single dose of 3×10^7 *P. falciparum* 7G8 pRBC treated with 50 nM TF-A (group A). **Figure S6.** Cytokine production in naïve and memory T lymphocytes in study participants inoculated with a single dose of 3×10^7 *P. falciparum* 7G8 pRBC treated with 50 nM TF-A (group A). **Figure S7.** Cytokine production in CD3[+] lymphocyte sub-populations in study participants inoculated with a single dose of 3×10^7 *P. falciparum* 7G8 pRBC treated with 50 nM TF-A (group A).

Abbreviations
A/L: Artemether-lumefantrine; BSA: Bovine serum albumin; CBA: Cytometric bead array; CCPM: Corrected counts per minute; CIPDD: Centre for Integrated Preclinical Drug Development; CM: Centanamycin; CPM: Counts per minute; ELISA: Enzyme-linked immunosorbent assay; EU: European Union; FBS: Foetal bovine serum; GMP: Good Manufacturing Practices; IFN: Interferon; IgG: Immunoglobulin G; IgM: Immunoglobulin M; IL: Interleukin; IU: International units; ng: Nanogram; nM: Nanomolar; PBMC: Peripheral blood mononuclear cells; PBS: Phosphate buffered saline; Pf: *Plasmodium falciparum*; PHA: Phytohaemagglutinin; PIC/S: Pharmaceutical Inspection Co-operation Scheme; pRBC: Parasitized red blood cells; qPCR: Quantitative polymerase chain reaction; RPMI: Roswell Park Memorial Institute medium; TF-A: Tafuramycin A; TMB: Tetramethylbenzidine; TNF: Tumour necrosis factor; U: Units; uRBC: Uninfected red blood cells

Acknowledgements
The authors gratefully acknowledge the study participants. We thank Tanya Forbes and Nicola Cocroft for regulatory support and Dr. Michael Batzloff and Dr. Chris Davis for advice and support throughout the study. We thank Ms. Maryna Brown for assistance with Project Management. We thank Dr. Peter Crompton for kindly providing plasma samples for positive controls for the ELISAs. We would like to thank Professor Dennis Shanks and Dr. Qin Cheng (Australian Army Malaria Institute) for kindly providing the *P. falciparum* 7G8 from which the *P. falciparum* 7G8 cell bank was derived. We would also like to thank Professor Shanks and Dr. Paul Griffin for serving on the Safety Review Team. We thank Dr. Stephanie Yanow for critically reviewing the manuscript.

Funding
Funding was provided by The Merchant Foundation, Atlantic Philanthropies and the National Health and Medical Research Council (NHMRC) of Australia (program grant to MFG, research fellowship to MFG). The funders had no role in the study design, data collection or analysis, decision to publish or preparation of manuscript.

Authors' contributions
DS planned and conducted the experiments, analysed/interpreted the data, managed the clinical study, manufactured the chemically treated inoculum and wrote the manuscript. JF, JM, SC, LG and JG were responsible for the clinical monitoring and management of the study participants. XL manufactured the chemically treated inoculum and assisted with laboratory sample processing and parasite culture for laboratory assays. IED manufactured the TF-A. IR, JP, NW, SD and MH assisted in the laboratory monitoring of study participants. SH supplied the *P. falciparum* NF54 parasite line used in the immunogenicity assays and provided regulatory and technical advice for the GMP-compliant production of the cell bank that was used to manufacture the vaccine. MG planned the experiments, contributed to the interpretation of the data and writing of the manuscript. All authors approved the final manuscript.

Competing interests
DS, XL, IED, IR, JP, NW, SD, MH and MG declare competing interests. At the time of this study, they were employees of Griffith University, which co-owns a patent family "Blood-Stage Malaria Vaccine". This patent family is related to the work described in this manuscript.

Author details
[1]Institute for Glycomics, Griffith University, Parklands Drive, Southport, Queensland, Australia. [2]Gold Coast University Hospital, 1 Hospital Blvd, Southport, Queensland, Australia. [3]Sanaria Inc., Gaithersburg, MD, USA.

References
1. World Health Organisation. World malaria report 2015. In: World Health Organisation, editor. ; 2015.
2. Sagara I, Dicko A, Ellis RD, Fay MP, Diawara SI, Assadou MH, Sissoko MS, Kone M, Diallo AI, Saye R, et al. A randomized controlled phase 2 trial of the blood stage AMA1-C1/Alhydrogel malaria vaccine in children in Mali. Vaccine. 2009;27(23):3090–8.
3. Ogutu BR, Apollo OJ, McKinney D, Okoth W, Siangla J, Dubovsky F, Tucker K, Waitumbi JN, Diggs C, Wittes J, et al. Blood stage malaria vaccine eliciting high antigen-specific antibody concentrations confers no protection to young children in Western Kenya. PLoS One. 2009;4(3):e4708.
4. Sirima SB, Cousens S, Druilhe P. Protection against malaria by MSP3 candidate vaccine. N Engl J Med. 2011;365(11):1062–4.
5. Olotu A, Fegan G, Wambua J, Nyangweso G, Awuondo KO, Leach A, Lievens M, Leboulleux D, Njuguna P, Peshu N, et al. Four-year efficacy of RTS, S/AS01E and its interaction with malaria exposure. N Engl J Med. 2013;368(12):1111–20.
6. Seder RA, Chang LJ, Enama ME, Zephir KL, Sarwar UN, Gordon IJ, Holman LA, James ER, Billingsley PF, Gunasekera A, et al. Protection against malaria by intravenous immunization with a nonreplicating sporozoite vaccine. Science. 2013;341(6152):1359–65.
7. Ishizuka AS, Lyke KE, DeZure A, Berry AA, Richie TL, Mendoza FH, Enama ME, Gordon IJ, Chang LJ, Sarwar UN, et al. Protection against malaria at 1 year and immune correlates following PfSPZ vaccination. Nat Med. 2016;22(6):614–23.
8. Sissoko MS, Healy SA, Katile A, Omaswa F, Zaidi I, Gabriel EE, Kamate B, Samake Y, Guindo MA, Dolo A, et al. Safety and efficacy of PfSPZ Vaccine against *Plasmodium falciparum* via direct venous inoculation in healthy malaria-exposed adults in Mali: a randomised, double-blind phase 1 trial. Lancet Infect Dis. 2017;17(5):498–509.
9. Lyke KE, Ishizuka AS, Berry AA, Chakravarty S, DeZure A, Enama ME, James ER, Billingsley PF, Gunasekera A, Manoj A, et al. Attenuated PfSPZ Vaccine induces strain-transcending T cells and durable protection against heterologous controlled human malaria infection. Proc Natl Acad Sci U S A. 2017;114(10):2711–6.
10. Epstein JE, Paolino KM, Richie TL, Sedegah M, Singer A, Ruben AJ, Chakravarty S, Stafford A, Ruck RC, Eappen AG, et al. Protection against *Plasmodium falciparum* malaria by PfSPZ Vaccine. JCI Insight. 2017;2(1):e89154.
11. Mordmuller B, Surat G, Lagler H, Chakravarty S, Ishizuka AS, Lalremruata A, Gmeiner M, Campo JJ, Esen M, Ruben AJ, et al. Sterile protection against human malaria by chemoattenuated PfSPZ vaccine. Nature. 2017;542(7642):445–9.
12. Stanisic DI, McCarthy JS, Good MF. Controlled human malaria infection: applications, advances, and challenges. Infect Immun. 2018;86(1):e00479–1.
13. Austin SC, Stolley PD, Lasky T. The history of malariotherapy for neurosyphilis. Modern parallels. JAMA. 1992;268(4):516–9.
14. Snounou G, Perignon JL. Malariotherapy--insanity at the service of malariology. Adv Parasitol. 2013;81:223–55.
15. Stanisic DI, Good MF. Whole organism blood stage vaccines against malaria. Vaccine. 2015;33(52):7469–75.
16. Purcell LA, Wong KA, Yanow SK, Lee M, Spithill TW, Rodriguez A. Chemically attenuated Plasmodium sporozoites induce specific immune responses, sterile immunity and cross-protection against heterologous challenge. Vaccine. 2008;26(38):4880–4.

17. Purcell LA, Yanow SK, Lee M, Spithill TW, Rodriguez A. Chemical attenuation of *Plasmodium berghei* sporozoites induces sterile immunity in mice. Infect Immun. 2008;76(3):1193–9.
18. Good MF, Reiman JM, Rodriguez IB, Ito K, Yanow SK, El-Deeb IM, Batzloff MR, Stanisic DI, Engwerda C, Spithill T, et al. Cross-species malaria immunity induced by chemically attenuated parasites. J Clin Invest. 2013;123:3353–62.
19. Raja AI, Cai Y, Reiman JM, Groves P, Chakravarty S, McPhun V, Doolan DL, Cockburn I, Hoffman SL, Stanisic DI, et al. Chemically attenuated blood-stage *Plasmodium yoelii* parasites induce long-lived and strain-transcending protection. Infect Immun. 2016;84(8):2274–88.
20. Reiman JM, Kumar S, Rodriguez IB, Gnidehou S, Ito K, Stanisic DI, Lee M, McPhun V, Majam V, Willemsen NM, et al. Induction of immunity following vaccination with a chemically attenuated malaria vaccine correlates with persistent antigenic stimulation. Clin Transl Immunol. 2018;7(4):e1015.
21. Sato A, McNulty L, Cox K, Kim S, Scott A, Daniell K, Summerville K, Price C, Hudson S, Kiakos K, et al. A novel class of in vivo active anticancer agents: achiral seco-amino- and seco-hydroxycyclopropylbenz[e]indolone (seco-CBI) analogues of the duocarmycins and CC-1065. J Med Chem. 2005;48(11):3903–18.
22. Su Z, Tam MF, Jankovic D, Stevenson MM. Vaccination with novel immunostimulatory adjuvants against blood-stage malaria in mice. Infect Immun. 2003;71(9):5178–87.
23. Demarta-Gatsi C, Smith L, Thiberge S, Peronet R, Commere PH, Matondo M, Apetoh L, Bruhns P, Menard R, Mecheri S. Protection against malaria in mice is induced by blood stage-arresting histamine-releasing factor (HRF)-deficient parasites. J Exp Med. 2016;213(8):1419–28.
24. Aly AS, Downie MJ, Mamoun CB, Kappe SH. Subpatent infection with nucleoside transporter 1-deficient Plasmodium blood stage parasites confers sterile protection against lethal malaria in mice. Cell Microbiol. 2010;12(7):930–8.
25. D'Ombrain MC, Robinson LJ, Stanisic DI, Taraika J, Bernard N, Michon P, Mueller I, Schofield L. Association of early interferon-gamma production with immunity to clinical malaria: a longitudinal study among Papua New Guinean children. Clin Infect Dis. 2008;47(11):1380–7.
26. Robinson L, D'Ombrain M, Stanisic D, Taraika J, Bernard N, Richards J, Beeson J, Tavul L, Michon P, Mueller I, et al. Cellular tumour necrosis factor, gamma interferon, and interleukin-6 responses as correlates of immunity and risk of clinical *Plasmodium falciparum* malaria in children from Papua New Guinea. Infect Immun. 2009;77(7):3033–43.
27. McCall MB, Hopman J, Daou M, Maiga B, Dara V, Ploemen I, Nganou-Makamdop K, Niangaly A, Tolo Y, Arama C, et al. Early interferon-gamma response against *Plasmodium falciparum* correlates with interethnic differences in susceptibility to parasitemia between sympatric Fulani and Dogon in Mali. J Infect Dis. 2010;201(1):142–52.
28. Luty AJ, Lell B, Schmidt-Ott R, Lehman LG, Luckner D, Greve B, Matousek P, Herbich K, Schmid D, Migot-Nabias F, et al. Interferon-gamma responses are associated with resistance to reinfection with *Plasmodium falciparum* in young African children. J Infect Dis. 1999;179(4):980–8.
29. Pombo DJ, Lawrence G, Hirunpetcharat C, Rzepczyk C, Bryden M, Cloonan N, Anderson K, Mahakunkijcharoen Y, Martin LB, Wilson D, et al. Immunity to malaria after administration of ultra-low doses of red cells infected with *Plasmodium falciparum*. Lancet. 2002;360(9333):610–7.
30. De SL, Stanisic DI, van Breda K, Bellete B, Harris I, McCallum F, Edstein MD, Good MF. Persistence and immunogenicity of chemically attenuated blood stage *Plasmodium falciparum* in Aotus monkeys. Int J Parasitol. 2016;46(9):581–91.
31. Stanisic DI, Liu XQ, De SL, Batzloff MR, Forbes T, Davis CB, Sekuloski S, Chavchich M, Chung W, Trenholme K, et al. Development of cultured *Plasmodium falciparum* blood-stage malaria cell banks for early phase in vivo clinical trial assessment of anti-malaria drugs and vaccines. Malar J. 2015;14:143.
32. Stanisic DI, Gerrard J, Fink J, Griffin PM, Liu XQ, Sundac L, Sekuloski S, Rodriguez IB, Pingnet J, Yang Y, et al. Infectivity of *Plasmodium falciparum* in malaria-naive individuals is related to knob expression and cytoadherence of the parasite. Infect Immun. 2016;84(9):2689–96.
33. Rockett RJ, Tozer SJ, Peatey C, Bialasiewicz S, Whiley DM, Nissen MD, Trenholme K, Mc Carthy JS, Sloots TP. A real-time, quantitative PCR method using hydrolysis probes for the monitoring of *Plasmodium falciparum* load in experimentally infected human volunteers. Malar J. 2011;10:48.
34. Padley DJ, Heath AB, Sutherland C, Chiodini PL, Baylis SA, Collaborative Study G: Establishment of the 1st World Health Organization International Standard for *Plasmodium falciparum* DNA for nucleic acid amplification technique (NAT)-based assays. Malar J 2008, 7:139.
35. Mosha JF, Sturrock HJ, Greenhouse B, Greenwood B, Sutherland CJ, Gadalla N, Atwal S, Drakeley C, Kibiki G, Bousema T, et al. Epidemiology of subpatent *Plasmodium falciparum* infection: implications for detection of hotspots with imperfect diagnostics. Malar J. 2013;12:221.
36. Currier J, Sattabongkot J, Good MF. 'Natural' T cells responsive to malaria: evidence implicating immunological cross-reactivity in the maintenance of TCR alpha beta+ malaria-specific responses from non-exposed donors. Int Immunol. 1992;4(9):985–94.
37. Kremsner PG, Winkler S, Brandts C, Wildling E, Jenne L, Graninger W, Prada J, Bienzle U, Juillard P, Grau GE. Prediction of accelerated cure in *Plasmodium falciparum* malaria by the elevated capacity of tumor necrosis factor production. Am J Trop Med Hyg. 1995;53(5):532–8.
38. Grau GE, Taylor TE, Molyneux ME, Wirima JJ, Vassalli P, Hommel M, Lambert PH. Tumor necrosis factor and disease severity in children with falciparum malaria. N Engl J Med. 1989;320(24):1586–91.
39. Kern P, Hemmer CJ, Van Damme J, Gruss HJ, Dietrich M. Elevated tumor necrosis factor alpha and interleukin-6 serum levels as markers for complicated *Plasmodium falciparum* malaria. Am J Med. 1989;87(2):139–43.
40. Day NP, Hien TT, Schollaardt T, Loc PP, Chuong LV, Chau TT, Mai NT, Phu NH, Sinh DX, White NJ, et al. The prognostic and pathophysiologic role of pro- and antiinflammatory cytokines in severe malaria. J Infect Dis. 1999;180(4):1288–97.
41. Freitas do Rosario AP, Langhorne J. T cell-derived IL-10 and its impact on the regulation of host responses during malaria. Int J Parasitol. 2012;42(6):549–55.
42. Lindenstrom T, Agger EM, Korsholm KS, Darrah PA, Aagaard C, Seder RA, Rosenkrands I, Andersen P. Tuberculosis subunit vaccination provides long-term protective immunity characterized by multifunctional CD4 memory T cells. J Immunol. 2009;182(12):8047–55.
43. Darrah PA, Patel DT, De Luca PM, Lindsay RW, Davey DF, Flynn BJ, Hoff ST, Andersen P, Reed SG, Morris SL, et al. Multifunctional TH1 cells define a correlate of vaccine-mediated protection against Leishmania major. Nat Med. 2007;13(7):843–50.
44. Roestenberg M, McCall M, Hopman J, Wiersma J, Luty AJ, van Gemert GJ, van de Vegte-Bolmer M, van Schaijk B, Teelen K, Arens T, et al. Protection against a malaria challenge by sporozoite inoculation. N Engl J Med. 2009;361(5):468–77.
45. Edstein MD, Kotecka BM, Anderson KL, Pombo DJ, Kyle DE, Rieckmann KH, Good MF. Lengthy antimalarial activity of atovaquone in human plasma following atovaquone-proguanil administration. Antimicrob Agents Chemother. 2005;49(10):4421–2.

Breaking bread: examining the impact of policy changes in access to state-funded provisions of gluten-free foods in England

Myles-Jay Linton[1,2*], Tim Jones[2], Amanda Owen-Smith[1,3], Rupert A. Payne[3], Joanna Coast[1,2], Joel Glynn[1] and William Hollingworth[1,2]

Abstract

Background: Coeliac disease affects approximately 1% of the population and is increasingly diagnosed in the United Kingdom. A nationwide consultation in England has recommend that state-funded provisions for gluten-free (GF) food should be restricted to bread and mixes but not banned, yet financial strain has prompted regions of England to begin partially or fully ceasing access to these provisions. The impact of these policy changes on different stakeholders remains unclear.

Methods: Prescription data were collected for general practice services across England ($n = 7176$) to explore changes in National Health Service (NHS) expenditure on GF foods over time (2012–2017). The effects of sex, age, deprivation and rurality on GF product expenditure were estimated using a multi-level gamma regression model. Spending rate within NHS regions that had introduced a 'complete ban' or a 'complete ban with age-related exceptions' was compared to spending in the same time periods amongst NHS regions which continued to fund prescriptions for GF products.

Results: Annual expenditure on GF products in 2012 (before bans were introduced in any area) was £25.1 million. Higher levels of GF product expenditure were found in general practices in areas with lower levels of deprivation, higher levels of rurality and higher proportions of patients aged under 18 and over 75. Expenditure on GF food within localities that introduced a 'complete ban' or a 'complete ban with age-related exceptions' were reduced by approximately 80% within the 3 months following policy changes. If all regions had introduced a 'complete ban' policy in 2014, the NHS in England would have made an annual cost-saving of £21.1 million (equivalent to 0.24% of the total primary care medicines expenditure), assuming no negative sequelae.

Conclusions: The introduction of more restrictive GF prescribing policies has been associated with 'quick wins' for NHS regions under extreme financial pressure. However, these initial savings will be largely negated if GF product policies revert to recently published national recommendations. Better evidence of the long-term impact of restricting GF prescribing on patient health, expenses and use of NHS services is needed to inform policy.

Keywords: Gluten-free, Coeliac disease, Prescriptions, Health expenditures, Primary health care, National Health Service, Deprivation, Clinical commission groups

---

* Correspondence: mj.linton@bristol.ac.uk
[1]Health Economics at Bristol, Population Health Sciences, Bristol Medical School, University of Bristol, Bristol, UK
[2]The National Institute for Health Research Collaboration for Leadership in Applied Health Research and Care West (NIHR CLAHRC West), University Hospitals Bristol NHS Foundation Trust, Bristol, UK
Full list of author information is available at the end of the article

Background

Healthcare services across Europe are under increasing financial pressure [1]. In 2015/2016 England's state-funded National Health Service (NHS) deficit reached £1.85 billion, the largest deficit in NHS history [2]. Despite a subsequent reduction in the deficit in 2016/2017 [3], there is ongoing pressure to achieve the NHS Five Year Forward View's target of finding savings of £22 billion by 2020 [4]. These financial difficulties prompt healthcare decision-makers to reconsider what the NHS can afford to provide. A widely noted reaction to this pressure has been the increasing prioritisation of cost-saving in the management of medicines, and subsequent disinvestment in prescribed items deemed to be of 'low clinical value' such as travel vaccines and homeopathy [5]. Another highly debated example is the prescription of gluten-free (GF) foods for people with gluten enteropathy, also known as coeliac disease (CD) [6].

CD is an autoimmune disease characterised by gastrointestinal symptoms following the ingestion of grains containing gluten (wheat, barley and rye) [7, 8], which affects approximately 1% of the population of Europe [9]. There was a four-fold increase in the incidence rate of CD recorded in the UK between 1990 and 2011, which was largely attributed to increased availability of routine diagnostic tests and greater awareness among clinicians and patients [10]. Like many autoimmune diseases [11], CD is diagnosed at a higher rate among women [10]. There is also evidence that the diagnosis of CD is higher within populations with lower levels of socioeconomic deprivation [12].

Unlike other autoimmune diseases, the only clinically effective treatment for CD is lifelong adherence to a GF diet [13], which is likely to be more financially burdensome than purchasing conventional products that contain gluten [14, 15]. Healthcare systems across the globe have approached this challenge in a variety of different ways. For example, people with CD in Canada are eligible for tax reductions to compensate for the additional costs of purchasing GF foods, while in Italy they are provided with a monthly cash allowance [16]. In the UK, the NHS has provided GF foods on prescription since the 1960s [17]. NHS prescriptions are available for a range of staple goods such as bread and pasta, along with sweet products such as cakes and biscuits [18]. A study into CD prevalence in the UK found that 80% of patients diagnosed with CD were in receipt of at least one GF prescription product through the NHS [10].

In February 2018, NHS England released the results of a nation-wide consultation and announced that prescriptions for GF foods should be restricted to bread and mixes (which can be used to make bread products such as rolls and loaves) [19]. The policy review was prompted by the increased accessibility of GF foods, in comparison to when GF food prescriptions were first introduced [20]. However, prior to this policy decision, an increasing number of NHS England's Clinical Commissioning Groups (CCGs) had already begun to fully or partially cease funding for prescriptions of GF products in some localities [21]. In sum, the prescription of clinically effective and widely available food products highlights a grey area concerning what should (and what should not) be considered 'medicine'.

The overarching aim of the study was to investigate the impact of potential policy changes on different stakeholders (patient groups and CCGs), by exploring three distinct objectives. First, we described changes in expenditure on GF products across all CCGs in England between 2012 and 2017. Next, we estimated GF food prescribing expenditure (for 2014) by general practitioner (GP) practice demographics, rurality and deprivation to identify groups of patients likely to be affected most by reduced prescribing of GF products. Finally, in a separate analysis, we compared the cost-savings made by CCGs which have switched to a 'complete ban' or a 'complete ban with age-related exceptions' with CCGs that have continued to provide GF product prescriptions.

Methods

Datasets

Prescribing data

Prescriptions for GF products were accessed through ' OpenPrescribing.net, EBM DataLab, University of Oxford, 2017', a resource that organises and presents the raw anonymised prescription data released by NHS Digital each month. These data are based on all NHS prescriptions dispensed in primary care pharmacies in England. For this study, OpenPrescribing provided us with a custom extract of the data containing the 'actual cost' of spending on GF products for all GP practices within England (grouped by CCG). NHS Digital defines 'actual cost' as the cost to the NHS, rather than the basic price of a drug or product (Net Ingredient Cost). The extract contained data on spending by each GP practice for each month from January 2012 through to June 2017. GF products were classified into three categories as bread products, staple products (e.g. flour and pasta) and other products (e.g. snacks and biscuits). A complete list of the products in each category is presented seperately (Additional file 1).

GP practice characteristics

We used data from NHS Digital from 2014 to calculate the percentage of registered patients who were female for each GP practice [22]. We used Public Health England's National General Practice Profiles (2014) to characterise GP practices in terms of, percentage of registered patients under 18 years of age, percentage of registered patients 75 years of age or older, population size (list size), Indices of Multiple Deprivation (IMD) score from 2015, and parent CCG [23]. By linking each GP practice postcode to a Lower Layer Super Output Area we were able to classify each GP practice by its level of rurality [24]. Specific Lower Layer Super Output Area rurality classifications were collated into broader categories as follows: Urban Conurbation (A1 and B1), Cities and Towns (C1 and C2), and Rural (D1, D2, E1 and E2). Finally, a spending rate was calculated for each GP practice as the total spend on GF prescriptions in 2014 per 1000 registered patients. We selected this time period as it was the year before most NHS CCGs began restricting their GF food policies. Of the 7596 practices in the 2014 GP prescribing data, 7176 (94%) had complete data once all datasets were linked on GP practice code. One further practice was excluded because more than 80% of its patients were aged above 75.

CCG policies

Data on CCG policies for GF prescribing were extracted from the Coeliac UK website [21]. After contacting all 207 CCGs, Coeliac UK reviewed policies for GF provisions as part of their 'Prescriptions Campaign'. This work resulted in an interactive web-based map containing CCG policies across England. Coeliac UK groups CCGs into four policy types, as (1) partial or complete withdrawal of prescriptions; (2) following national prescribing guidelines; (3) restricting products and/or units; and (4) policy or GF prescribing under review. Within this study these policy types were re-categorised into (1) complete ban on prescriptions, (2) complete ban on prescriptions (with age-related exceptions), (3) no ban on prescriptions, (4) partial restrictions on products and/or units, and (5) policy under review. The rationale for re-classifying the policies, particularly '(1) partial or complete withdrawal of prescriptions' was to recognise the meaningful difference between a restriction and a complete withdrawal of provisions. Verification of Coeliac UK's policy data against the information available on CCG websites was conducted for a small, random selection of CCGs ($n = 21$, 10%). For each of these CCGs, Coeliac UK's data accurately reflected the policy arrangements stated in official statements on CCG websites.

The mapping between these policies is presented separately (Additional file 2). All policy data were extracted by the research team (on 05/09/2017) and stored in a spreadsheet. A summary table of the frequency of the five policy types is presented in Table 1. The highest number of CCGs followed a 'partially restricted' policy, limiting the number of units and products available for prescription (70/207, 34%).

Over one-quarter of CCGs had introduced a 'complete ban' or 'complete ban with age-related exceptions' (58/207, 28%). Due to the variability in policy details among CCGs with partial restrictions, and

Table 1 Summary of Clinical Commissioning Group gluten-free prescribing policies in 2017

Policy type	Frequency (%)
Partial restrictions on products and/or units[a]	70 (34%)
No ban	61 (29%)
Complete ban	46 (22%)
Policy under review	18 (9%)
Complete ban (with age-related exceptions)[b]	12 (6%)

[a]Prescribing was limited to a lower number of monthly units or a restricted set of products which was largely dependent on the individual Clinical Commissioning Group
[b]Gluten-free products still prescribed for children/adolescents under the age of 18 or 19, and in some cases pregnant women

availability of data on CCGs with policies under review, this study focused on CCGs with no ban, a complete ban, or a complete ban (with age-related exceptions). Five bans were introduced in 2015 (complete bans = 4, complete ban with age-related exceptions = 1), 22 in 2016 (complete bans = 17, complete ban with age-related exceptions = 5), and 28 were introduced in the first two-quarters of 2017 (complete bans = 16, Complete ban with age-related exceptions = 12).

Statistical analysis

Total spending for each quarter was calculated across all CCGs ($N = 207$) in England between 2012 (Quarter 1 – January, February and March) and 2017 (Quarter 2 – April, May and June). Total spending was split into the three main product categories (bread products, staple products and other products).

To estimate GF prescribing expenditure by GP practice demographics, rurality and deprivation, GP practices with complete data (for 2014) were entered into a multi-level gamma regression, using the 'meglm' command in Stata (version 14.2) with a gamma distribution and log link function. We estimated how spending rate varied with the following predictors: percentage of women, percentage of population aged under 18, percentage of population aged 75+, IMD 2015 (classified into quintiles, where 1 = least deprived), and rural/urban classification. GP practices were clustered by their parent CCG in the model.

To be eligible for inclusion in the examination of policy impacts on spending rates we required CCGs to have GF spending data for at least 3 months following policy changes. Given that the latest available data were for June 2017, CCGs were eligible if they had switched to a complete ban ($n = 24$) or partial ban with age-related exceptions ($n = 8$) prior to April 2017. The process undertaken to match these CCGs to CCGs with a 'no ban' policy types was based on annual expenditure in 2014 and is outlined in separately (Additional file 3).

Results

Spending on GF products in the past 5 years

Annual expenditure on GF products in 2012 (pre-policy bans) was £25.1 million (Fig. 1). Throughout the study period, 'Bread products' accounted for the largest proportion (64–67%) of spending. Spending began to decline in 2015 when some CCGs introduced policies to restrict prescribing. The lowest quarterly spending rate (£3.96 million) was observed for 2017 (Quarter 2). This is equivalent to a 39% reduction (quarterly saving of £2.58 million) in overall expenditure since spending on GF products peaked in the fourth quarter of 2014 (£6.54 million).

The impact of sex, age, rurality and deprivation on GF spending

Regression results for GP practices with complete data in 2014 ($n = 7175$) demonstrated deprivation had a strong association with expenditure (Table 2). GP practices in the most deprived areas (IMD 5th quintile) had the lowest spending rates on GF products (adjusted point estimate 0.77, 95% confidence interval (CI) 0.72–0.83). Incremental reductions in deprivation (lower quintiles) were associated with incrementally higher spending rates on GF products. GP practices in urban conurbations had the lowest spending rates among the three levels of rurality (adjusted point estimate 0.85, 95% CI 0.78–0.93). GP practices with a higher percentage of patients under 18 (adjusted point estimate 1.02, 95% CI 1.02–1.03) and over 75 (adjusted point estimate 1.07, 95% CI 1.06–1.07) had higher spending on GF prescriptions. Sex was not associated with spending on GF prescriptions after adjusting for the remaining variables in the model (adjusted point estimate 1.00, 95% CI 0.99–1.01). As a sensitivity analysis, we examined whether there was an interaction between rurality and deprivation, yet the interaction term was not found to be statistically significant (Additional file 4).

Trends in expenditure on GF products within CCGs with alternative GF prescription policies

The average total monthly spending rates within CCGs with a 'complete ban' policy, were compared to matched CCGs that had 'no ban' on GF prescriptions, and to CCGs with 'complete ban with age-related exceptions' (Fig. 2). Further details on the spread of these data are presented in Additional file 5. Over time, spending within CCGs with no ban on GF prescribing remained unchanged. In contrast, CCGs that introduced a complete ban saw an average reduction in spending of approximately 80% (equivalent to £9100–£9400 savings per CCG per month). The effect of the policy change had an immediate impact on spending and the reduction in spending levelled off around the second month following policy change. A comparable drop in spending was observed between CCGs which introduced a complete ban and those which had introduced a complete ban for adults only. Despite matching CCGs on their annual expenditure in 2014, expenditure was slightly lower in the 'no ban' CCGs in the

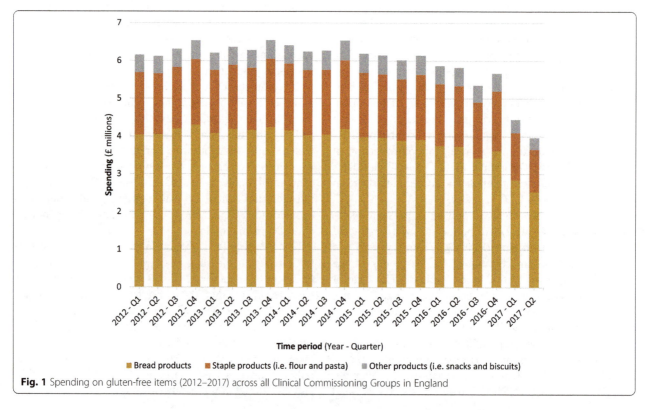

Fig. 1 Spending on gluten-free items (2012–2017) across all Clinical Commissioning Groups in England

Table 2 Modelling spending rate (in 2014), clustered by Clinical Commissioning Group, sex/age variables

Model predictors	Unadjusted point estimate (95% confidence interval)	Adjusted[a] point estimate (95% confidence interval)
Sex		
Change per % increase in female patients	1.03 (1.02–1.04)	1.00 (0.99–1.01)
Age		
Change per % increase in patients ≤ 18 years	0.99 (0.99–1.00)	1.02 (1.02–1.03)
Change per % increase in patients ≥ 75 years	1.06 (1.05–1.07)	1.07 (1.06–1.07)
Level of rurality		
Baseline: Rural	1	1
Towns and Cities	0.85 (0.81–0.90)	0.93 (0.89–0.98)
Urban Conurbation	0.73 (0.67–0.80)	0.85 (0.78–0.93)
Level of deprivation		
Baseline: 1 – Least Deprived	1	1
2	0.88 (0.83–0.92)	0.93 (0.88–0.98)
3	0.80 (0.76–0.85)	0.88 (0.83–0.93)
4	0.71 (0.67–0.75)	0.80 (0.75–0.85)
5 – Most Deprived	0.67 (0.63–0.71)	0.77 (0.72–0.83)

[a]Adjusted for all other predictors in the model

3 months leading up to the ban, which might reflect the fact that policy reforms in some areas took some years to implement. If all CCGs had introduced a complete ban on GF prescriptions in 2014, and spending rates followed the 82.9% reduction observed in this study, the NHS in England would have saved £21.1 million on GF products that year. This figure is equivalent to 0.24% of the total expenditure on medicines in primary care for 2014/2015 (£8.7 billion) [25].

Discussion
Main findings
We found that expenditure on GF products was reduced by an average of approximately 80% within the 3 months after CCGs introduced a 'complete ban' or 'complete ban with age-related exceptions' on GF prescriptions. Spending on GF products peaked in the fourth quarter of 2014 (2014 Q4: £6.54 million) and has since fallen by approximately one-third (2017 Q2: £3.96 million). We estimate that if all CCGs had introduced a 'complete ban' policy for 2014 the NHS would have made an annual cost-saving of £21.1 million. The policies are likely to have the largest impact on spending among GP practices in the least deprived areas, most rural locations and with the highest proportion of patients over the age of 75.

Strengths and weaknesses of the study
To our knowledge, this is the first study to examine the impact of GF product prescription policy changes on cost-savings. As such, our work provides timely insight into the financial implications of recent NHS England GF prescription policy options. This study is comprehensive and representative due to its use of prescription data from all 207 CCGs in England. We explored the cost-savings associated with introducing a 'complete ban' or 'complete ban with age-related exceptions' compared to CCGs with a 'no ban' policy. Differences in the specific criteria used by CCGs with a 'partial restriction on products and/or units' meant that they were not examined in this analysis. Further, we did not have access to data on the number of people with diagnosed CD in each GP practice. Given our focus on prescription data, this work presents one part of a larger story. For example, it is unclear what the impact of policy changes might be on the frequency of consultations, medications or referral rates for gastrointestinal symptoms.

Comparison with other studies
In line with evidence that CD is diagnosed at a higher rate among more affluent patients [12], this study found that spending on GF prescriptions was highest in GP practices with the lowest levels of deprivation. One explanation for this may be that symptom recognition and care seeking is higher among people in higher socioeconomic positions [26]. We also found that GF product expenditure was higher within GP practices with higher proportions of patients over the age of 75 and under the age of 18. In England, patients in both of these age categories are exempt from prescription charges, and therefore this observation is expected [27]. Finally, although CD is diagnosed in more women than men [10], having a higher proportion of female patients within GP practices was not associated with greater expenditure on GF products (when controlling for rurality, age and deprivation).

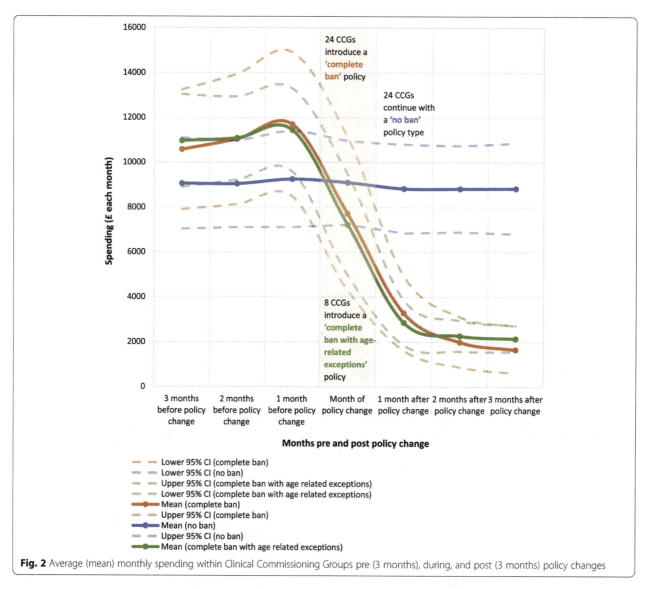

Fig. 2 Average (mean) monthly spending within Clinical Commissioning Groups pre (3 months), during, and post (3 months) policy changes

Implications for patients, clinicians and policymakers

The results of this study demonstrate that policy-driven restrictions on GF prescriptions have been a quick and effective strategy for CCGs to reduce their expenditure. Given our findings, new national recommendations that endorse the prescription of GF bread and mix products are unlikely to yield meaningful cost savings for CCGs [19]. Additionally, the publication of national recommendations 3 years after CCGs began acting unilaterally is likely to create further confusion amongst patients. These changes may be particularly confusing within localities that previously ceased funding for GF products which may now decide to reintroduce them to be in accordance with national recommendations. The higher price paid by the NHS for similar products that would cost less for patients to buy in retail outlets remains a contentious topic [6]: however, higher savings might be yielded if improvements were made to the procurement processes currently in place.

While GF products may be increasingly available in retail stores, they are not necessarily nutritionally equivalent to the products prescribed currently through the NHS. Prescribed products through specialist suppliers such as Juvela [28] and Glutafin [29] are fortified with calcium, iron, folic acid and B vitamins, nutrients that CD patients are commonly deficient in due to malabsorption in the intestines [30]. In the UK, retail wheat flour is typically fortified, yet this is not necessarily the case with GF substitute products [31]. If policy changes result in CD patients switching to retail suppliers for their GF products, they may need to complement their diet with additional nutritional supplements, which may impose additional costs.

Despite technological advancements in the diagnosis of CD, patients often wait many years (mean 5.8 years) following their first GP consultation to receive a formal diagnosis of CD [32], during which there is evidence of increased costs to the NHS [33]. If prescription policies tighten, patients who have faced delayed diagnoses will face the additional obstacle of no access to NHS prescribed treatment.

Restricting GF prescribing may in fact be a false economy. If patients are unable to achieve a GF diet when they do not have GF prescriptions [34], and this leads to an increase in symptoms, then the policies will have a negative effect on NHS resources and health outcomes in the medium term. In addition, the restriction of GF prescribing will have financial consequences for people with CD. Although this study found that spending on GF prescriptions has been highest amongst GP practices in the least deprived areas, those less affluent patients who do access GF prescriptions may be the most likely to struggle with the added financial strain of adhering to a GF diet in the absence of prescriptions [14]. To address this knowledge gap, a qualitative examination into the impact of these policy changes on patients would provide useful insight into how the withdrawal of prescriptions might influence compliance with a GF diet.

In the face of this mismatch between CCG policies and national recommendations, a grey area concerning the extent to which 'food' products are considered 'healthcare' is revealed. While the link between food and health is widely noted [35–37], including food items such as GF bread alongside pharmaceutical products on the national formulary is, and will continue to be, controversial. This is particularly so given that prescription rates are highest among GPs in more affluent areas, suggesting that GF product prescriptions may not be reducing health inequalities. In the longer term, the solution in England might be for greater cooperation between the government, food manufacturers and the retail industry to make GF products more affordable and widely available.

Future research

Despite many CCGs already opting to limit the prescription of GF products [21], our understanding of the wider impact of these policy changes remains incomplete. This study explored the short-term financial consequence of policy restrictions, but there is a need to also conduct medium- and longer-term analyses to explore the resource implications of these policy changes in terms of GP consultations, hospital admissions and other forms of healthcare utilisation. Similarly, the impact of policy changes on health outcomes could be highlighted by investigating increases in the use of vitamin and mineral supplements, and gastrointestinal drugs such as anti-diarrhoeals to combat gluten-induced symptoms. Several studies have indicated that GF foods can cost up to four-times as much as gluten-containing alternatives [14, 15]; therefore, there is a need to investigate the financial burden that more restrictive GF food policies shift onto patients.

Interestingly, NHS regions (CCGs) that implemented a complete ban policy did not see a full reduction in expenditure on GF products. Within the 3-month period studied, spending within these CCGs decreased by approximately 80%, yet this also reveals that GF products were still being prescribed and supplied while they were banned. All of the CCGs (apart from one CCG at 2 months post-policy change) reported that expenditure on GF products had not been completely reduced. One explanation for this finding is that there may have been slow or, in some cases, incomplete implementation of policies within CCGs. Further exploration is needed into the personal perspectives of GPs [38], and the exceptional circumstances that might be used as rationale for prescribing banned products. As in other clinical settings, there is a need to further explore the interplay between policy-level decision-making and prescribing decisions made at the patient level [39].

Conclusions

The introduction of more restrictive GF prescribing policies has been associated with 'quick wins' for CCGs under extreme financial pressure. However, these initial savings will be largely negated if CCGs revert to recently published national recommendations. Better evidence of the long-term impact of restricting GF prescribing on patient health, expenses and use of NHS services is needed to inform policy.

Additional files

Additional file 1: List of gluten-free products in each product category.

Additional file 2: Mapping between policy types.

Additional file 3: Matching process used for examination into policy-related cost-savings.

Additional file 4: Modelling Spending Rate (in 2014), clustered by CCG, sex/age variables.

Additional file 5: Mean and standard deviations for expenditure on GF products among CCGs with three policy types.

Abbreviations

CCG: Clinical Commissioning Group; CD: coeliac disease; CI: confidence interval; GF: gluten free; GP: general practitioner; IMD: indices of multiple deprivation; NHS: National Health Service

Acknowledgements

The research is supported by the National Institute for Health Research (NIHR) Collaboration for Leadership in Applied Health Research and Care West (CLAHRC West) at University Hospitals Bristol NHS Foundation Trust. The views expressed are those of the authors and not necessarily those of the NHS, the NIHR or the Department of Health. We also acknowledge OpenPrescribing.net (EBM DataLab, University of Oxford) for providing our study with prescription data.

Funding
This research was funded by the National Institute for Health Research (NIHR) Collaboration for Leadership in Applied Health Research and Care West (NIHR CLAHRC West). The views expressed in this article are those of the author(s) and not necessarily those of the NHS, the NIHR, or the Department of Health and Social Care.

Authors' contributions
WH initiated the study. ML, TJ and WH conceptualised and designed the analysis plan. ML and TJ acquired, cleaned and analysed the data. ML, TJ, WH, AS, RP, JC and JG aided in the interpretation of the results. ML prepared and drafted the first version of the manuscript. Each of the authors was individually involved in the drafting process, approved the final version of the manuscript, and agreed to be accountable for all aspects of the work.

Competing interests
The authors declare that they have no competing interests.

Author details
[1]Health Economics at Bristol, Population Health Sciences, Bristol Medical School, University of Bristol, Bristol, UK. [2]The National Institute for Health Research Collaboration for Leadership in Applied Health Research and Care West (NIHR CLAHRC West), University Hospitals Bristol NHS Foundation Trust, Bristol, UK. [3]Centre for Academic Primary Care, Population Health Sciences, Bristol Medical School, University of Bristol, Bristol, UK.

References
1. Reeves A, McKee M, Basu S, Stuckler D. The political economy of austerity and healthcare: Cross-national analysis of expenditure changes in 27 European nations 1995–2011. Health Policy. 2014;115(1):1–8.
2. Dunn P, McKenna H, Murray R. Deficits in the NHS 2016. London: The King's Fund; 2016.
3. NHS Improvement: Monitor: Annual Report and Accounts 2016/17. 2017. https://www.gov.uk/government/publications/nhs-improvement-annual-report-and-accounts-201617. Accessed 24 Jan 2018.
4. NHS. NHS Five Year Forward View. London: NHS; 2014.
5. Dowden A. Do we need guidance on prescribing low-value medicines? Prescriber. 2017;28(10):39–43.
6. Kurien M, Sleet S, Sanders DS, Cave J. Should gluten-free foods be available on prescription? BMJ. 2017;356:i6810.
7. Lammers KM, Vasagar B, Fasano A. Definition of celiac disease and gluten sensitivity. In: Celiac Disease: Springer; 2014. p. 13–25. https://www.england.nhs.uk/publication/nhs-five-year-forward-view/. Accessed 24 Jan 2018.
8. Sapone A, Bai JC, Ciacci C, Dolinsek J, Green PH, Hadjivassiliou M, Kaukinen K, Rostami K, Sanders DS, Schumann M. Spectrum of gluten-related disorders: consensus on new nomenclature and classification. BMC Med. 2012;10(1):13.
9. Mustalahti K, Catassi C, Reunanen A, Fabiani E, Heier M, McMillan S, Murray L, Metzger M-H, Gasparin M, Bravi E. The prevalence of celiac disease in Europe: results of a centralized, international mass screening project. Ann Med. 2010;42(8):587–95.
10. West J, Fleming KM, Tata LJ, Card TR, Crooks CJ. Incidence and prevalence of celiac disease and dermatitis herpetiformis in the UK over two decades: population-based study. Am J Gastroenterol. 2014;109(5):757–68.
11. Ngo S, Steyn F, McCombe P. Sex differences in autoimmune disease. Front Neuroendocrinol. 2014;35(3):347–69.
12. Zingone F, West J, Crooks CJ, Fleming KM, Card TR, Ciacci C, Tata LJ. Socioeconomic variation in the incidence of childhood coeliac disease in the UK. Arch Dis Child. 2015;100(5):466–73.
13. Tack GJ, Verbeek WH, Schreurs MW, Mulder CJ. The spectrum of celiac disease: epidemiology, clinical aspects and treatment. Nat Rev Gastroenterol Hepatol. 2010;7(4):204–13.
14. Burden M, Mooney PD, Blanshard RJ, White WL, Cambray-Deakin DR, Sanders DS. Cost and availability of gluten-free food in the UK: in store and online. Postgrad Med J. 2015;91(1081):622–6.
15. Fry L, Madden A, Fallaize R. An investigation into the nutritional composition and cost of gluten-free versus regular food products in the UK. J Hum Nutr Diet. 2017;31(1):108–20.
16. Pinto-Sánchez MI, Bercik P, Verdu EF, Bai JC. Extraintestinal manifestations of celiac disease. Dig Dis. 2015;33(2):147–54.
17. Tighe M, Sleet S, Currell S, Martin J, Puntis J. Gluten-free food prescriptions for children with coeliac disease: should families have to pay? Br J Gen Pract. 2017;67(661):348–9.
18. Martin U, Mercer S. A comparison of general practitioners prescribing of gluten-free foods for the treatment of coeliac disease with national prescribing guidelines. J Hum Nutr Diet. 2014;27(1):96–104.
19. Department of Health and Social Care. Report of Responses Following the Public Consultation on Gluten Free Prescribing. United Kingdom: Department of Health and Social Care; 2018. https://www.gov.uk/government/consultations/availability-of-gluten-free-foods-on-nhs-prescription. Accessed 1 Feb 2018.
20. Department of Health and Social Care. A Consultation on the Availability of Gluten Free Foods on Prescription in Primary Care. United Kingdom: Department of Health and Social Care; 2017. https://www.gov.uk/government/consultations/availability-of-gluten-free-foods-on-nhs-prescription. Accessed 1 Feb 2018.
21. Coeliac UK: Prescription policies. Coeliac UK; 2017. https://www.coeliac.org.uk/gluten-free-diet-and-lifestyle/prescriptions/prescription-policies/. Accessed 5 Sept 2017.
22. NHS Digital: Numbers of Patients Registered at a GP Practice-Oct 2014. NHS Digital; 2017. https://data.gov.uk/dataset/numbers_of_patients_registered_at_a_gp_practice. Accessed 15 Sept 2017.
23. Public Health England: National General Practice Profiles. Public Health England; 2017. https://fingertips.phe.org.uk/profile/general-practice/data. Accessed 15 Sept 2017.
24. Rural Urban Classification (2011) of Lower Layer Super Output Areas in England and Wales. https://ons.maps.arcgis.com/home/item.html?id=9855221596994bde8363a685cb3dd58a. Accessed 15 Sept 2017.
25. Health and Social Care Information Centre: Prescribing Costs in Hospitals and the Community England 2014–15. 2015. https://digital.nhs.uk/data-and-information/publications/statistical/prescribing-costs-in-hospitals-and-the-community/2014-15. Accessed 27 Nov 2017.
26. Olén O, Bihagen E, Rasmussen F, Ludvigsson JF. Socioeconomic position and education in patients with coeliac disease. Dig Liver Dis. 2012;44(6):471–6.
27. Hassell K, Atella V, Schafheutle EI, Weiss MC, Noyce PR. Cost to the patient or cost to the healthcare system? Which one matters the most for GP prescribing decisions? A UK–Italy comparison. Eur J Public Health. 2003;13(1):18–23.
28. Juvela: Juvela FAQs. Juvela; 2017. https://www.juvela.co.uk/faqs/. Accessed 19 Apr 2018.
29. Glutafin: Glutafin fabulous five. 2017.https://www.glutafin.co.uk/blog/glutafin-fabulous-five/. Accessed 19 Apr 2018.
30. García-Manzanares Á, Lucendo AJ. Nutritional and dietary aspects of celiac disease. Nutr Clin Pract. 2011;26(2):163–73.
31. Robins G, Akobeng A, McGough N, Merrikin E, Kirk E. A systematic literature review on the nutritional adequacy of a typical gluten-free diet with particular reference to iron, calcium, folate and B vitamins. UK: Food Standards Agency Report; 2009. https://www.food.gov.uk/sites/default/files/media/document/research-report-gluten-free.pdf. Accessed 20 Apr 2018.
32. Norström F, Lindholm L, Sandström O, Nordyke K, Ivarsson A. Delay to celiac disease diagnosis and its implications for health-related quality of life. BMC Gastroenterol. 2011;11(1):118.
33. Violato M, Gray A, Papanicolas I, Ouellet M. Resource use and costs associated with coeliac disease before and after diagnosis in 3,646 cases: results of a UK primary care database analysis. PLoS One. 2012;7(7):e41308.
34. Muhammad H, Reeves S, Ishaq S, Mayberry J, Jeanes YM. Adherence to a Gluten Free Diet Is Associated with Receiving Gluten Free Foods on Prescription and Understanding Food Labelling. Nutrients. 2017;9(7):705.
35. James WPT, Nelson M, Ralph A, Leather S. Socioeconomic determinants of health: the contribution of nutrition to inequalities in health. BMJ. 1997;314(7093):1545.
36. Mytton OT, Clarke D, Rayner M. Taxing unhealthy food and drinks to improve health. BMJ: Br Med J (Online). 2012;344. https://www.bmj.com/content/344/bmj.e2931.long.
37. Robertson A, Tirado C, Lobstein T, Jermini M, Knai C, Jensen JH, Ferro-Luzzi A, James W. Food and health in Europe: a new basis for action. WHO Reg Publ Eur Ser. 2004;(96):i–xvi. 1-385, back cover
38. Thistlethwaite J, Ajjawi R. The decision to prescribe: influences and choice. InnovAiT. 2010;3(4):237–43.

Pretreatment chest x-ray severity and its relation to bacterial burden in smear positive pulmonary tuberculosis

S. E. Murthy[1*], F. Chatterjee[2], A. Crook[3], R. Dawson[4], C. Mendel[5], M. E. Murphy[1], S. R. Murray[5], A. J. Nunn[3], P. P. J. Phillips[3], Kasha P. Singh[1], T. D. McHugh[1], and S. H. Gillespie[6*] On behalf of the REMoxTB Consortium

Abstract

Background: Chest radiographs are used for diagnosis and severity assessment in tuberculosis (TB). The extent of disease as determined by smear grade and cavitation as a binary measure can predict 2-month smear results, but little has been done to determine whether radiological severity reflects the bacterial burden at diagnosis.

Methods: Pre-treatment chest x-rays from 1837 participants with smear-positive pulmonary TB enrolled into the REMoxTB trial (Gillespie et al., N Engl J Med 371:1577–87, 2014) were retrospectively reviewed. Two clinicians blinded to clinical details using the Ralph scoring system performed separate readings. An independent reader reviewed discrepant results for quality assessment and cavity presence. Cavitation presence was plotted against time to positivity (TTP) of sputum liquid cultures (MGIT 960). The Wilcoxon rank sum test was performed to calculate the difference in average TTP for these groups. The average lung field affected was compared to $\log_{10}$ TTP by linear regression. Baseline markers of disease severity and patient characteristics were added in univariable regression analysis against radiological severity and a multivariable regression model was created to explore their relationship.

Results: For 1354 participants, the median TTP was 117 h (4.88 days), being 26 h longer (95% CI 16–30, $p < 0.001$) in patients without cavitation compared to those with cavitation. The median percentage of lung-field affected was 18.1% (IQR 11.3–28.8%). For every 10-fold increase in TTP, the area of lung field affected decreased by 11.4%. Multivariable models showed that serum albumin decreased significantly as the percentage of lung field area increased in both those with and without cavitation. In addition, BMI and logged TTP had a small but significant effect in those with cavitation and the number of severe TB symptoms in the non-cavitation group also had a small effect, whilst other factors found to be significant on univariable analysis lost this effect in the model.

Conclusions: The radiological severity of disease on chest x-ray prior to treatment in smear positive pulmonary TB patients is weakly associated with the bacterial burden. When compared against other variables at diagnosis, this effect is lost in those without cavitation. Radiological severity does reflect the overall disease severity in smear positive pulmonary TB, but we suggest that clinicians should be cautious in over-interpreting the significance of radiological disease extent at diagnosis.

Keywords: Pulmonary tuberculosis, chest x-ray, cavitation, pretreatment

---

* Correspondence: s.murthy@ucl.ac.uk; shg3@st-andrews.ac.uk
[1]UCL Centre for Clinical Microbiology, Department of Infection, University College London, Royal Free Campus, Rowland Hill Street, London NW3 2PF, UK
[6]Medical and Biological Sciences, School of Medicine, University of St Andrews, North Haugh, St Andrews KY16 9TF, UK
Full list of author information is available at the end of the article

Background

Since their introduction in routine clinical practice in the 1920s, chest radiographs have been used as a primary tool to diagnose and manage pulmonary tuberculosis (PTB) [1–3]. To date, despite their limitations and the availability of computed tomography, they remain the most commonly used tool in PTB diagnosis and management worldwide [4–6]. The chest x-ray (CXR) has been used not only as a diagnostic tool, but also to estimate disease severity in multiple TB studies and clinical trials [7–9].

There are several methods of grading the radiological severity of disease by estimating the extent of lung field that is 'abnormal', including the WHO grading system [10] or the US National Tuberculosis and Respiratory Disease Association classification [11]. In 2010, Ralph et al. [12] created a simple validated scoring system (using a score out of 140) from findings that the proportion of lung fields affected by disease at diagnosis of PTB was associated with a greater acid fast bacilli (AFB) smear grade and that the presence of cavitation (but not number or size of cavitation), along with the percentage of lung field affected on CXR, predicted 2-month smear positivity on treatment. This has gained some currency in studies describing radiological severity [13–15] and in a subsequent study that validated this approach [16].

The relationship between radiological appearance and disease severity has been assessed by comparison with measures of bacterial load such as smear microscopy and culture [17–21]. At diagnosis, the presence of cavitation visible on CXR has been associated with a higher sputum AFB smear grade [12, 17, 22]. The time taken for specimens in automated liquid culture to signal positive is inversely related to bacterial load [13, 23, 24]. Using this concept, a study of 95 images showed that the presence of cavitation on CXR was associated with a shorter time to positivity (TTP) [21]. More recently, some studies have shown that patients with cavitation have a higher bacterial load as judged by TTP in liquid culture [23, 24]. Another study of 244 patients with radiographic assessment of cavitation found that the colony forming units per milliliter were significantly higher in those with cavitation; this was also true using TTP as a marker for bacterial load [22].

In his seminal review of post mortem examinations of patients with TB, Canetti [25] described a difference in the number of bacteria in lung tissue of samples with cavities compared to those with caseous necrotic tissue only and areas of alveolitis. He found that tubercle bacilli were abundant in the inner layer of a cavity, abundant but less so in a solid area of caseous tissue, and rare within areas of inflammatory tissue. As Canetti described bacilli-rich areas as well as areas of inflammatory change, one would think that the host's inflammatory response in addition to the bacterial load should affect the findings on the CXR prior to treatment. We look at a number of patient factors that may affect this host response and which have been associated with radiological findings in other studies, such as on HIV status [26], diabetes mellitus status [27, 28], age [29], ethnicity [30, 31], and gender [32], to investigate what host factors affect radiological severity. Hypoalbuminemia at diagnosis of PTB and low body mass index (BMI) are surrogates of disease severity known to lower survival rates [33, 34]. TB symptoms at diagnosis have been associated with worse burden of disease [35].

With so much weight put on the extent of radiological findings, little is known about what this reflects. We use the REMoxTB database [36] of patients from Africa and Asia with PTB to determine whether radiological extent of disease judged by the CXR severity score correlates with *M. tuberculosis* bacterial load as measured by Mycobacteria-Growth-Indicator-Tube (MGIT) TTP.

Methods

Study sites and patients

Data were collected from the REMoxTB clinical trial, which compared the use of two 4-month moxifloxacin-containing regimens to the standard 6 month first line treatment for PTB [36]. Between 2007 and 2012, 1931 patients were enrolled from 51 sites across 8 countries in Africa and Asia and the protocol mandated pre-treatment postero-anterior CXRs, sputum sampling for AFB smear and culture, and routine blood tests (including liver function tests, albumin levels and HIV testing). During the trial, study patients were excluded if they had severe medical comorbidities or were already taking antiretroviral treatment for HIV prior to study enrollment. In this study, all patients were adults aged 18 years or more, who had smear- and culture-positive PTB by molecular speciation.

CXR scoring

The CXR images were taken at the clinical sites by a radiographer and either uploaded as a digital image (DICOM file) or presented to the clinical site staff as a plain film. Plain films were digitalized with digital photography using a standard protocol to ensure images were of an adequate quality. An early assessment of 'readability' was performed and, where films were judged poor, sites were asked to re-take the images. All images were converted into DICOM files for evaluation.

The digital images were read independently by two clinicians (SHG and SEM) using the Osirix medical imaging software on Apple iMAC computers with at least 1920 × 1080 pixel screens, and readers were encouraged to take regular breaks during the reading process. Images were sent to readers by study site and were read in the same order.

Both readers followed standardized criteria to establish whether an image was of sufficient quality for analysis (Table 1). If deemed satisfactory, the image was assessed for the presence of cavitation and a measure of percentage of abnormal lung field. In the case of discrepant results on readability or presence of cavitation, a third reader blinded to the primary assessment reviewed the film (FC). Only those images that the first two readers agreed on for readability or those that the third reader deemed readable were used in the final analysis. The final result for cavity presence was based on agreement between the primary readers or, if discrepant, the majority result including the third reading. The percentage of lung field affected was calculated using the method described by Ralph et al. [12], where the reader divides the lung fields into quadrants and by observation scores each quadrant by its percentage of abnormal opacification. The scores are then added together and divided by four to produce a total percentage of lung field affected by disease.

Microbiological and clinical data

Sputum samples and demographic data were collected as part of the clinical trial protocol at screening and baseline visits, prior to starting treatment. Sputum samples were either early morning samples or spot samples, none of which were induced. The samples were processed by standard methodology and graded as described in the trial report. Samples that were re-treated due to contamination were not included in the analysis as this process altered the calculated TTP and, thus, could not guarantee an accurate quantification result. As part of the pre-treatment assessment, participants were tested for HIV and were asked about a history of diabetes mellitus. In addition, a series of questions about symptoms were asked and symptoms graded by severity using the modified Division of AIDS system [37] (Table 2).

Statistical analysis

The inter-reader variability was presented on a Bland–Altman plot using the final severity scores from readers 1 and 2. The average of the two readers' calculation of the percentage of lung field affected was used with the final results of cavity assessment. Images where readers disagreed by 1.96 standard deviations or more were not included in the analysis to ensure accuracy in the average percentage value. The presence or absence of cavitation was plotted against TTP and a Wilcoxon rank sum test to calculate the difference in average TTP for each of the two groups was performed. The average percentage area of lung field affected was compared to $\log_{10}$TTP using linear regression and plotted on a scatterplot.

Baseline clinical and biochemical findings (age, sex, ethnicity, BMI, serum albumin, number of grade 3 or 4 TB symptoms, HIV status and type II diabetes status) and radiological severity score were included in a univariable regression analysis. Those found to be significant ($p < 0.05$) were used to create a multivariable regression model to determine the relationship of these characteristics with the radiological severity score. For this process the participants were put into two groups; those with cavitation and those without. Wilcoxon rank sum tests and χ^2 tests were used to compare both groups. All statistical analysis was performed using R statistical software [38].

Ethical approval

This study was performed within the scope of the approvals provided for the REMoxTB clinical trial [36].

Results

Out of 1931 patients randomized for the trial, 1837 had CXRs taken within the required protocol time frame. Following the three-reader quality assessment, 1713 images were deemed readable. Taking into account available data required for analysis, including non-retreated culture results with TTP data, the total number of cases was 1354 from 47 study sites (Fig. 1). The baseline characteristics and findings for the 1354 cases with available matching data are shown in Table 3 and breakdown of participants by site in Table 4. A comparison of the characteristics between the included and excluded cohort are also shown to ensure sampling bias was not an issue (Table 5).

Reader agreement

There was agreement for 1394 (76%) of the 1837 images available for either their readable quality or the presence or absence of cavitation. Agreement between the two readers on cavitation presence was 0.495 by Cohen's Kappa score (95% CI 0.45–0.54, $p < 0.001$), where a value of < 0.4 is poor, 0.4–0.75 is fair to good, and > 0.75 to 1 is excellent [39]. The level of agreement when assessing the percentage of the area of lung field affected was illustrated using a Bland–Altman plot (Fig. 2).

Table 1 Inclusion and exclusion criteria for deeming an image of sufficient quality for reading

Inclusion	Exclusion
Postero-anterior film	Artefacts obscuring the view of the lung fields
A full view of lung fields – the whole thorax with the first rib, lateral ribs and costophrenic angles in view	Images acquired more than 4 weeks prior to pretreatment visit or more than 3 weeks after this
Adequate penetration of film to allow ribs and lung parenchyma to be distinguished	

Table 2 Division of AIDS (DAIDS) grading of adverse event (AE) severity (modified version). This describes the grading system referred to in this study to describe the severity of TB symptoms such as cough, night sweats, weight loss, and hemoptysis

Parameter	Grade 1	Grade 2	Grade 3	Grade 4
Clinical AE NOT identified elsewhere in this DAIDS AE grading table	Symptoms causing no or minimal interference with usual social and functional activities	Symptoms causing greater than minimal interference with usual social and functional activities	Symptoms causing inability to perform usual social and functional activities	Symptoms causing inability to perform basic self-care functions OR Medical or operative intervention indicated to prevent permanent impairment, persistent disability, or death
e.g., Unintentional weight loss	NA	5–9% loss in body weight from baseline	10–19% loss in body weight from baseline	≥ 20% loss in body weight from baseline OR aggressive intervention indicated (e.g., tube feeding or total parenteral nutrition)

Cavity presence and bacterial load

The number of images confirmed to have cavitation visible was 1049 (77.5%) of 1354. The median TTP for MGIT samples from all 1354 patients was 117 h (4.88 days) with an interquartile range of 89 h (3.7 days) to 153 h (6.4 days). Figure 3 shows a boxplot of distribution of TTP between those without and with cavitation on CXR at baseline. This demonstrates that the median TTP is 26 h greater in those patients without compared to those with cavitation (95% CI 16–30, $p < 0.001$, Wilcoxon rank sum test).

Extent of radiological disease and bacterial load

The median percentage of lung fields affected on the chest radiographs was 18.1% (interquartile range 11.3–27.5%). Figure 4 shows a scatterplot of the percentage of lung field affected against the sputum culture $\log_{10}$TTP values for the 1354 patients. Using linear regression for every 10-fold increase in TTP, the area affected decreases by 11.4% ($p < 0.001$, 95% CI 14.9–7.9%).

Multivariable regression model: pre-treatment factors and baseline radiological severity

The percentage of lung fields affected was compared to other parameters in two groups; those with cavity presence and those without cavitation. Characteristics of these two groups are shown in Table 6, with both groups showing statistical differences in albumin levels (lower albumin levels in the cavity group), ethnicity (African participants having a higher level of cavitation and Asians with a greater number without cavitation), TTP (lower TTP in the cavity group), and percentage of lung field affected (greater in the cavity group). HIV status, diabetes status, culture TTP ($\log_{10}$TTP), serum albumin, number of grade 3 or 4 TB symptoms, BMI, age, and ethnicity were found to have a statistically significant

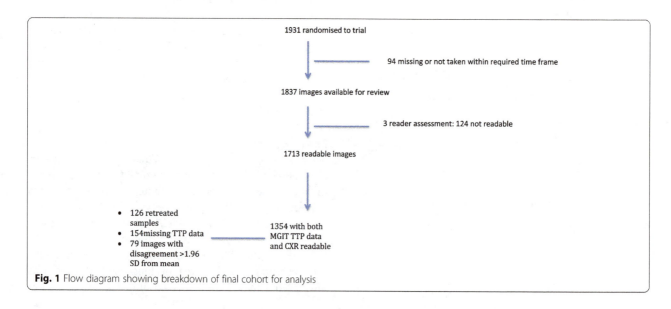

Fig. 1 Flow diagram showing breakdown of final cohort for analysis

Table 3 Baseline characteristics of final 1354 subjects

Baseline characteristic	N (%)	Median	IQR (1st, 3rd quartile)
Age (years)		31.6	24.1, 41.9
Sex			
Male	959 (70.8%)		
Female	395 (29.2%)		
Ethnicity			
African	924 (68.2%)		
Asian	430 (31.8%)		
Diabetes			
Yes	69 (5%)		
No	1285 (95%)		
HIV			
Yes	104 (7.7%)		
No	1250 (92.3%)		
Albumin (g/L)		34	30, 38
Body mass index (kg/m^2)		18.5	16.9, 20.3
Grade 3+ tuberculosis symptoms			
0	1271 (93.9%)		
1	60 (4.4%)		
2	16 (1.2%)		
3	7 (0.5%)		
4	1 (0.07%)		
Time to positivity (hours)		117	89, 153
Cavity			
Yes	1049 (77.5%)		
No	305 (22.5%)		
Average area affected (%)		18.13	11.25, 27.5

Table 4 The 47 sites across 8 countries where the participants (1354) were recruited

COUNTRY	SITE	N (total 1354)
South Africa	Stellenbosch	325
	Cape Town	221
	Durban	36
	Johannesburg	73
	Durban 2	7
	Soweto	1
	Ukzn	4
	Brits	48
	Tembisa	4
Tanzania	Moshi	57
	Mbeya	72
Zambia	Lusaka	40
Kenya	Nairobi	36
Thailand (2 sites)	Bangkok	104
Malaysia	Kuala Lumpur	56
China	Tianjin	18
India (29 sites)	Dehli, Agra, Jaipur	252

effect on the radiological severity of chest images by univariable analysis in the group with cavity disease (Table 7). In the non-cavitatory disease group, only ethnicity, serum albumin, and number of grade 3 symptoms were statistically significant on univariable analysis. Putting these significant variables in a multivariable regression model (Table 8) in those patients with cavitatory disease, the factors found to have a significant effect on the area of lung field affected were BMI, serum albumin, and $\log_{10}$TTP. In those without cavitatory disease, the factors found to have a significant effect on area of lung field affected were the number of grade 3 and 4 symptoms and serum albumin.

Discussion and conclusions

The REMoxTB study provided a unique opportunity to address important questions about the role of radiology in the diagnosis and evaluation of severity of TB infection in a large group of smear- and culture-positive patients with PTB that spanned two continents. The subjectivity of CXR interpretation has been a longstanding concern in clinical practice and there have been multiple attempts to develop methods to standardize image reading in order to reduce reader variability [12, 40–42]. This study shows that agreement between readers in cavity assessment was moderate (Kappa score 0.495), comparable to other studies that found a Kappa agreement variation on cavity presence from 0.24 to 0.7 [43–48]. The clustering of scores across the x-axis and '0' line of full agreement on the Bland–Altman plot (Fig. 2) confirms that the assessment of area of lung field affected is reproducible.

A high proportion of patients in this study had radiological evidence of cavitation (78%), compared with 72% in a study of 800 Turkish patients [20], 53.1% in a study of 893 USA-based patients [48], and 51% in a recent multicenter trial of 1692 patients in African sites [49]. Previous reports have suggested that the presence and number of cavities is related to bacterial load [12, 19–22, 50], but most of these studies were small, with an average of 138 patients (a range of 61–244). Using this large sample of patients we were able to show that there is a statistically significant reduction in the TTP (our surrogate for bacterial load) in patients with cavities compared to those without, with a median reduction of 26 h ($p < 0.001$). The large number of patients in this study provides the statistical power to demonstrate this unequivocally. It would, however, be reasonable to assume that such a reduction in TTP is of modest clinical significance, given that the replication rate of *M. tuberculosis* is approximately 14–24 h.

Table 5 A comparison of the included and excluded cohorts. Using χ^2 tests and Wilcoxon rank sum test p values are provided

Baseline characteristic	Included (n = 1354)			Excluded (n = 359)			p value
	N (%)	Median	IQR (1st, 3rd quartile)	N (%)	Median	IQR (1st, 3rd quartile)	
Age (years)		31.6	24.1, 41.9		29.8	24.2, 40.8	0.39
Body mass index (kg/m²)		18.5	16.9, 20.3		18.2	16.3, 20.3	0.06
Sex							0.32
Male	959 (70.8%)			244 (68%)			
Female	395 (29.2%)			115 (32%)			
Ethnicity							1.0
African	924 (68.2%)			245 (68.2%)			
Asian	430 (31.8%)			114 (31.8%)			
Diabetes							0.30
Yes	69 (5%)			13 (3.6%)			
No	1285 (95%)			346 (96.4%)			
HIV							0.10
Yes	104 (7.7%)			18 (5%)			
No	1250 (92.3%)			341 (95%)			
Albumin (g/L)		34	30, 38		35	30, 39.3	0.19
Time to positivity (hours)		117	89, 153	(n = 79 with values)	105	85.5, 140.5	0.10
Cavity							1.0
Yes	1049 (77.5%)			278 (77.4%)			
No	305 (22.5%)			81 (22.6%)			
Average area affected		18.13	11.3, 27.5		21.88	11.9, 32.5	0.001

Looking at the two groups of cavity and no cavity, the cavity group had lower albumin, TTP, and greater area affected suggesting that those with cavities appear to have other markers of 'severe' disease.

More cavities were proportionately found in the African cohort than in the Asian cohort. This raises the question of whether ethnicity plays a role in cavity

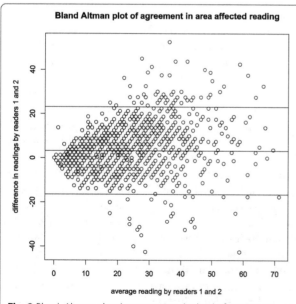

Fig. 2 Bland–Altman plot demonstrating the level of agreement between readers 1 and 2 in scoring the 1713 images for radiological severity (x axis: the mean average numerical score between readers 1 and 2, y axis: the difference in scores for each image between readers 1 and 2). Horizontal lines show the mean ± 1.96 standard deviations; 3.34 (23.11–16.44) (SD = 10.10)

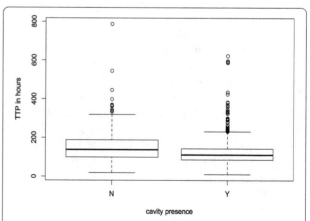

Fig. 3 Boxplot of TTP distribution comparing subjects without and those with cavitation present on CXR. Thick black horizontal lines represent the median values with the interquartile range being the horizontal edges of the boxes. The overall range lies out with these and extreme outliers above the plots

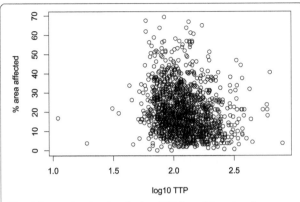

Fig. 4 Scatterplot showing the $\log_{10}$TTP (hours) from baseline sputum cultures against the percentage of lung field affected on the CXRs

formation and the immune response to TB addressed in previous studies [29–31]. A recent study suggests that the pattern of radiological presentation at diagnosis is associated with certain inflammatory profiles in patients [30]. Significant differences between the cytokine response of Africans and Eurasian patients rather than *Mycobacterial* strain type have been demonstrated [30, 31]. This may be a contributing factor to the radiological severity of patients at presentation as we also noted a small but significant difference through univariate analysis of radiological score between patients of African origin and those of south and southeast Asian origin that was lost when put into a multivariable analysis.

The study also shows a relationship between overall area of lung field affected on radiograph and bacterial load with a very shallow association seen on the scatterplot presented (Fig. 4). The association described that it would require a 10-fold increase in TTP to change the area affected by 11%, suggesting that patients with a higher bacterial load do have greater radiological severity but the effect of this association is small.

Our study addresses the effect of variables such as ethnicity, initial bacterial load, nutritional status, HIV status, sex, age, symptom severity, and diabetic status by multivariable-regression analysis on radiological severity. When weighted against each other in a model, bacterial load does not have a statistically significant effect on the degree of diseased lung field on CXR in the group with non-cavitatory disease and, again, a modest effect in those with cavitation. This fits with the autopsy findings that Canetti described, where higher bacillary burden was found within cavities and their surrounding tissues but was much lower within the inflammatory, non-cavitating tissue alone [25].

The only variable found to be related to the severity of the CXR at diagnosis is the serum albumin level in both the cavity and non-cavity groups. Poor nutritional status of patients with TB, using pre-treatment albumin levels and BMI as surrogate markers of nutritional status [33, 34, 51], has been associated with poorer treatment outcomes and death. In our study, patients with low serum albumin concentration at diagnosis (at a level of 15 g/L at the lowest) had a contributing effect to the radiological severity, but again to a modest degree, with a 0.65% and 0.48% decrease in area affected for every 1 g/L increase in serum albumin at baseline in the cavitatory and non-cavitatory groups, respectively (Fig. 5).

Through this analysis, our findings show that the factors affecting the appearance of the radiograph are likely to be multifactorial and to include host parameters such as ethnicity, age, co-morbidities, the bacterial load, and degree of disease progression. The interaction of the factors affecting the inflammatory response of an individual to PTB infection is being explored in other research.

We included those with HIV and type II diabetes mellitus in our cohort and found no significant effect on the radiological severity. This may be due to our HIV cohort being a select group with CD4 counts > 250 at PTB diagnosis without preceding anti-retrovirals and those with diabetes with less severe disease as a requirement for the clinical trial. They may, therefore, not reflect the full spectrum of morbidity and its effects on CXR severity.

In summary, our study is the largest review of radiology in a well characterized patient group with smear- and culture-positive PTB and suggests that, although CXR is a valuable tool for diagnosis, its use for judging the bacterial burden of disease has limited value. This is not unexpected, as the radiological image appears to be a composite of the interaction of disease pathology caused by the organism, the severity of the immune response and the nutritional status of the patient. The statistical power of this large study has enabled us to

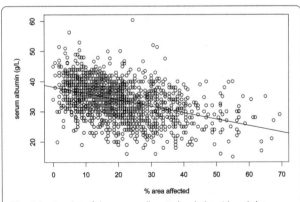

Fig. 5 Scatterplot of the serum albumin levels (x-axis) and the percentage of lung field affected on the CXR (y-axis) for all 1354 participants. A linear regression line shows a steady decrease in serum albumin as more area is affected by disease

Table 6 Characteristics of those with and without cavitation used in the analysis comparing other baseline factors and radiological severity on CXR at diagnosis

Baseline characteristic	WITH CAVITY (n = 1049)			WITHOUT CAVITY (n = 305)			p value
	n	Median	IQR (1st, 3rd quartile)	n	Median	IQR	
Age (years)		31.4	23.7, 41.0		32.1	25.2, 44.2	0.03
Sex							0.95
Male	742 (70.7%)			217 (71.1%)			
Female	307 (29.3%)			88 (28.9%)			
Ethnicity							
African	742 (70.7%)			182 (59.7%)			< 0.01
Asian	307 (29.3%)			123 (40.3%)			
Diabetes							
Yes	50 (4.5%)			19 (6.2%)			0.38
No	1049 (95.5%)			286 (93.8%)			
HIV							0.79
Yes	81 (7%)			25 (8.2%)			
No	1081 (93%)			280 (91.8%)			
No. of Grade 3 + symptoms	68			16			0.51
Albumin (g/L)		33.5	9.0, 37.8		37	32.0, 40.0	< 0.01
Body mass index (kg/m^2)		18.3	16.9, 20.1		19.0	17.3, 21.1	< 0.01
Time to positivity (hours)		112	86.0, 144.0		138	100, 188	< 0.01
Average area affected		20	13.75, 30		10	6.25, 16.9	< 0.01

precisely measure the associations between CXR severity and other factors measured. The effect of serum albumin level on the radiological severity serves as an indicator that hypo-albuminemia is a marker of disease severity, as shown in other studies where it has been indicated to predict poor outcome in PTB [52]. The full value of CXR as a prognostic marker is yet to be seen and warrants further analysis. Although the associations between CXR severity and other factors conform with our expectations that patients with higher bacterial burden have more extensive disease, the small size of the effect and the finding that, in a multivariable

Table 7 Results of univariable analysis. The β-coefficient represents the change in percentage area of lung field affected for every 1 unit increase in variable. For Log$_{10}$TTP, this is the change in percentage area affected for every 10-fold increase in TTP

	With cavity			Without cavity		
	β-coefficient	95% CI	p value	β-coefficient	95% CI	p value
Age	0.09	(0.03, 0.15)	0.003	−0.0004	(−0.07, 0.07)	0.90
Sex						
Male vs. female	0.91	(−0.71, 2.5)	0.27	−0.41	(−2.49, 1.68)	0.70
Ethnicity						
Asia vs. Africa	−2.33	(−3.95, −0.73)	0.004	−2.5	(−4.41, −0.59)	0.01
Diabetes	1.17	(−2.27, 4.63)	0.05	1.86	(−2.04, 5.77)	0.39
Positive vs. negative						
HIV						0.14
Positive vs. negative	2.11	(−0.67, 4.89)	0.01	−2.78	(−6.21, 0.65)	0.11
Albumin (g/L)	−0.72	(−0.82, −0.61)	< 0.001	−0.53	(−0.68, −0.38)	< 0.001
Body mass index	−0.55	(−0.76, −0.33)	< 0.001	−0.13	(−0.41, 0.19)	0.40
MGIT Log$_{10}$ttp (hours)	−8.87	(−13.08, −4.67)	< 0.001	−2.41	(−7.10, 2.29)	0.31
Grade 3+ tuberculosis symptoms	2.17	(0.33, 4.02)	0.02	5.03	(1.88, 8.17)	0.002

Table 8 Multivariable regression analysis using variables found significant in univariate analysis. The β-coefficient represents the change in percentage area affected for every 1 unit rise in variables for albumin, BMI, number of grade 3/4 symptoms, and age. For log$_{10}$TTP, this represents the change in percentage area affected for a 10-fold increase in TTP. For ethnicity, HIV, and diabetes this indicates the percentage difference in area affected between the two groups (for example, compared to the African cohort, Asians had 0.67% less area affected on the CXR than the African cohort)

	With cavity			Without cavity		
	β-coefficient	95% CI	p value	β-coefficient	95% CI	p value
Log$_{10}$TTP (hours)	−4.72	(−8.73, 0.72)	0.02			
Albumin (g/L)	−0.65	(−0.76, −0.53)	< 0.001	−0.48	(−0.64, −0.32)	< 0.001
Grade 3 + Symptoms	0.05	(−1.68, 1.79)	0.95	3.13	(0.11, 6.15)	0.04
Body mass index	−0.50	(−0.72, −0.27)	< 0.001	−0.07	(−0.33, 0.19)	0.63
Ethnicity						
Asia vs. Africa	−0.67	(−2.33, 0.98)	0.43	−0.90	(−2.80, 1.00)	0.35
Age	0.05	(−0.01, 0.11)	0.13			
HIV						
Positive vs. Negative	0.54	(−2.09, 3.17)	0.69			
Diabetes						
Positive vs. Negative	3.03	(−0.33, 6.40)	0.07			

model, it is outweighed by other patient factors in those without cavitation and is modest in those with cavitation would suggest that clinicians should be cautious in over-interpreting cause of radiological disease extent at diagnosis.

Abbreviations
AFB: acid fast bacilli; BMI: body mass index; CXR: chest x-ray; DICOM: digital imaging and communications in medicine; MGIT: mycobacteria-growth-indicator-tube; PTB: pulmonary tuberculosis; TB: tuberculosis; TTP: time-to-positivity

Acknowledgements
We thank all participants in the REMoxTB clinical trial, without whom this study would not have been possible, and the study clinicians and nursing staff, and all staff involved in the REMoxTB study at all of our study sites. The REMoxTB Consortium: Task Applied Sciences and Stellenbosch University, South Africa – Andreas Diacon, Madeleine Hanekom, Amour Venter; University of Cape Town, South Africa – Kimberley Narunsky; Mbeya Medical Research Programme, Tanzania – B. Mtafya, N. Elias Ntinginya, Andrea Rachow; Centre for Respiratory Disease Research at KEMRI, Kenya – Evans Amukoye, B. Miheso, M. Njoroje; Kilimanjaro Christian Medical Center, Tanzania – Noel Sam, D. Damas, Alphonce Liyoyo; Institute of Respiratory Medicine Jalan Pahang, Malaysia – A. Ahmad Mahayiddin; Chest Disease Institute, Thailand – C. Chuchottaworn, J. Boonyasopun, B. Saipan; University of Zambia & University Teaching Hospital, Zambia – Shabir Lakhi, D. Chanda, J. Mcyeze; Medical Research Council, South Africa – Alexander Pym, N. Ngcobo; Madibeng Centre for Research, South Africa – Cheryl Louw, H. Veldsman; Hospital General de Occidente de la Secretaría de Salud del Estado de Jalisco, Mexico – Gerardo Amaya-Tapia, T. Vejar Aguirre; Dr. D. K. Chauhan Clinic, India – D. K. Chauhan; Dr. R. K. Garg's Clinic, India – R. K. Garg; Dr. Nirmal Kumar Jain Clinic, India – N. K. Jain; Indra Nursing Home and Maternity Centre, India – A. Aggarwal; Mahatma Gandhi Medical College & Hospital, India 302022 – M. Mishra; Dr. Sanjay Teotia Clinic, India – S. Teotia; Aurum, Tembisa Hospital, South Africa – S. Charalambous, N. Hattidge, L. Pretorious; University of KwaZulu Natal, South Africa (ACTG Site) – N. Padayachi; Perinatal HIV Research Unit, Chris Hani Baragwanath Hospital, South Africa (ACTG Site) – L. Mohapi; Beijing Tuberculosis and Thoracic Tumor Research Institute, China – M. Gao, X. Li, L. Zhang; Shanghai Pulmonary Hospital, China – Q. Zhang; Siddharth Nursing Home, India – S. Aggarwal; TB Alliance – K. Belizaire, M. Benhayoun, D. Everitt, A. Ginsberg, M. Laurenzi, B. Rawls, C. Ridali, M. Spigelman, A. Uys, C. van Niekerk; University College London – A. L. C. Bateson, M. Betteridge, S. Birkby, E. Bongard, M. Brown, H. Ciesielczuk, C. Cook, E. Cunningham, J. Huggett, R. Hunt, C. Ling, M. Lipman, P. Mee, F. M. R. Perrin, R. Shorten, K. Smith, V. Yorke-Edwards, A. Zumla.

Funding
Supported by the Global Alliance for TB Drug Development with support from the Bill and Melinda Gates Foundation, the European and Developing Countries Clinical Trials Partnership (grant IP.2007.32011.011), US Agency for International Development, UK Department for International Development, Directorate General for International Cooperation of the Netherlands, Irish Aid, Australia Department of Foreign Affairs and Trade, and National Institutes of Health, AIDS Clinical Trials Group. Further, it was supported by grants from the National Institute of Allergy and Infectious Diseases (NIAID) (UM1AI068634, UM1 AI068636, and UM1AI106701), NIAID grants to the University of KwaZulu Natal, South Africa, AIDS Clinical Trials Group (ACTG) site 31422 (1U01AI069469), to the Perinatal HIV Research Unit, Chris Hani Baragwanath Hospital, South Africa, ACTG site 12301 (1U01AI069453), and to the Durban International Clinical Trials Unit, South Africa, ACTG site 11201 (1U01AI069426), as well as by Bayer Healthcare through the donation of moxifloxacin and Sanofi through the donation of rifampin. Andrew Nunn's salary came through core funding MC_UU_12023/27 Tuberculosis Treatment Trials.

Authors' contributions
SEM and SHG designed the study, performed data analysis and data interpretation, and wrote the manuscript. SEM, SHG, and FC analyzed the chest x-rays. SHG and TMH contributed to study design and analyses and supervised the study. PPJP, AJN, SRM, AC, CM, MEM, KPS, and RD all also contributed to interpretation of data and to the final submitted manuscript. MEM, KS, and SEM were instrumental in supervising and collecting the images. All authors read and approve the final manuscript.

Authors' information
SEM is a clinician and research associate at University College London (UCL). FC is a radiology consultant at Barts Health trust, NHS, UK. AC is a Medical Research Council (MRC) senior statistician. RD is an associate professor at University of Cape Town Lung Institute. MM is a clinician and research associate at UCL. SRM is Senior Medical Officer at TB Alliance. AJN is Associate Director and Chair of Infection Research at MRC. PPJP is a senior statistician at MRC. CM is Senior VP of Research and Development at TB Alliance. KPS is a clinician and research associate at UCL. TDM is Professor of Clinical Microbiology at UCL and Director of the UCL Centre for Clinical Microbiology. SHG is the Sir James Black Professor of Medicine at the University of St Andrews.

Competing interests
The authors declare that they have no competing interests.

Author details
[1]UCL Centre for Clinical Microbiology, Department of Infection, University College London, Royal Free Campus, Rowland Hill Street, London NW3 2PF, UK. [2]Department of Radiology, Barts Health NHS Trust, The Royal London Hospital, Whitechapel Road, London E1 1BB, UK. [3]Medical Research Council UK Clinical Trials Unit at University College London, Aviation House, 125 Kingsway, London WC2B 6NH, UK. [4]University of Cape Town Lung Institute, George Street, Mowbray, Cape Town, South Africa. [5]Global Alliance for Tuberculosis Drug Development, New York, NY 10005, USA. [6]Medical and Biological Sciences, School of Medicine, University of St Andrews, North Haugh, St Andrews KY16 9TF, UK.

References
1. Garland LH. Conditions to be differentiated in the roentgen diagnosis of pulmonary tuberculosis. Ann Intern Med. 1948;29(5):878–80.
2. Cardinale L, Parlatano D, Boccuzzi F, Onoscuri M, Volpicelli G, Veltri A. The imaging spectrum of pulmonary tuberculosis. Acta Radiol. 2015;56(5):557–64.
3. Tattevin P. The validity of medical history, classic symptoms, and chest radiographs in predicting pulmonary tuberculosis*: derivation of a pulmonary tuberculosis prediction model. Chest J. 1999;115(5):1248.
4. Skoura E, Zumla A, Bomanji J. Imaging in tuberculosis. Int J Infect Dis. 2015;32:87–93.
5. World Health Organization. Systematic Screening for Active Tuberculosis: Principles and Recommendations. Geneva: WHO; 2013.
6. World Health Organization. Chest radiography in tuberculosis detection: summary of current WHO recommendations and guidance on programmatic approaches. World Health Organization. 2016. http://www.who.int/iris/handle/10665/252424. ISBN 9789241511506.
7. Burman WJ, Goldberg S, Johnson JL, Muzanye G, Engle M, Mosher AW, et al. Moxifloxacin versus ethambutol in the first 2 months of treatment for pulmonary tuberculosis. Am J Respir Crit Care Med. 2006;174(3):331–8.
8. Benator D, Bhattacharya M, Bozeman L, Burman W, Cantazaro A, Chaisson R, et al. Rifapentine and isoniazid once a week versus rifampicin and isoniazid twice a week for treatment of drug-susceptible pulmonary tuberculosis in HIV-negative patients: a randomised clinical trial. Lancet. 2002;360(9332):528–34.
9. Simon G. Radiology in epidemiological studies and some therapeutic trials. Br Med J. 1966;2(5512):491–4.
10. Fox AJ. Classification of radiological appearance and the derivation of a numerical score. Br J Ind Med. 1975;32(4):273–82.
11. National Tuberculosis and Respiratory Disease Association. Diagnostic Standards and Classification of Tuberculosis. New York: National Tuberculosis and Respiratory Disease Association; 1969. p. 94.
12. Ralph AP, Ardian M, Wiguna A, Maguire GP, Becker NG, Drogumuller G, et al. A simple, valid, numerical score for grading chest x-ray severity in adult smear-positive pulmonary tuberculosis. Thorax. 2010;65(10):863–9.
13. Olaru ID, Heyckendorf J, Grossmann S, Lange C. Time to culture positivity and sputum smear microscopy during tuberculosis therapy. PLoS One. 2014;9(8):e106075. Delogu G, editor
14. Padayatchi N, Gopal M, Naidoo R, Werner L, Naidoo K, Master I, et al. Clofazimine in the treatment of extensively drug-resistant tuberculosis with HIV coinfection in South Africa: a retrospective cohort study. J Antimicrob Chemother. 2014;69(11):3103–7.
15. Kenangalem E, Waramori G, Pontororing GJ, Sandjaja, Tjitra E, Maguire G, et al. Tuberculosis outcomes in Papua, Indonesia: the relationship with different body mass index characteristics between Papuan and non-Papuan ethnic groups. PLoS One. 2013;8(9):e76077. da Silva Nunes M, editor
16. Pinto LM, Dheda K, Theron G, Allwood B, Calligaro G, van Zyl-Smit R, et al. Development of a simple reliable radiographic scoring system to aid the diagnosis of pulmonary tuberculosis. PLoS One. 2013;8(1):e54235.
17. Rathman G, Sillah J, Hill PC, Murray JF, Adegbola R, Corrah T, et al. Clinical and radiological presentation of 340 adults with smear-positive tuberculosis in The Gambia. Int J Tuberc Lung Dis. 2003;7(10):942–7.
18. Brust JCM, Berman AR, Zalta B, Haramati LB, Ning Y, Heo M, et al. Chest radiograph findings and time to culture conversion in patients with multidrug-resistant tuberculosis and HIV in Tugela Ferry, South Africa. PLoS One. 2013;8(9):e73975.
19. Matsuoka S, Uchiyama K, Shima H, Suzuki K, Shimura A, Sasaki Y, et al. Relationship between CT findings of pulmonary tuberculosis and the number of acid-fast bacilli on sputum smears. Clin Imaging. 2004;28(2):119–23.
20. Ozsahin SL, Arslan S, Epozturk K, Remziye E, Dogan OT. Chest X-ray and bacteriology in the initial phase of treatment of 800 male patients with pulmonary tuberculosis. J Bras Pneumol. 2011;37(3):294–301.
21. Perrin FMR, Woodward N, Phillips PPJ, McHugh TD, Nunn AJ, Lipman MCI, et al. Radiological cavitation, sputum mycobacterial load and treatment response in pulmonary tuberculosis. Int J Tuberc Lung Dis. 2010;14(12):1596–602.
22. Palaci M, Dietze R, Hadad DJ, Ribeiro FKC, Peres RL, Vinhas SA, et al. Cavitary disease and quantitative sputum bacillary load in cases of pulmonary tuberculosis. J Clin Microbiol. 2007;45(12):4064–6.
23. O'Sullivan DM, Sander C, Shorten RJ, Gillespie SH, Hill AVS, McHugh TD, et al. Evaluation of liquid culture for quantitation of Mycobacterium tuberculosis in murine models. Vaccine. 2007;25(49):8203–5.
24. Pheiffer C, Carroll NM, Beyers N, Donald P, Duncan K, Uys P, et al. Time to detection of Mycobacterium tuberculosis in BACTEC systems as a viable alternative to colony counting. Int J Tuberc Lung Dis. 2008;12(7):792–8.
25. Canetti G. The Tubercle Bacillus in the Pulmonary Lesion of Man. Inc. New York: Springer Publishing Company; 1955.
26. Aderaye G, Bruchfeld J, Assefa G, Feleke D, Källenius G, Baat M, et al. The relationship between disease pattern and disease burden by chest radiography, M. tuberculosis load, and HIV status in patients with pulmonary tuberculosis in Addis Ababa. Infection. 2004;32(6):333–8.
27. Dooley KE, Chaisson RE. Tuberculosis and diabetes mellitus: convergence of two epidemics. Lancet Infect Dis. 2009;9(12):737–46.
28. Pérez-Guzman C, Torres-Cruz A, Villarreal-Velarde H, Salazar-Lezama MA, Vargas MH. Atypical radiological images of pulmonary tuberculosis in 192 diabetic patients: a comparative study. Int J Tuberc Lung Dis. 2001;5(5):455–61.
29. Morris CD. The radiography, haematology and biochemistry of pulmonary tuberculosis in the aged. Q J Med. 1989;71(266):529–36.
30. Coussens AK, Wilkinson RJ, Nikolayevskyy V, Elkington PT, Hanifa Y, Islam K, et al. Ethnic variation in inflammatory profile in tuberculosis. PLoS Pathog. 2013;9(7):e1003468.
31. Pareek M, Evans J, Innes J, Smith G, Hingley-Wilson S, Lougheed KE, et al. Ethnicity and mycobacterial lineage as determinants of tuberculosis disease phenotype. Thorax. 2013;68(3):221–9.
32. Thorson A, Long NH, Larsson LO. Chest X-ray findings in relation to gender and symptoms: a study of patients with smear positive tuberculosis in Vietnam. Scand J Infect Dis. 2007;39(1):33–7.
33. Matos ED, Moreira Lemos AC. Association between serum albumin levels and in-hospital deaths due to tuberculosis. Int J Tuberc Lung Dis. 2006;10(12):1360–6.

34. Kim H-J, Lee C-H, Shin S, Lee JH, Kim YW, Chung HS, et al. The impact of nutritional deficit on mortality of in-patients with pulmonary tuberculosis. Int J Tuberc Lung Dis. 2010;14(1):79–85.
35. Hales CM, Heilig CM, Chaisson R, Leung CC, Chang KC, Goldberg SV, et al. The association between symptoms and microbiologically defined response to tuberculosis treatment. Ann Am Thorac Soc. 2013;10(1):18–25.
36. Gillespie SH, Crook AM, McHugh TD, Mendel CM, Meredith SK, Murray SR, et al. Four-month moxifloxacin-based regimens for drug-sensitive tuberculosis. N Engl J Med. 2014;371(17):1577–87.
37. World Health Organization. Antiretroviral Therapy for HIV Infection in Infants and Children: Towards Universal Access. Recommendations for a Public Health Approach. 2010. ISBN 9789241599801.
38. R Development Core Team. R: A Language and Environment for Statistical Computing. Vienna: R Foundation for Statistical Computing; 2014. https://www.r-project.org/.
39. Mandrekar JN. Measures of interrater agreement. J Thorac Oncol. 2011;6(1):6–7.
40. Stout JE, Kosinski AS, Hamilton CD, Goodman PC, Mosher A, Menzies D, et al. Effect of improving the quality of radiographic interpretation on the ability to predict pulmonary tuberculosis relapse. Acad Radiol. 2010;17(2):157–62.
41. Bossuyt PM. The STARD Statement for Reporting Studies of Diagnostic Accuracy: explanation and elaboration. Clin Chem. 2003;49(1):7–18.
42. Whiting P, Rutjes AWS, Reitsma JB, Bossuyt PMM, Kleijnen J. The development of QUADAS: a tool for the quality assessment of studies of diagnostic accuracy included in systematic reviews. BMC Med Res Methodol. 2003;3:25.
43. Balabanova Y, Coker R, Fedorin I, Zakharova S, Plavinskij S, Krukov N, et al. Variability in interpretation of chest radiographs among Russian clinicians and implications for screening programmes: observational study. BMJ. 2005;331(7513):379–82.
44. Abubakar I, Story A, Lipman M, Bothamley G, van Hest R, Andrews N, et al. Diagnostic accuracy of digital chest radiography for pulmonary tuberculosis in a UK urban population. Eur Respir J. 2010;35(3):689–92.
45. Dawson R, Masuka P, Edwards DJ, Bateman ED, Bekker L-G, Wood R, et al. Chest radiograph reading and recording system: evaluation for tuberculosis screening in patients with advanced HIV. Int J Tuberc Lung Dis. 2010;14(1):52–8.
46. Tudor GR, Finlay D, Taub N. An assessment of inter-observer agreement and accuracy when reporting plain radiographs. Clin Radiol. 1997;52(3):235–8.
47. Zellweger JP, Heinzer R, Touray M, Vidondo B, Altpeter E. Intra-observer and overall agreement in the radiological assessment of tuberculosis. Int J Tuberc Lung Dis. 2006;10(10):1123–6.
48. Hamilton CD, Stout JE, Goodman PC, Mosher A, Menzies R, Schluger NW, et al. The value of end-of-treatment chest radiograph in predicting pulmonary tuberculosis relapse. Int J Tuberc Lung Dis. 2008;12(9):1059–64.
49. Merle CS, Fielding K, Sow OB, Gninafon M, Lo MB, Mthiyane T, et al. A four-month gatifloxacin-containing regimen for treating tuberculosis. N Engl J Med. 2014;371(17):1588–98.
50. Ors F, Deniz O, Bozlar U, Gumus S, Tasar M, Tozkoparan E, et al. High-resolution CT findings in patients with pulmonary tuberculosis: correlation with the degree of smear positivity. J Thorac Imaging. 2007;22(2):154–9.
51. Khan A, Sterling TR, Reves R, Vernon A, Horsburgh CR, the Tuberculosis Trials Consortium. Lack of weight gain and relapse risk in a large tuberculosis treatment trial. Am J Respir Crit Care Med. 2006;174(3):344–8.
52. Kim S, Kim H, Kim WJ, Lee S-J, Hong Y, Lee H-Y, et al. Mortality and predictors in pulmonary tuberculosis with respiratory failure requiring mechanical ventilation. Int J Tuberc Lung Dis. 2016;20(4):524–9.

Complex interactions between malaria and malnutrition: a systematic literature review

D Das[1,2], R F Grais[4], E A Okiro[7], K Stepniewska[1,2], R Mansoor[1,2], S van der Kam[5], D J Terlouw[6,10,11], J Tarning[1,2,3], K I Barnes[8,9] and P J Guerin[1,2*]

Abstract

Background: Despite substantial improvement in the control of malaria and decreased prevalence of malnutrition over the past two decades, both conditions remain heavy burdens that cause hundreds of thousands of deaths in children in resource-poor countries every year. Better understanding of the complex interactions between malaria and malnutrition is crucial for optimally targeting interventions where both conditions co-exist. This systematic review aimed to assess the evidence of the interplay between malaria and malnutrition.

Methods: Database searches were conducted in PubMed, Global Health and Cochrane Libraries and articles published in English, French or Spanish between Jan 1980 and Feb 2018 were accessed and screened. The methodological quality of the included studies was assessed using the Newcastle-Ottawa Scale and the risk of bias across studies was assessed using the GRADE approach. The preferred reporting items for systematic reviews and meta-analyses (PRISMA) guideline were followed.

Results: Of 2945 articles screened from databases, a total of 33 articles were identified looking at the association between malnutrition and risk of malaria and/or the impact of malnutrition in antimalarial treatment efficacy. Large methodological heterogeneity of studies precluded conducting meaningful aggregated data meta-analysis. Divergent results were reported on the effect of malnutrition on malaria risk. While no consistent association between risk of malaria and acute malnutrition was found, chronic malnutrition was relatively consistently associated with severity of malaria such as high-density parasitemia and anaemia. Furthermore, there is little information on the effect of malnutrition on therapeutic responses to artemisinin combination therapies (ACTs) and their pharmacokinetic properties in malnourished children in published literature.

Conclusions: The evidence on the effect of malnutrition on malaria risk remains inconclusive. Further analyses using individual patient data could provide an important opportunity to better understand the variability observed in publications by standardising both malaria and nutritional metrics. Our findings highlight the need to improve our understanding of the pharmacodynamics and pharmacokinetics of ACTs in malnourished children. Further clarification on malaria-malnutrition interactions would also serve as a basis for designing future trials and provide an opportunity to optimise antimalarial treatment for this large, vulnerable and neglected population.

Keywords: Malaria, Anthropometry, Stunting, Wasting, Underweight

---

* Correspondence: philippe.guerin@wwarn.org
[1]WorldWide Antimalarial Resistance Network (WWARN), Oxford, UK
[2]Centre for Tropical Medicine and Global Health, Nuffield Department of Clinical Medicine, University of Oxford, Oxford, UK
Full list of author information is available at the end of the article

Background

Malaria and malnutrition in children (refers to all forms of undernutrition) are reported independently to be major causes of morbidity and mortality in low- and middle-income countries. About 3.2 billion people remained at risk of malaria with an estimated 216 million new cases (95% confidence interval 196–263 million) and 445,000 deaths worldwide in 2016; the majority of deaths occur in children under 5 years in sub-Saharan Africa [1]. Approximately 3.1 million deaths in children under five are attributed to malnutrition each year, representing 45% of all childhood deaths [2]. The interaction between malaria and childhood malnutrition has been studied for many years and complex interactions between these high-burden conditions are now increasingly recognised. Understanding the consequences of malnutrition on malaria and vice versa is crucial and may help guide the choice of public health interventions and research priorities where significant co-morbidity exists.

Malnutrition is a complex phenomenon due to its multifactorial aetiology and diverse clinical presentation. Acute malnutrition manifests with wasting (low weight for height) and chronic malnutrition as stunting (low height for age). Being underweight (low weight for age) can result from either chronic or acute malnutrition or both. Assessment of malnourishment can be conducted using anthropometric indicators which compare child's weight and height to the standardised age- and sex-specific growth reference derived from the international reference population of children between 6 and 59 months of age (World Health Organization (WHO) Child Growth Standards 2006) [3]. The anthropometric indicators are expressed as a number of standard deviations (SDs) below or above the reference mean or median value, Z-score. Cutoffs of − 3 are used to indicate severe malnutrition and values between − 2 and − 3 are considered to be moderate malnutrition. Weight-for-height Z-score (WHZ) is the indicator used to classify a child with wasting. Mid-Upper Arm Circumference (MUAC) is another frequently used indicator for wasting. Severe acute malnutrition (SAM) is defined as MUAC < 115 mm and/or WHZ < − 3 and/or bilateral pitting oedema. Stunting is defined by the measure of height-for-age Z-score (HAZ) and a child is considered as being underweight based on low weight-for-age Z-score (WAZ). These definitions do not take micronutrient malnutrition into account, which can occur even if the person is getting enough energy and they are not thin or short.

The exact relationship between childhood malnutrition and malaria remains complex, controversial, and poorly understood. One of the key questions is, to what extent the burden of malaria is attributable to wasting and stunting? In regard to the impact of malaria on malnutrition, some evidence suggests malaria has adverse effects on nutritional status of young children [4–9]. On the other hand, whether and how malnutrition influences malaria morbidity and mortality is debated. Some studies have reported that malnutrition is associated with a higher risk of malaria [10–13], others have suggested a protective effect [14–17], or no differential risk [18, 19]. Similarly, there is very limited evidence on the relationship between nutritional status and antimalarial drug efficacy. Clinical efficacy of the current first-line malaria treatment, the artemisinin combination therapies (ACTs), in malnourished children has been rarely explored [20–22]. Understanding the complex relationship of the immune response of individuals infected with malaria and suffering of malnutrition is crucial to guide specific antimalarial therapeutic approaches in this vulnerable sub-population. There are key knowledge gaps in defining the complex relationship between malnutrition and malaria, which need to be identified and addressed. We aimed to conduct a systematic review of the current understanding of interactions between acute or chronic malnutrition and the risk of developing malarial infection. A further objective was to explore published literature on the impact of malnutrition on the efficacy of antimalarial treatment.

Methods

We conducted a systematic literature review of manuscripts published between Jan 1, 1980, and Feb 19, 2018. PubMed, Global Health and Cochrane Libraries were searched using key terms (Additional file 1), and articles published in English, French or Spanish were accessed. Two reviewers identified relevant articles of interest, as per criteria listed below, by screening titles and abstracts of publications retrieved. The preferred reporting items for systematic reviews and meta-analyses (PRISMA) guideline [23] was followed. The PRISMA checklist is provided as Additional file 2 and the review is registered in international prospective register of systematic reviews (PROSPERO Registration No. CRD42017056934).

Eligibility screening

For the selected articles, full text was obtained and assessed for relevance to any of the following topics of interest: (1) association between malnutrition and risk of malaria and (2) malnutrition and antimalarial treatment efficacy. We excluded studies primarily focused on non-malarial conditions such as TB, HIV, neglected tropical diseases, pneumonia or diarrhoeal diseases; non-clinical studies (systematic reviews, opinion pieces, editorials, modelling studies, economic evaluations, guidelines, protocols, book chapters) and in vitro, animal, plant or molecular studies; studies on malaria in pregnancy and placental malaria; demographic and health surveys, mortality surveys, qualitative studies; case reports or series; vaccine studies; and studies primarily focused only on malaria or malnutrition or micronutrient deficiencies or anaemia. For this review, observational and interventional studies in non-pregnant populations with malnutrition assessed by anthropometric measurements as exposure and risk of malaria infection (whether asymptomatic parasitemia or uncomplicated malaria) as outcome were included.

Data extraction
From each of the included studies in this review, the following variables were extracted: authors, year of publication, country, study design, age (range or median/mean), sex (ratio), sample size, growth standards, malaria transmission intensity, definition of malaria and the reported risk estimates. The methodological quality of the included studies was assessed using the Newcastle-Ottawa Scale (NOS) [24] and the risk of bias across studies was assessed using the GRADE approach [25]. The risk of bias assessment within and across studies is presented as Additional file 3.

Analysis
Aggregated data meta-analysis was not possible due to the heterogeneity of studies in respect to study design, definition of malnutrition, definition of malaria, study population, e.g. age group target, analysis conducted and effect measures presented. Only summaries of study findings are presented in this review. Association between malnutrition and risk of malaria was deemed to be statistically significant if either the P value was < 0.05 and/or the 95% confidence intervals (CIs) did not include 1. The risk of malaria was classified as "increased" or "decreased" according to the interpretation of the effect estimates provided (i.e. incidence risk ratio (IRR), odds ratio (OR), risk ratio (RR) or hazard ratio (HR)) if statistical significance was achieved as described above.

Results
The literature search identified 2945 articles. A total of 32 articles identified through the search and 1 article obtained through citation tracking were included, describing cross-sectional surveys ($n = 16$), longitudinal studies ($n = 12$), interventional studies ($n = 3$), case-control study ($n = 1$) and individual patient data meta-analysis ($n = 1$) (Fig. 1). Details of the 33 studies included in this review are given in Table 1, while the study characteristics are summarised in Additional file 4.

Association between malnutrition and risk of malaria
In total, 29 studies assessed the association between malnutrition and risk of malaria (Tables 2, 3 and 4).

Risk of malaria infection in children with stunting (chronic malnutrition)
Twenty-three studies explored the relationship between stunting and risk of malaria infection (Table 2). Overall results were conflicting, with 15 studies showing that

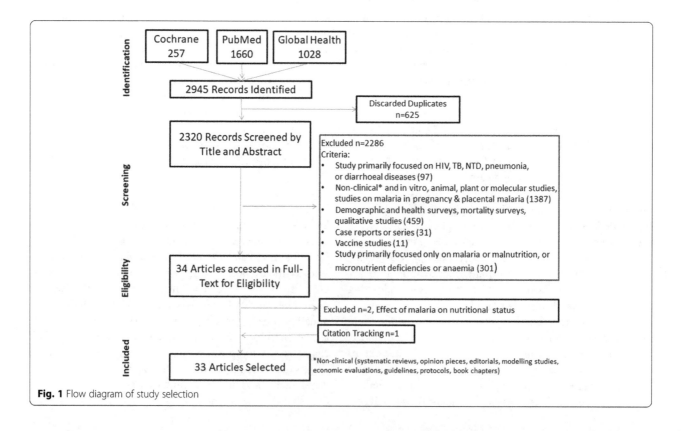

Fig. 1 Flow diagram of study selection

Table 1 Details of the studies included (N = 33)

Author, year, reference	Country	Region	Study design	Topics of interest*
Akiyama 2016 [46]	Lao PDR	South East Asia	Cross-sectional	1a, 1c
Alexandre 2015 [47]	Brazilian Amazon	Latin America	Longitudinal	1a
Arinaitwe 2012 [48]	Uganda	Africa	Longitudinal	1a, 1c
Ayana 2015 [49]	Ethiopia	Africa	Retrospective cohort	1a, 1b, 1c
Bilal Shikur 2016 [28]	Ethiopia	Africa	Case-control	1b
Crookston 2010 [50]	Ghana	Africa	Cross-sectional	1a
Custodio 2009 [30]	Equatorial Guinea	Africa	Survey	1a, 1b, 1c
Deen 2002 [10]	Gambia	Africa	Longitudinal	1a, 1b, 1c
Denoeud-Ndam 2016 [35]	Mali, Niger	Africa	Non-randomised comparative trial	2
Deribew 2010 [51]	Ethiopia	Africa	Cross-sectional	1a, 1b, 1c
Ehrhardt 2006 [11]	Ghana	Africa	Survey	1b, 1c
El Samani 1987 [52]	Sudan	Africa	Cross-sectional	1c
Fillol 2009 [27]	Senegal	Africa	Longitudinal	1a, 1b, 1c
Friedman 2005 [26]	Kenya	Africa	Survey	1a, 1b
Genton 1998 [14]	Papua New Guinea	Oceania	Longitudinal	1a, 1b
Jeremiah 2007 [53]	Nigeria	Africa	Cross-sectional	1c
Kateera 2015 [54]	Rwanda	Africa	Cross-sectional	1a, 1b, 1c
Maketa 2015 [55]	Democratic Republic of Congo (DRC)	Africa	Cross-sectional	1a
Mamiro 2005 [56]	Tanzania	Africa	Cross-sectional	1a
Mitangala 2012 [34]	Democratic Republic of Congo (DRC)	Africa	Therapeutic efficacy study	2
Mitangala 2013 [21]	Democratic Republic of Congo (DRC)	Africa	Survey	1a, 1b, 1c
Muller 2003 [18]	Burkina Faso	Africa	Longitudinal	1a, 1b, 1c
Nyakeriga 2004 [6]	Kenya	Africa	Longitudinal	1a, 1c
Obua 2008 [33]	Uganda	Africa	Therapeutic efficacy study	2
Snow 1991 [17]	Gambia	Africa	Longitudinal	1a, 1b, 1c
Sumbele 2015 [57]	Cameroon	Africa	Cross-sectional	1a, 1b, 1c
Takakura 2001 [29]	Lao PDR	South East Asia	Survey	1b
Tonglet 1999 [32]	Democratic Republic of Congo (DRC)	Africa	Longitudinal	1a, 1c
Uscategui Penuela 2009 [58]	Colombia	Latin America	Cross-sectional	1a, 1b
Verhoef 2002 [13]	Kenya	Africa	Survey	1a, 1b
Verret 2011 [22]	Uganda	Africa	Longitudinal	1a, 1c, 2
William 1997 [31]	Vanuatu	Oceania	Longitudinal	1b, 1c
WWARN Lumefantrine PK/PD Study Group 2015 [36]	Multiple	Multiple	Individual patient data meta-analysis	2

*Topics of Interest: Risk of malaria infection in children with (1a) stunting, (1b) wasting, (1c) underweight; (2) malnutrition and anti-malarial drug efficacy

Table 2 Relationship between chronic malnutrition (stunting) and risk of malarial infection ($N = 23$)

Author, Year, Reference	HAZ cutoff	Malaria outcome	Risk estimate comparing children below and above HAZ cutoff	Risk
Akiyama 2016 [46]	≤ -2	Asymptomatic malaria confirmed by PCR	OR = 3.34 (95% CI = 1.25–8.93)	Increased
Alexandre 2015 [47]	< -2	Fever and thick blood smear	HR = 0.31 (95% CI = 0.10–0.99), $P = 0.049$	Decreased
Arinaitwe 2012 [48]	-1 and -2	Pf malaria, fever and a positive blood smear	IRR = 1.24 (95% CI 1.06–1.46), $P = 0.008$	Increased
	< -2	Pf malaria, fever and a positive blood smear	IRR = 1.24 (95% CI 1.03–1.48), $P = 0.02$	Increased
Ayana 2015 [49]	< -2	Malaria by RDT	HR = 2.50 (95% CI = 1.4–5.1)	Increased
Crookston 2010 [50]	≥ -2 and < -1	Asymptomatic malaria confirmed by PCR	OR = 2.23 (95% CI = 0.99–5.02)	No impact
	≥ -3 and < -2	Asymptomatic malaria confirmed by PCR	OR = 0.56 (95% CI = 0.16–1.69)	No impact
	< -3	Asymptomatic malaria confirmed by PCR	OR = 1.02 (95% CI = 0.20–3.76)	No impact
Custodio 2009 [30]	< -2	Pf malaria parasitemia prevalence	OR = 3.07 (95% CI = 1.40–6.73)	Increased
Deen 2002 [10]	< -2	Malaria episode (fever ≥ 37.5 °C or parasitemia $> 5000/\mu L$)	RR = 1.35 (95% CI = 1.08–1.69), $P = 0.01$	Increased
Deribew 2010 [51]	< -2	Pf malaria (any parasitemia)	AOR = 0.9 (95% CI = 0.7–1.2), $P = 0.85$	No impact
Fillol 2009 [27]	< -2	Clinical malaria (fever ≥ 37.5 °C plus parasitemia $\geq 3000/\mu L$)	"Non-significant association" reported	No impact
	< -2	High density parasitemia (geometric mean $\geq 300/\mu L$)	AOR = 2.42 (95% CI = 1.12–5.24), $P = 0.03$	Increased
Friedman 2005 [26]	< -2	Concurrent malaria (any parasitemia)	AOR = 1.98, $P < 0.0001$	Increased
	< -2	High density parasitemia (any species, > 1500–$7000/\mu L$)	AOR = 1.84, $P < 0.0001$	Increased
	< -2	Clinical malaria (fever plus high density parasitemia)	AOR = 1.77, $P = 0.06$	Increased
	< -2	Severe anaemia (Haemoglobin < 7 g/dL)	AOR = 2.65, $P < 0.0001$*	–
Genton 1998 [14]	< -2	Pf malaria (fever plus any parasitemia)	Adj. Rate ratio = 1.13 (95% CI = 0.98–1.29), $P = 0.09$	No impact
	< -2	Pf malaria (fever plus parasitemia $\geq 5 \times 10^9/L$)	Adj. Rate ratio = 1.19 (95% CI = 1.01–1.40), $P = 0.03$	Increased
	< -2	Pf malaria (fever plus parasitemia $\geq 10 \times 10^9/L$)	Adj. Rate ratio = 1.18 (95% CI = 0.98–1.41), $P = 0.08$	No impact
Kateera 2015 [54]	< -2	Pf malaria (any parasitemia)	"Non-significant association" reported	No impact
Maketa 2015 [55]	≤ -2	Asymptomatic malaria by blood smear	AOR = 1.8, $P = 0.01$	Increased
Mamiro 2005 [56]	< -2	Malaria by blood smear	AOR = 1.9 (95% CI = 1.1–3.2), $P = 0.02$	Increased
Mitangala 2013 [21]	< -2	Pf malaria parasitemia ($\geq 5000/\mu L$)	AOR = 0.72 (95% CI = 0.37–1.40)	No impact
	< -3	Pf malaria parasitemia ($\geq 5000/\mu L$)	AOR = 0.48 (95% CI = 0.25–0.91)	Decreased
Muller 2003 [18]	≤ -2	Pf malaria (fever plus parasitemia $\geq 1/\mu L$)	RR = 1.0 (95% CI = 0.9–1.1), $P = 0.87$	No impact
	≤ -2	Pf malaria (fever plus parasitemia $\geq 5000/\mu L$)	RR = 1.0 (95% CI = 0.9–1.2), $P = 0.59$	No impact
	≤ -2	Pf malaria (fever plus parasitemia $\geq 100,000/\mu L$)	RR = 0.8 (95% CI = 0.5–1.4), $P = 0.44$	No impact
Nyakeriga 2004 [6]	< -2	Pf malaria (fever plus any parasitemia)	Adj. IRR = 1.89 (95% CI = 1.01–3.53), $P = 0.05$	Increased
	< -2	Pf malaria (fever plus any para < 1 year, $> 2500/\mu L > 1$ year)	Adj. IRR = 1.93 (95% CI = 0.9–4.16), $P = 0.09$	Increased

Table 2 Relationship between chronic malnutrition (stunting) and risk of malarial infection (N = 23) (Continued)

Author, Year, Reference	HAZ cutoff	Malaria outcome	Risk estimate comparing children below and above HAZ cutoff	Risk
Snow 1991 [17]	< −2	Clinical malaria (fever plus any parasitemia)	"Non-significant association" reported	No impact
	< −2	Asymptomatic malaria parasitemia	"Non-significant association" reported	No impact
Sumbele 2015 [57]	< −2	Clinical malaria parasitemia	Stunted vs. Non-stunted: 16.9% vs. 7.5%, $P = 0.01$	Increased
	< −2	Asymptomatic malaria parasitemia	Stunted vs. Non-stunted: 26.0% vs. 26.2%, $P = 0.91$	No impact
Tonglet 1999 [32]	< −2	Clinical malaria without lab confirmation in < 9 m	AOR = 1.16 (95% CI = 0.54–1.77)	Increased
	< −2	Clinical malaria without lab confirmation in ≥ 9 m	AOR = 0.71 (95% CI = 0.28–1.14)	No impact
Uscategui Penuela 2009 [58]	< −2	Malaria infection	OR = 1.94 (95% CI = 1.07–3.50), $P = 0.023$	Increased
Verhoef 2002 [13]	< −2	Laboratory confirmed malaria	OR = 0.87 (95% CI = 0.69–1.09), $P = 0.23$	No impact
Verret 2011 [22]	≥ −1 and < 0	Pf malaria risk of recurrent parasitemia	HR = 2.35 (95% CI = 0.85–6.48), $P = 0.099$	No impact
	≥ −2 and < −1	Pf malaria risk of recurrent parasitemia	HR = 2.89 (95% CI = 1.06–7.89), $P = 0.039$	Increased
	< −2	Pf malaria risk of recurrent parasitemia	HR = 3.18 (95% CI = 1.18–8.56), $P = 0.022$	Increased

Pf Plasmodium falciparum, HAZ height-for-age Z-scores, CI confidence interval, OR odds ratio, HR hazard ratio, RR risk ratio, IRR incidence rate ratio, AOR adjusted odds ratio
*Limited to anaemia

stunting was associated with an increased malaria risk, 11 studies showing no association and 2 studies showing a protective effect of stunting (Table 2).

A prospective cohort study of 487 children under 5 years of age in rural Gambia by Deen et al. reported that being stunted increased the risk of malaria infection significantly (RR = 1.35 (95% CI = 1.08–1.69)) [10]. The authors hypothesised that the observed association between malnutrition and malaria infection might be influenced by confounding factors such as HIV co-infection or socio-economic factors. Similarly, in a cross-sectional survey in children < 3 years in Kenya, Friedman and colleagues found an increased malaria risk in stunted children, showing a trend towards an increased risk of clinical malaria (OR = 1.77, $P = 0.06$), and significantly increased risk of any malaria parasitemia (OR = 1.98, $P < 0.0001$), high-density parasitemia (any species, > 1500–7000/μL; OR = 1.84, $P < 0.0001$) and severe anaemia (OR = 2.65, $P < 0.0001$) [26]. In contrast, a longitudinal study from the Gambia by Snow et al. in children aged 1–4 years reported only a minor (non-significant) impact of stunting on clinical and asymptomatic malaria episodes [17]. Two longitudinal malaria surveillance reports, one in Senegal with 874 children aged 12 months–5 years and the other in Burkina Faso with 685 children aged 6–30 months did not show any association between a low HAZ and subsequent malaria attacks [18, 27]. Similarly, Verhoef et al. in Kenya did not observe an association between being stunted and the risk of malaria infection; however, they showed that stunting might determine the severity of malaria-associated anaemia in African children [13]. Verret et al. found that in chronically malnourished children in a high-transmission setting in Uganda, children with mild (HAZ [≥ − 2 and < − 1]) to moderate (HAZ < − 2) stunting not given trimethoprim-sulfamethoxazole prophylaxis were at higher risk for recurrent parasitemia [22]. Contrary to this, in a cohort survey of 790 children under 5 years in the Kivu province, Democratic Republic of Congo (DRC), Mitangala and colleagues found that being severely stunted was protective of subsequent malaria parasitemia [21]. This finding was supported by Genton et al. in a prospective cohort of 136 children aged 10–120 months in Papua New Guinea showing that lower HAZ had a protective effect against *falciparum* malaria [14].

Risk of malaria infection in children with wasting

Eighteen studies explored the relationship between wasting and risk of malaria infection (Table 3). Overall, results were again conflicting, with three studies showing that wasting was associated with an increased malaria risk, two studies showing a protective effect and most studies showing no association (Table 3).

Takakura et al. [29], Ehrhardt et al. [11] and Shikur et al. [28] found an increased risk of *P. falciparum* malaria in children with wasting. In a case-control study involving 428 under-five children in Ethiopia, Shikur and colleagues found that severely wasted children were three

Table 3 Relationship between acute malnutrition (wasting) and risk of malarial infection (N = 18)

Author, Year, Reference	WHZ cutoff	Malaria outcome	Risk estimate comparing children below and above WHZ cutoff	Risk
Ayana 2015 [49]	< −2	Malaria by RDT	"Non-significant association" reported	No impact
Bilal Shikur 2016 [28]	< −2	Malaria by RDT or blood film	AOR = 0.66 (95% CI = 0.21–2.03)	No impact
	< −3	Malaria by RDT or blood film	AOR = 2.90 (95% CI = 1.14–7.61), $P = 0.025$	Increased
Custodio 2009 [30]	< −2	Pf malaria parasitemia prevalence	"Non-significant association" reported	No impact
Deen 2002 [10]	< −2	Malaria episode (fever ≥ 37.5 °C or parasitemia > 5000/μL)	RR = 0.87 (95% CI = 0.69–1.10)	No impact
Deribew 2010 [51]	< −2	Pf malaria (any parasitemia)	AOR = 0.6 (95% CI = 0.2–1.3), $P = 0.18$	No impact
Ehrhardt 2006 [11]	< −2	Fever	OR = 1.74 (95% CI = 1.16–2.60), $P = 0.004$	.
	< −2	Clinical malaria (fever ≥ 37.5 °C plus any parasitemia)	OR = 1.86 (95% CI = 1.14–3.02), $P = 0.007$	Increased
Fillol 2009 [27]	< −2	Clinical malaria (fever ≥ 37.5 °C plus parasitemia ≥ 3000/μL)	OR = 0.33 (95% CI = 0.13–0.81), $P = 0.02$	Decreased
	< −2	High-density parasitemia (geometric mean ≥ 300/μL)	AOR = 0.48 (95% CI = 0.04–5.34), $P = 0.55$	No impact
Friedman 2005 [26]	< −2	Concurrent malaria (any parasitemia)	AOR = 0.75, $P = 0.18$	No impact
	< −2	High-density parasitemia (any species, > 1500–7000/μL)	AOR = 0.96, $P = 0.88$	No impact
	< −2	Clinical malaria (fever plus high-density parasitemia)	AOR = 1.11, $P = 0.86$	No impact
	< −2	Severe anaemia (Haemoglobin < 7 g/dL)	AOR = 2.00, $P = 0.04$*	.
Genton 1998 [14]	< −2	Pf malaria (fever plus any parasitemia)	Adj. rate ratio = 0.92 (95% CI = 0.77–1.11), $P = 0.4$	No impact
	< −2	Pf malaria (fever plus parasitemia ≥ 5 × 10^9/L)	Adj. rate ratio = 0.96 (95% CI = 0.77–1.19), $P = 0.69$	No impact
	< −2	Pf malaria (fever plus parasitemia ≥ 10 × 10^9/L)	Adj. rate ratio = 0.97 (95% CI = 0.75–1.24), $P = 0.78$	No impact
Kateera 2015 [54]	< −2	Pf malaria (any parasitemia)	"Non-significant association" reported	No impact
Mitangala 2013 [21]	< −2	Pf malaria parasitemia (≥ 5000/μL)	AOR = 0.34 (95% CI = 0.08–1.45), $P = 0.15$	No impact
Muller 2003 [18]	< −2	Pf malaria (fever plus parasitemia ≥ 1/μL)	RR = 1.0 (95% CI = 0.9–1.2), $P = 0.99$	No impact
	< −2	Pf malaria (fever plus parasitemia ≥ 5000/μL)	RR = 1.0 (95% CI = 0.9–1.2), $P = 0.58$	No impact
	< −2	Pf malaria (fever plus parasitemia ≥ 100,000/μL)	RR = 1.0 (95% CI = 0.5–1.8), $P = 0.94$	No impact
Snow 1991 [17]	< −2	Clinical malaria (fever plus any parasitemia)	"Non-significant association" reported	No impact
	< −2	Asymptomatic malaria parasitemia	"Non-significant association" reported	No impact
Sumbele 2015 [57]	< −2	Clinical malaria parasitemia	Wasted vs. Non-wasted: 6.5% vs. 9.7%, $P = 0.78$	No impact
	< −2	Asymptomatic malaria parasitemia	Wasted vs. Non-wasted: 22.6% vs. 26.7%, $P = 0.77$	No impact
Takakura 2001 [29]	< −2	Pf malaria	Wasted vs. Non-wasted: 17% vs. 4%, $P < 0.05$	Increased
	< −2	P. vivax malaria	"Non-significant association" reported	No impact

Table 3 Relationship between acute malnutrition (wasting) and risk of malarial infection (N = 18) (Continued)

Author, Year, Reference	WHZ cutoff	Malaria outcome	Risk estimate comparing children below and above WHZ cutoff	Risk
Uscategui Penuela 2009 [58]	< −2	Malaria infection	OR = 2.64 (95% CI = 0.30–23.02), P = 0.38	No impact
Verhoef 2002 [13]	< −2	Laboratory confirmed malaria	OR = 0.78 (95% CI = 0.58–1.05), P = 0.1	No impact
William 1997 [31]	< −2	Clinical malaria (fever plus para ≥ 1000/μL)	"Non-significant association" reported	No impact
	< −2	P. vivax malaria	"Non-significant association" reported	No impact

Pf Plasmodium falciparum, WHZ weight-for-height Z-scores, CI confidence interval, OR odds ratio, HR hazard ratio, RR risk ratio, IRR incidence rate ratio, AOR adjusted odds ratio
*Limited to anaemia

times more likely to have malaria episode than non-wasted children (adjusted OR = 2.90 (95% CI = 1.14–7.61) [28]. In 2006, Ehrhardt et al. reported a survey involving 2905 children in Ghana aged 6–108 months in which wasting was significantly associated with a higher risk of clinical malaria (OR = 1.86, 95% CI = 1.14–3.02) [11]. Takakura et al. in a cross-sectional study of 309 children and adolescents (aged 2 to 18 years) in the Lao PDR showed that P. falciparum infection was associated with wasting [29]. However, Fillol and colleagues reported a significant protective association between being wasted (WHZ < − 2) at the onset of the rainy season and the risk of a clinical malaria episode (OR = 0.33, 95% CI = 0.13–0.81) in 874 preschool children (between 12 months and 5 years of age) in Senegal [27]. Similarly, in a cross-sectional survey of 1862 very young children (from 0 to 36 months age) in western Kenya, Friedman et al. showed that wasting decreased the risk of concurrent malaria (OR = 0.75, P = 0.18) and high-density parasitemia (OR = 0.96, P = 0.88), although increased the risk of severe malarial anaemia (OR = 2.0, P = 0.04) [26]. In contrast, two other longitudinal studies conducted in the Gambia [17] and in Burkina Faso [18] and a few cross-sectional surveys from Equatorial Guinea [30], Eastern Kenya [13] and Ghana [11] reported no association between being wasted and the risk of malaria infections.

Risk of malaria infection in underweight children

Nineteen studies explored the relationship between being underweight-for-age and risk of malaria infection (Table 4). Overall, results were again conflicting, with five studies showing that underweight children carried a higher malaria risk, and the remaining studies showing no association (Table 4).

In 2006, Ehrhardt et al. using cross-sectional surveys in Ghana found that being underweight was significantly associated with a higher risk of having fever of any cause (OR = 1.59, 95% CI = 1.13–2.23), clinical malaria (OR = 1.67, 95% CI = 1.10–2.50) and anaemia (OR = 1.68, 95% CI = 1.38–2.04) [11]. This was confirmed by Sumbele et al. [57] who found that 21.6% of underweight children but only 8.2% of adequately nourished children developed clinical malaria (P = 0.007) in Cameroon. In a series of cross-sectional surveys conducted in the South Pacific island of Vanuatu in 1997, Williams et al. found a strong association between the incidence of P. vivax malaria and subsequently becoming underweight (IRR = 2.6, 95% CI = 1.5–4.4) but no significant effect of P. falciparum malaria (IRR = 1.1, 95% CI = 0.57–2.1) [31]. On the other hand, Tonglet et al. reported a non-significant protective association between being underweight and the risk of clinical malaria in children between 9 months and 2 years of age in the DRC (OR = 0.68, 95% CI = 0.24–1.11) [32].

Malnutrition and anti-malarial drug efficacy

Limited data exist on the effect of malnutrition on response to antimalarial drugs, in particular ACTs. Only five studies were identified in our literature search, and results were again contradictory.

In 2008, Obua et al. explored the impact of nutritional status on the dose, drug concentrations and treatment outcome with co-packaged chloroquine plus sulfadoxine-pyrimethamine in 83 children (6 months–5 years) with uncomplicated falciparum malaria [33]. The authors found that stunting (height-for-age Z-score < − 2) was associated with higher bodyweight-adjusted (mg/kg) doses of chloroquine and sulfadoxine-pyrimethamine, higher sulfadoxine concentrations on day 1 and chloroquine concentrations on day 3, and better cure rates (P = 0.046).

In a longitudinal study of 292 infants (aged 4–12 months) in Uganda, a high malaria transmission intensity setting, ACTs (artemether-lumefantrine and dihydroartemisinin-piperaquine) were generally efficacious with a good early parasitological response (99% of study participants cleared parasites by day 3) for treatment of P. falciparum malaria, including in 43% chronically malnourished children [22]. However, in this study, stunted children (height-for-age Z-score < − 2) in the dihydroartemisinin-piperaquine arm who were not taking trimethoprim-sulfamethoxazole prophylaxis (given to all

Table 4 Relationship between being underweight and risk of malarial infection ($N = 19$)

Author, year, reference	WAZ cutoff	Malaria outcome	Risk estimate comparing children below and above WAZ cutoff	Risk
Akiyama 2016 [46]	≤ −2	Asymptomatic malaria confirmed by PCR	OR = 1.33 (95% CI = 0.53–3.30)	No impact
Arinaitwe 2012 [48]	−1 and −2	Pf malaria, fever and a positive blood smear	IRR = 1.09 (95% CI 0.95–1.25), $P = 0.24$	No impact
	< −2	Pf malaria, fever and a positive blood smear	IRR = 1.12 (95% CI 0.86–1.46), $P = 0.39$	No impact
Ayana 2015 [49]	< −2	Malaria by RDT	"Non-significant association" reported	No impact
Custodio 2009 [30]	< −2	Pf malaria parasitemia prevalence	"Non-significant association" reported	No impact
Deen 2002 [10]	< −2	Malaria episode (fever ≥ 37.5 °C or parasitemia > 5000/μL)	RR = 1.01 (95% CI = 0.82–1.26)	No impact
Deribew 2010 [51]	< −2	Pf malaria (any parasitemia)	AOR = 0.9 (95% CI = 0.7–1.2), $P = 0.90$	No impact
Ehrhardt 2006 [11]	< −2	Fever	AOR = 1.59 (95% CI = 1.13–2.23), $P = 0.008$	Increased
	< −2	Clinical malaria (fever ≥ 37.5 °C plus any parasitemia)	AOR = 1.67 (95% CI = 1.10–2.50), $P = 0.009$	Increased
	< −2	Anaemia (Haemoglobin < 11 g/dL)	AOR = 1.68 (95% CI = 1.38–2.04), $P < 0.0001^{\varphi}$	.
El Samani 1987 [52]	Weight-for-age 75–89% (mild)	History of malaria in past 2 months	AOR = 1.20 (95% CI = 0.70–2.00)	No impact
	Weight-for-age < 75% (moderate)	History of malaria in past 2 months	AOR = 2.10, (95% CI = 1.10–4.00)	Increased
Fillol 2009 [27]	< −2	Clinical malaria (fever ≥ 37.5 °C plus parasitemia ≥ 3000/μL)	"Non-significant association" reported	No impact
	< −2	High density parasitemia (geometric mean ≥ 300/μL)	AOR = 0.96 (95% CI = 0.35–2.66), $P = 0.94$	No impact
Jeremiah 2007 [53]	< −2	Malaria by blood smear	RR = 1.02 (95% CI = 0.34–2.37), $P < 0.02$	Increased
Kateera 2015 [54]	< −2	Pf malaria (any parasitemia)	"Non-significant association" reported	No impact
Mitangala 2013 [21]	< −2	Pf malaria parasitemia (≥ 5000/μL)	AOR = 0.85 (95% CI = 0.53–1.35), $P = 0.49$	No impact
Muller 2003 [18]	≤ −2	Pf malaria (fever plus parasitemia ≥ 1/μL)	RR = 1.0 (95% CI = 0.9–1.1), $P = 0.98$	No impact
	≤ −2	Pf malaria (fever plus parasitemia ≥ 5000/μL)	RR = 1.0 (95% CI = 0.9–1.2), $P = 0.68$	No impact
	≤ −2	Pf malaria (fever plus parasitemia ≥ 100,000/μL)	RR = 0.8 (95% CI = 0.5–1.4), $P = 0.49$	No impact
Nyakeriga 2004 [6]	< −2	Pf malaria (fever plus any parasitemia)	IRR = 1.33 (95% CI = 0.64–2.70), $P = 0.44$	No impact
	< −2	Pf malaria (fever plus any para < 1 year, > 2500/μL > 1 year)	IRR = 0.28 (95% CI = 0.51–3.17), $P = 0.60$	No impact
Snow 1991 [17]	< −2	Clinical malaria (fever plus any parasitemia)	"Non-significant association" reported	No impact
	< −2	Asymptomatic malaria parasitemia	"Non-significant association" reported	No impact
Sumbele 2015 [57]	< −2	Clinical malaria parasitemia	Underweight vs. Non: 21.6% vs. 8.2%, $P = 0.007$	Increased
	< −2	Asymptomatic malaria parasitemia	Underweight vs. Non: 21.6% vs. 27.5%, $P = 0.44$	No impact

Table 4 Relationship between being underweight and risk of malarial infection (N = 19) (Continued)

Author, year, reference	WAZ cutoff	Malaria outcome	Risk estimate comparing children below and above WAZ cutoff	Risk
Tonglet 1999 [32]	< − 2	Clinical malaria without lab confirmation in < 9 m	AOR = 1.31 (95% CI = 0.68–1.94)	No impact
	< − 2	Clinical malaria without lab confirmation in ≥ 9 m	AOR = 0.68 (95% CI = 0.24–1.11)	No impact
Verret 2011 [22]	(≥ − 1 and < 0)	Pf malaria risk of recurrent parasitemia	HR = 0.65 (95% CI = 0.37–1.15), $P = 0.137$	No impact
	(≥ − 2 and < − 1)	Pf malaria risk of recurrent parasitemia	HR = 0.86 (95% CI = 0.45–1.62), $P = 0.636$	No impact
	< − 2	Pf malaria risk of recurrent parasitemia	HR = 1.01 (95% CI = 0.54–1.89), $P = 0.969$	No impact
William 1997 [31]	< − 2	Clinical malaria (fever plus parasitemia ≥ 1000/μL)	IRR = 1.1 (95% CI = 0.57–2.1)*, $P = 0.8$	No impact
	< − 2	Clinical malaria (fever plus parasitemia ≥ 1000/μL)	IRR = 1.3 (95% CI = 0.9–1.9)**, $P = 0.2$	No impact
	< − 2	P. vivax malaria	IRR = 2.6 (95% CI = 1.5–4.4)*, $P < 0.0001$;	Increased
	< − 2	P. vivax malaria	IRR = 1.3 (95% CI = 0.9–2.0)**, $P = 0.2$	No impact

Pf Plasmodium falciparum, WAZ weight-for-age Z-scores, CI confidence interval, OR odds ratio, HR hazard ratio, RR risk ratio, IRR incidence rate ratio, AOR adjusted odds ratio
φLimited to anaemia;*6 months preceding anthropometric assessment; **6 months following anthropometric assessment

HIV-infected and exposed infants) were at higher risk for recurrent parasitaemia (HR 3.18 (95% CI 1.18–8.56); $P = 0.022$). Another study carried out in the DRC in 445 children, comparing the efficacy of standard doses of artesunate-amodiaquine between children with and without severe acute malnutrition (SAM), observed no evidence of reduced efficacy in children with SAM, which had an adequate clinical and parasitological cure rate, ACPR, of 91.4% [34]. A recent multi-centre (Mali and Niger), open-label trial compared the efficacy and pharmacokinetics of artemether-lumefantrine in 399 children with or without SAM. The results of this study showed adequate therapeutic efficacy in both SAM and non-SAM groups (day 42 ACPR 100% vs. 98.3% respectively) with no early treatment failures and no difference in parasite clearance reported. However, a higher risk of re-infection in children older than 21 months suffering from SAM was evident (AHR 2.10 (1.04–4.22); $P = 0.038$) [35]. Similarly in a large pooled analysis of individual pharmacokinetic-pharmacodynamic (PK-PD) data from 2787 patients treated with artemether-lumefantrine for uncomplicated Pf malaria, the WorldWide Antimalarial Resistance Network (WWARN) demonstrated that among children 1–4 years of age in high-transmission areas, the risk of reinfection increased with a decrease in WAZ with a HR of 1.63 (95% CI 1.09 to 2.44) for a child with WAZ of − 3 compared to an adequately nourished child (WAZ = 0) [36].

Information on the pharmacokinetic properties of ACTs in malnourished children is critically lacking in the published literature. Our search retrieved a study published in 2016 which assessed the efficacy of AL in relation to drug exposure in children with SAM vs. non-SAM in Mali and Niger [35]. This study measured lumefantrine concentration and showed that despite the administration of 92 g fat with dosing of SAM children (compared to 15 mL milk in non-SAM children), day 7 lumefantrine concentrations were lower in children with SAM compared to non-SAM (median 251 vs. 365 ng/mL, $P = 0.049$). In the WWARN pooled analysis of individual PK-PD data from patients treated with artemether-lumefantrine for uncomplicated Pf malaria, underweight-for-age young children (< 3 years) had 23% (95% CI − 1 to 41%) lower day 7 lumefantrine concentrations than adequately nourished children of same age [36].

Discussion

The evidence on the effect of malnutrition on malaria risk remains controversial and in many instances contradictory. The current review highlights some key limitations in the way the interaction between malaria and malnutrition has been assessed and reported. First, differences in methodology, study populations, the variability in measures used to define malnutrition (e.g. different growth references, different cut off thresholds), and the heterogeneous malaria transmission intensities with different levels of host immunity within the different studies make the comparison challenging. Second, there is a paucity of information on the effect of malnutrition on therapeutic responses to ACTs and their pharmacokinetic properties in malnourished children in published literature. Generally, vulnerable populations with common co-morbidities such as malnutrition, obesity, HIV or tuberculosis co-infection are excluded from or under-represented in antimalarial drug efficacy trials [37]. Although weight is documented, height is rarely recorded in ACT efficacy trials (< 20% of 250 trials currently included in the WWARN repository, personal communication Kasia Stepniewska), restricting the possibilities for secondary analyses. Another useful metric, mid-upper arm circumference (MUAC) is also rarely documented in malaria clinical trials despite being relatively easy to measure and low MUAC shown to be associated with increased malaria risk [38] and decreased lumefantrine bioavailability [39]. Several confounding factors and effect modifiers have been suggested such as age, co-morbidities (e.g. HIV, tuberculosis co-infection and drug interactions), immunity, socio-economic status, or refeeding practices. However, these confounding factors are poorly documented and controlled for in most of the reported studies in this review.

This review has several limitations. First, one third of the studies included in this review recruited individuals of all ages, and disaggregating observations by the age of individuals (below and above 5 years) was not possible. Methodologically, the temporal relationship between malnutrition and risk of malaria (and progression from infection to symptomatic malaria) could not be assessed because of cross-sectional study design (50% included studies). It is also limited by the extent to which important confounders (such as differential micronutrient deficiencies, ecological and genetic factors) are measured and reported in the included articles. Finally, the heterogeneity of the selected studies (presented as Additional file 5) including variations in measurement of nutritional status, definition of malaria, and statistical approaches adopted in deriving the risk estimates restricted plausible aggregated data meta-analysis in this review.

Interestingly, while no consistent association between risk of malaria and acute malnutrition was found, chronic malnutrition was relatively consistently associated with severity of malaria such as high-density parasitemia and anaemia [10, 26, 27]. The mechanism behind the higher risk of recurrent parasitemia could be explained partially by the impact of chronic malnutrition on the immune system and/or lower antimalarial bioavailability. Likewise, the apparent protection of wasted children from clinical malaria might be caused by their being administered a higher mg/kg antimalarial dose and/or a modulation of their immune response and thus an absence of symptoms, e.g. fever usually associated with malaria as opposed to an absence of malaria infection. Friedman et al. showed high-density parasitemia as a predictor for chronic malnutrition [26]. Nevertheless, the role of malaria in the aetiology of malnutrition remains unclear. The effect of malaria on nutritional status appeared to be greatest during the first 2 years of life and age acted as an effect modifier in the association between malaria episodes and malnutrition [6].

ACTs are now recommended for the treatment of uncomplicated falciparum malaria in almost all malaria-endemic countries and the number of children exposed to these antimalarial agents is increasing. A priority area is to identify gaps in our current knowledge in regard to the pharmacokinetic properties of artemisinins and partner drugs in malnourished paediatric populations to optimise dosing in order to ensure efficacy, safety and avoid the selection of parasite resistance [40]. Exposing pathogens to sub-therapeutic levels of active ingredients is a major driver of resistance. Protein-energy malnutrition, defined as insufficient calorie and protein intake, may have potential physiological effects on the absorption, distribution and metabolism of ACTs and subsequently affect the efficacy and safety of ACTs. Severe acute malnutrition can cause pathophysiological changes, including increasing total body water, leading to greater volume of distribution of drugs, which in turn may cause sub-optimal drug exposure when ACTs are given at standard doses [35, 41]. This could be further compounded by malnutrition in paediatric patients leading to dosing inaccuracies of ACTs when dose is calculated by age (over-dosing for actual body weight) or weight (under-dosing for age). Malnutrition can also be associated with intestinal malabsorption and villous atrophy of the jejunal mucosa which may cause impaired drug absorption [42]. The reduced absorption of lipids and fats has the potential to specifically affect the lipid-soluble ACTs [43]. The hepatic metabolism of the ACTs may be compromised in malnourished children. For instance, in case of quinine, hepatic metabolism is decreased in protein deficiency and increased in global malnutrition [44]. Thus, hepatic metabolised drugs should be carefully monitored in children with malnutrition. A recent individual patient data (IPD) meta-analysis conducted by the WWARN to investigate the effect of dosing strategy on efficacy of artemether-lumefantrine showed that the risk of treatment failure was greatest in malnourished children aged 1–3 years in Africa (PCR-adjusted efficacy 94.3%, 95% CI 92.3–96.3) [45]. Another large WWARN IPD meta-analysis of individual PK-PD data from patients treated with artemether-lumefantrine (AL) for uncomplicated malaria, showed day 7 concentrations adjusted for mg/kg dose were lowest in very young children (< 3 years), among whom underweight-for-age children had 23% (95% CI – 1 to 41%) lower concentrations than adequately nourished children of the same age and 53% (95% CI 37 to 65%) lower concentrations than adults [36]. This raises the question of whether an adapted dosing regimen is needed in malnourished young children. The PK-PD evaluation of artemisinins and longer-acting partner antimalarials for the treatment of malaria in paediatric populations and the effect of malnutrition on the pharmacological activity of ACTs is a priority area to identify and address key knowledge gaps.

Conclusions

A summary of the remaining knowledge gaps is presented to serve as the basis for prioritising future research strategies and highlights the need for standardising measures and reporting of nutritional status. Further analyses using individual patient data could provide an important opportunity to better understand the variability observed in publications by standardising both malaria nutritional metrics. In an era of emergence and spread of antimalarial drug resistance, it is imperative to improve our understanding of the pharmacodynamics and pharmacokinetics of ACTs in malnourished children to optimise antimalarial treatment of this very large vulnerable population. Pooled analysis, gap analysis and carefully designed prospective, randomised controlled clinical trials can provide strong evidence on the outstanding questions raised in this review related to malaria-malnutrition interactions.

Additional files

Additional file 1: PubMed, Global Health, Cochrane database search terms

Additional file 2: PRISMA checklist

Additional file 3: The methodological quality of the included studies

Additional file 4: Characteristics of the selected studies (N = 33) (XLSX 12 kb)

Additional file 5: Graphical presentation of reported risk estimates by nutritional status

Abbreviations

ACT: Artemisinin combination therapy; AOR: Adjusted odds ratio; CI: Confidence interval; DRC: Democratic Republic of Congo; GRADE: Grading of Recommendations Assessment, Development, and Evaluation; HAZ: Height-for-age Z-score; HR: Hazard ratio; IPD: Individual patient data; IRR: Incidence risk ratio; MUAC: Mid-Upper Arm Circumference; NOS: Newcastle-Ottawa Scale; OR: Odds ratio; Pf: *Plasmodium falciparum*; PK-PD: Pharmacokinetic-pharmacodynamic; RR: Risk ratio; SAM: Severe acute malnutrition; SD: Standard deviation; WAZ: Weight-for-age Z-score; WHO: World Health Organization; WHZ: Weight-for-height Z-score; WWARN: WorldWide Antimalarial Resistance Network

Acknowledgements

The authors gratefully acknowledge the assistance of Eli Harriss with database searches and Per Olav Vandvik for reviewing the methods of the manuscript. The authors are also very grateful to Prabin Dahal, Makoto Saito, Andrea Stewart and Alex Gardiner for their valuable comments on the manuscript.

Funding

WorldWide Antimalarial Resistance Network (WWARN) is funded by the Bill and Melinda Gates Foundation. EAO is supported by the Wellcome as an Intermediary Fellow (# 201866) and also acknowledge the support of the Wellcome to the Kenya Major Overseas Programme (# 077092 and 203077).

Authors contributions

PJG conceived the concept of the review and supervised and coordinated the project. DD and RM reviewed literatures and extracted data. KS and RM reviewed the methodology and data analysis. DD drafted the manuscript. KIB, RFG, EO, SK, KS and PJG reviewed and edited drafts of the manuscript. DJT and JT provided intellectual input on the review. All authors read and approved the final version of the manuscript.

Competing interests

The authors declare that they have no competing interests.

Author details

[1]WorldWide Antimalarial Resistance Network (WWARN), Oxford, UK. [2]Centre for Tropical Medicine and Global Health, Nuffield Department of Clinical Medicine, University of Oxford, Oxford, UK. [3]Mahidol Oxford Tropical Medicine Research Unit, Faculty of Tropical Medicine, Mahidol University, Bangkok, Thailand. [4]Epicentre, Paris, France. [5]Médecins Sans Frontières, Amsterdam, Netherlands. [6]Liverpool School of Tropical Medicine, Liverpool, UK. [7]Kemri Wellcome Trust Research Programme, Kilifi, Kenya. [8]Division of Clinical Pharmacology, Department of Medicine, University of Cape Town, Cape Town, South Africa. [9]WorldWide Antimalarial Resistance Network (WWARN) Pharmacology, University of Cape Town, Cape Town, South Africa. [10]Malawi-Liverpool Wellcome Trust Clinical Research Programme, Blantyre, Malawi. [11]College of Medicine, University of Malawi, Blantyre, Malawi.

References

1. World Malaria Report 2016. Geneva: World Health Organization; 2016. http://www.who.int/malaria/publications/world-malaria-report-2016/report/en/.
2. Black RE, Victora CG, Walker SP, Bhutta ZA, Christian P, de Onis M, Ezzati M, Grantham-McGregor S, Katz J, Martorell R, et al. Maternal and child undernutrition and overweight in low-income and middle-income countries. Lancet. 2013;382(9890):427–51.
3. WHOMGRS. WHO child growth standards based on length/height, weight and age. Acta Paediatr Suppl. 2006;450:76–85.
4. Bradley-Moore AM, Greenwood BM, Bradley AK, Kirkwood BR, Gilles HM. Malaria chemoprophylaxis with chloroquine in young Nigerian children. III Its effect on nutrition. Ann Trop Med Parasitol. 1985;79(6):575–84.
5. Colbourne MJ. The effect of malaria suppression in a group of Accra school children. Trans R Soc Trop Med Hyg. 1955;49(4):556–69.
6. Nyakeriga AM, Troye-Blomberg M, Chemtai AK, Marsh K, Williams TN. Malaria and nutritional status in children living on the coast of Kenya. Am J Clin Nutr. 2004;80(6):1604–10.
7. Snow RW, Molyneux CS, Njeru EK, Omumbo J, Nevill CG, Muniu E, Marsh K. The effects of malaria control on nutritional status in infancy. Acta Trop. 1997;65(1):1–10.
8. ter Kuile FO, Terlouw DJ, Kariuki SK, Phillips-Howard PA, Mirel LB, Hawley WA, Friedman JF, Shi YP, Kolczak MS, Lal AA, et al. Impact of permethrin-treated bed nets on malaria, anemia, and growth in infants in an area of intense perennial malaria transmission in western Kenya. Am J Trop Med Hyg. 2003;68(4 Suppl):68–77.
9. ter Kuile FO, Terlouw DJ, Phillips-Howard PA, Hawley WA, Friedman JF, Kolczak MS, Kariuki SK, Shi YP, Kwena AM, Vulule JM, et al. Impact of

permethrin-treated bed nets on malaria and all-cause morbidity in young children in an area of intense perennial malaria transmission in western Kenya: cross-sectional survey. Am J Trop Med Hyg. 2003;68(4 Suppl):100–7.
10. Deen JL, Walraven GEL, von Seidlein L. Increased risk for malaria in chronically malnourished children under 5 years of age in rural Gambia. J Trop Pediatr. 2002;48(2):78–83.
11. Ehrhardt S, Burchard GD, Mantel C, Cramer JP, Kaiser S, Kubo M, Otchwemah RN, Bienzle U, Mockenhaupt FP. Malaria, anemia, and malnutrition in african children--defining intervention priorities. J Infect Dis. 2006;194(1):108–14.
12. Man WD, Weber M, Palmer A, Schneider G, Wadda R, Jaffar S, Mulholland EK, Greenwood BM. Nutritional status of children admitted to hospital with different diseases and its relationship to outcome in the Gambia, West Africa. Tropical Med Int Health. 1998;3(8):678–86.
13. Verhoef H, West CE, Veenemans J, Beguin Y, Kok FJ. Stunting may determine the severity of malaria-associated anemia in African children. Pediatrics. 2002;110(4):e48.
14. Genton B, Al-Yaman F, Ginny M, Taraika J, Alpers MP. Relation of anthropometry to malaria morbidity and immunity in Papua new Guinean children. Am J Clin Nutr. 1998;68(3):734–41.
15. Hendrickse RG, Hasan AH, Olumide LO, Akinkunmi A. Malaria in early childhood. An investigation of five hundred seriously ill children in whom a "clinical" diagnosis of malaria was made on admission to the children's emergency room at University College Hospital, Ibadan. Ann Trop Med Parasitol. 1971;65(1):1–20.
16. Murray MJ, Murray AB, Murray NJ, Murray MB. Diet and cerebral malaria: the effect of famine and refeeding. Am J Clin Nutr. 1978;31(1):57–61.
17. Snow RW, Byass P, Shenton FC, Greenwood BM. The relationship between anthropometric measurements and measurements of iron status and susceptibility to malaria in Gambian children. Trans R Soc Trop Med Hyg. 1991;85(5):584–9.
18. Muller O, Garenne M, Kouyate B, Becher H. The association between protein-energy malnutrition, malaria morbidity and all-cause mortality in west African children. Tropical Med Int Health. 2003;8(6):507–11.
19. Tshikuka JG, Gray-Donald K, Scott M, Olela KN. Relationship of childhood protein-energy malnutrition and parasite infections in an urban African setting. Tropical Med Int Health. 1997;2(4):374–82.
20. Hess FI, Nukuro E, Judson L, Rodgers J, Nothdurft HD, Rieckmann KH. Anti-malarial drug resistance, malnutrition and socio-economic status. Tropical Med Int Health. 1997;2(8):721–8.
21. Mitangala PN, D'Alessandro U, Donnen P, Hennart P, Porignon D, Bisimwa Balaluka G, Zozo Nyarukweba D, Cobohwa Mbiribindi N, Dramaix Wilmet M. Malaria infection and nutritional status: results from a cohort survey of children from 6-59 months old in the Kivu province, Democratic Republic of the Congo. Revue d'epidemiologie et de sante publique. 2013;61(2):111–20.
22. Verret WJ, Arinaitwe E, Wanzira H, Bigira V, Kakuru A, Kamya M, Tappero JW, Sandison T, Dorsey G. Effect of nutritional status on response to treatment with artemisinin-based combination therapy in young Ugandan children with malaria. Antimicrob Agents Chemother. 2011;55(6):2629–35.
23. Moher D, Liberati A, Tetzlaff J, Altman DG, Group P. Preferred reporting items for systematic reviews and meta-analyses: the PRISMA statement. BMJ (Clinical research ed). 2009;339:b2535.
24. Well GASB, O'Connell D, Peterson J. The Newcastle-Ottawa scale (NOS) for assessing the quality of non-randomised studies in meta-analyses. Ottawa: Ottawa Hospital Research Institute; 2011.
25. Guyatt GHOA, Vist G, Kunz R, Brozek J. GRADE guidelines: 4. Rating the quality of evidence--study limitations (risk of bias). J Clin Epidemiol. 2011;64(4):407–15.
26. Friedman JF, Kwena AM, Mirel LB, Kariuki SK, Terlouw DJ, Phillips-Howard PA, Hawley WA, Nahlen BL, Shi YP, ter Kuile FO. Malaria and nutritional status among pre-school children: results from cross-sectional surveys in western Kenya. Am J Trop Med Hyg. 2005;73(4):698–704.
27. Fillol F, Cournil A, Boulanger D, Cisse B, Sokhna C, Targett G, Trape JF, Simondon F, Greenwood B, Simondon KB. Influence of wasting and stunting at the onset of the rainy season on subsequent malaria morbidity among rural preschool children in Senegal. Am J Trop Med Hyg. 2009;80(2):202–8.
28. Shikur B, Deressa W, Lindtjørn B. Association between malaria and malnutrition among children aged under-five years in Adami Tulu District, south-Central Ethiopia: a case-control study. BMC Public Health. 2016;16(1):174.
29. Takakura M, Uza M, Sasaki Y, Nagahama N, Phommpida S, Bounyadeth S, Kobayashi J, Toma T, Miyagi I. The relationship between anthropometric indicators of nutritional status and malaria infection among youths in Khammouane Province, Lao PDR. Southeast Asian J Trop Med Public Health. 2001;32(2):262–7.
30. Custodio E, Descalzo MA, Villamor E, Molina L, Sanchez I, Lwanga M, Bernis C, Benito A, Roche J. Nutritional and socio-economic factors associated with Plasmodium falciparum infection in children from Equatorial Guinea: results from a nationally representative survey. Malar J. 2009;8:225.
31. Williams TN, Maitland K, Phelps L, Bennett S, Peto TE, Viji J, Timothy R, Clegg JB, Weatherall DJ, Bowden DK. Plasmodium vivax: a cause of malnutrition in young children. QJM. 1997;90(12):751–7.
32. Tonglet R, Mahangaiko Lembo E, Zihindula PM, Wodon A, Dramaix M, Hennart P. How useful are anthropometric, clinical and dietary measurements of nutritional status as predictors of morbidity of young children in Central Africa? Trop Med Int Health. 1999;4(2):120–30.
33. Obua C, MNJWO-OLLGUH, Petzold MG. Impact of nutritional status on fixed-dose chloroquine and sulfadoxine/pyrimethamine combination treatment of malaria in Ugandan children. Int J Trop Med. 2008;3(3):53–9.
34. MitanIgala NP, D'Alessandro U, Hennart P, Donnen P, Porignon D. Efficacy of Artesunate plus Amodiaquine for treatment of uncomplicated clinical falciparum malaria in severely malnourished children aged 6–59 months, Democratic Republic of Congo. J Clin Exp Pathol. 2012;S3:005.
35. Denoeud-Ndam L, Dicko A, Baudin E, Guindo O, Grandesso F, Diawara H, Sissoko S, Sanogo K, Traoré S, Keita S, et al. Efficacy of artemether-lumefantrine in relation to drug exposure in children with and without severe acute malnutrition: an open comparative intervention study in Mali and Niger. BMC Med. 2016;14(1):167.
36. WorldWide Antimalarial Resistance Network Lumefantrine PKPDSG. Artemether-lumefantrine treatment of uncomplicated Plasmodium falciparum malaria: a systematic review and meta-analysis of day 7 lumefantrine concentrations and therapeutic response using individual patient data. BMC Med. 2015;13:227.
37. Barnes KI, Lindegardh N, Ogundahunsi O, Olliaro P, Plowe CV, Randrianarivelojosia M, Gbotosho GO, Watkins WM, Sibley CH, White NJ. World antimalarial resistance network (WARN) IV: clinical pharmacology. Malar J. 2007;6:122.
38. Gahutu J-B, Steininger C, Shyirambere C, Zeile I, Cwinya-Ay N, Danquah I, Larsen CH, Eggelte TA, Uwimana A, Karema C, et al. Prevalence and risk factors of malaria among children in southern highland Rwanda. Malar J. 2011;10(1):134.
39. Chotsiri P, Denoeud-Ndam L, Charunwatthana P, Dicko A: Population pharmacokinetic and time-to-event modelling of the antimalarial drug lumefantrine in young children with severe acute malnutrition. In: Available from: https://www.page-meeting.org/pdf_assets/6574-20170608_PAGE_poster_LF_SAM_children_print.pdf.
40. Mercer AE, Sarr Sallah M. The pharmacokinetic evaluation of artemisinin drugs for the treatment of malaria in paediatric populations. Expert Opin Drug Metab Toxicol. 2011;7(4):427–39.
41. Oshikoya KA, Sammons HM, Choonara I. A systematic review of pharmacokinetics studies in children with protein-energy malnutrition. Eur J Clin Pharmacol. 2010;66(10):1025–35.
42. Oshikoya KA, Senbanjo IO. Pathophysiological changes that affect drug disposition in protein-energy malnourished children. Nutr Metab. 2009;6:50.
43. Murphy JL, Badaloo AV, Chambers B, Forrester TE, Wootton SA, Jackson AA. Maldigestion and malabsorption of dietary lipid during severe childhood malnutrition. Arch Dis Child. 2002;87(6):522–5.
44. Treluyer JM, Roux A, Mugnier C, Flouvat B, Lagardere B. Metabolism of quinine in children with global malnutrition. Pediatr Res. 1996;40(4):558–63.
45. Worldwide Antimalarial Resistance Network ALDISG. The effect of dose on the antimalarial efficacy of artemether-lumefantrine: a systematic review and pooled analysis of individual patient data. Lancet Infect Dis. 2015;15(6):692–702.
46. Akiyama T, Pongvongsa T, Phrommala S, Taniguchi T, Inamine Y, Takeuchi R, Watanabe T, Nishimoto F, Moji K, Kano S, et al. Asymptomatic malaria, growth status, and anaemia among children in Lao People's Democratic Republic: a cross-sectional study. Malar J. 2016;15(1):499.
47. Alexandre MAA, Benzecry SG, Siqueira AM, Vitor-Silva S, Melo GC, Monteiro WM, Leite HP, Lacerda MVG, Alecrim MGC. The association between nutritional status and malaria in children from a rural community in the Amazonian region: a longitudinal study. PLoS Negl Trop Dis. 2015;9(4):e0003743.
48. Arinaitwe E, Gasasira A, Verret W, Homsy J, Wanzira H, Kakuru A, Sandison TG, Young S, Tappero JW, Kamya MR, et al. The association between malnutrition and the incidence of malaria among young HIV-infected and -uninfected Ugandan children: a prospective study. Malar J. 2012;11(1):90.

49. Ayana TG, Solomon T, Atsbeha H, Shumbulo EL, Amente WD, Lindtjorn B. Malnutrition and malaria infection in children 6-59 months: a cohort study in Adami Tulu District, Ethiopia. Trop Med Int Health. 2015;20(Suppl. 1):294.
50. Crookston BT, Alder SC, Boakye I, Merrill RM, Amuasi JH, Porucznik CA, Stanford JB, Dickerson TT, Dearden KA, Hale DC, et al. Exploring the relationship between chronic undernutrition and asymptomatic malaria in Ghanaian children. Malar J. 2010;9(1):39.
51. Deribew A, Alemseged F, Tessema F, Sena L, Birhanu Z, Zeynudin A, Sudhakar M, Abdo N, Deribe K, Biadgilign S. Malaria and under-nutrition: a community based study among under-five children at risk of malaria, south-West Ethiopia. PLoS One. 2010;5(5):e10775.
52. el Samani FZ, Willett WC, Ware JH. Nutritional and socio-demographic risk indicators of malaria in children under five: a cross-sectional study in a Sudanese rural community. J Trop Med Hyg. 1987;90(2):69–78.
53. Jeremiah ZA, Uko EK. Childhood asymptomatic malaria and nutritional status among Port Harcourt children. East Afr J Public Health. 2007;4(2):55–8.
54. Kateera F, Ingabire CM, Hakizimana E, Kalinda P, Mens PF, Grobusch MP, Mutesa L, van Vugt M. Malaria, anaemia and under-nutrition: three frequently co-existing conditions among preschool children in rural Rwanda. Malar J. 2015;14(1):440.
55. Maketa V, Mavoko HM, da Luz RI, Zanga J, Lubiba J, Kalonji A, Lutumba P, Van Geertruyden J-P. The relationship between Plasmodium infection, anaemia and nutritional status in asymptomatic children aged under five years living in stable transmission zones in Kinshasa, Democratic Republic of Congo. Malar J. 2015;14(1):83.
56. Mamiro PS, Kolsteren P, Roberfroid D, Tatala S, Opsomer AS, Van Camp JH. Feeding practices and factors contributing to wasting, stunting, and iron-deficiency anaemia among 3-23-month old children in Kilosa district, rural Tanzania. J Health Popul Nutr. 2005;23(3):222–30.
57. Sumbele IUN, Bopda OSM, Kimbi HK, Ning TR, Nkuo-Akenji T. Nutritional status of children in a malaria meso endemic area: cross sectional study on prevalence, intensity, predictors, influence on malaria parasitaemia and anaemia severity. BMC Public Health. 2015;15(1):1099.
58. Uscategui Penuela RM, Perez Tamayo EM, Corrales Agudelo LV, Correa Botero A, Estrada Restrepo A, Carmona Fonseca J. Relationship between malaria, malnutrition, food insecurity and low socioeconomical conditions in children of Turbo, Colombia. Perspectivas en Nutricion Humana. 2009;11:153–64.

How are health-related behaviours influenced by a diagnosis of pre-diabetes? A meta-narrative review

Eleanor Barry[*], Trisha Greenhalgh and Nicholas Fahy

Abstract

Background: Several countries, including England, have recently introduced lifestyle-focused diabetes prevention programmes. These aim to reduce the risk of individuals with pre-diabetes developing type 2 diabetes. We sought to summarise research on how socio-cultural influences and risk perception affect people's behaviour (such as engagement in lifestyle interventions) after being told that they have pre-diabetes.

Methods: Using the RAMESES standards for meta-narrative systematic reviews, we identified studies from database searches and citation-tracking. Studies were grouped according to underlying theorisations of pre-diabetes. Following a descriptive analysis, the studies were synthesised with reference to Cockerham's health lifestyle theory.

Results: In total, 961 titles were scanned, 110 abstracts assessed and 35 full papers reviewed. Of 15 studies included in the final analysis, 11 were based on individual interviews, focus groups or ethnography and five on structured questionnaires or surveys. Three meta-narratives emerged. The first, which we called biomedical, characterised pre-diabetes as the first stage in a recognised pathophysiological illness trajectory and sought to intervene with lifestyle changes to prevent its progression. The second, which we called psychological, focused on the theory-informed study of the knowledge, attitudes and behaviours in people with pre-diabetes. These studies found that participants generally had an accurate perception of their risk of developing diabetes, but this knowledge did not directly lead to behavioural change. Some psychological studies incorporated wider social factors in their theoretical models and sought to address these through action at the individual level. The third meta-narrative we termed social realist. These studies conceptualised pre-diabetes as the product of social determinants of health and they applied sociological theories to explore the interplay between individual agency and societal influences, such as the socio-cultural context and material and economic circumstances. They recommended measures to address these structural influences on lifestyle choices.

Conclusions: The study of pre-diabetes to date has involved at least three research disciplines (biomedicine, psychology and sociology), which up to now have operated largely independently of one another. Behavioural science and sociology are increasing our understanding of how personal, social, cultural and economic aspects influence health-related behaviours. An interdisciplinary approach with theoretically informed multi-level studies could potentially improve the success of diabetes prevention strategies.

Keywords: Diabetes prevention, Socio-cultural influences, Risk perception, Systematic review

---

* Correspondence: Eleanor.barry@phc.ox.ac.uk
Nuffield Department of Primary Care Health Sciences, University of Oxford, Radcliffe Primary Care Building, Radcliffe Observatory Quarter Woodstock Road, Oxford OX2 6GG, UK

Background

In the UK, there are 4 million people diagnosed with diabetes, 95% of whom have type 2 diabetes mellitus (T2DM). This has a major impact on the health of the individuals through microvascular disease (diabetic retinopathy, diabetic nephropathy and neuropathy), macrovascular disease (heart attacks and strokes) and mental health problems [1]. T2DM has a huge financial impact on the National Health Service (NHS) with 10% of its budget being spent on treating diabetes. The total cost of diabetes (direct and indirect costs) is estimated to be £23.7 billion and is expected to rise to £39.8 billion by 2035/36 [1]. As a consequence, diabetes prevention has become a national health priority [2].

Current UK diabetes prevention policy is based on using probability scores to identify those at high risk of T2DM and offer them a blood test screen [3]. The term 'pre-diabetes' has been created to encapsulate all individuals who have abnormal glycaemic blood tests but have not reached diabetic thresholds. The aim of the at-risk categorisation is to identify, monitor and refer people to interventions or medical treatment to prevent the development of T2DM [3]. These interventions are based on randomised controlled trials, which show that lifestyle measures and medication can reduce diabetes incidence and delay diabetes onset in those with pre-diabetes [4, 5]. Another high-risk group is women with a history of gestational diabetes (GDM – diabetes developing during pregnancy); 70% of such women progress to T2DM within 10 years [6].

NHS England recently commissioned a national Diabetes Prevention Programme (DPP) [7] in which those identified as pre-diabetic are offered a lifestyle intervention programme. Patients diagnosed with pre-diabetes will generally experience no illness and may never go on to develop diabetes [8]. As part of the DPP, their weight, glycaemic control (HbA1c) and blood pressure are monitored annually [3]. Our recent quantitative systematic review [9] revealed that only about one-third of individuals identified by screening programmes as pre-diabetic actually attend intervention programmes. There is limited research on the reasons for this low uptake.

The emergence of diabetes prevention programmes directed at people at risk of diabetes raises important concerns of how this labelling alters a person's health-related behaviour. Being invited to a lifestyle education programme may not automatically result in behavioural change. A diagnosis of pre-diabetes may increase motivation for individuals to change their behaviour, but it may also cause harm by inducing anxiety over a condition that may never develop [8, 9]. Lifestyles targeted by policy interventions are more than just behaviours; they are social practices that are socially and culturally shaped. Social practices develop to coordinate with daily routines (such as cooking, eating and family interactions) and cannot be meaningfully studied in isolation. They link with other social practices in bundles [10], creating a complex web of interdependent activity. Exploring the interactions between social practices (for example, through individual narrative interviews or ethnography) can help identify the wider determinants of health [10].

In this study, we sought to review the published literature on how a diagnosis of pre-diabetes influences behaviour, taking account of influences at both the individual and social levels. To cover as broad a range of the literature as possible, we sought a methodology that would allow us to combine both qualitative and quantitative studies from a range of different disciplines.

Aim, research questions and objectives

The aim of the study was to inform diabetes prevention policies by exploring how individual perceptions and wider socio-cultural influences shape individual health behaviours in response to a pre-diabetes diagnosis (or equivalent).

The specific research questions were:

A. How do individuals with pre-diabetes understand what it means to be at risk of developing diabetes?
B. Do people believe that their wider socio-cultural environment will affect their ability to make lifestyle changes? If so, in what ways?
C. What are the implications of these findings for the design and delivery of diabetes prevention programmes?

Specifically, we sought to:

- Identify primary studies that had explored health-related behaviours in populations at risk of diabetes
- Develop a taxonomy of these studies in terms of their epistemological assumptions and methodological approaches
- Extract and analyse data on risk perception, health-related lifestyle changes and individual and socio-cultural influences on these
- Synthesise findings from studies across disciplines, using seemingly conflicting data to draw out higher-order insights
- Draw conclusions on implications for the design and refinement of diabetes prevention programmes

Methods

The study was undertaken as part of a MSc in public health and as background to a doctoral study in which the experience of pre-diabetes will be studied qualitatively. As desk research, this review did not require research ethics approval. The work was part of a wider programme of research that included a quantitative systematic review of screening programmes for pre-diabetes and the efficacy of lifestyle interventions and metformin in reducing progression to T2DM [9].

Choice of approach

An initial browsing search revealed that empirical studies on how pre-diabetes influences behaviour had been undertaken from multiple perspectives and published in a wide range of journals, resulting in at least two separate literatures with little dialogue between them. Both quantitative (survey) and qualitative (interview, focus group and ethnography) studies had been undertaken, with different underlying assumptions about what pre-diabetes was and how human behaviour should be studied. Seeking to embrace all previous research on the topic, we initially began a mixed-studies review as described by Pluye et al. [11].

However, it quickly became apparent that the key challenge in this review would be synthesising data from studies that had different ontological and epistemological starting points. For this reason, we adopted the meta-narrative approach originally proposed by Greenhalgh et al. and developed further as the RAMESES standards [12]. A meta-narrative review takes as its unit of analysis the research tradition, which is a linked set of studies from a common (but evolving) set of conceptual assumptions and theoretical approaches. Scientists in one research tradition tend to build on (and/or seek to refute) the work of previous scientists in the same tradition but pay less attention to researchers outside that tradition. The methodology aims to highlight—and generate higher-order data from—the contrasting ways in which different research traditions have studied the same topic.

Meta-narrative review is an interpretive review methodology based on six principles: pragmatism (when working with a large and heterogeneous literature, select sources that appear most relevant to a particular problem), pluralism (acknowledge and celebrate that different researchers have examined a topic in different ways), historicity (consider which earlier studies influenced which later ones), contestation (use conflicting findings to drive the search for richer explanations), reflexivity (critically examine your own assumptions, methods and emerging findings) and peer review (present emerging findings periodically to external audiences and take account of their feedback). It has much in common with other interpretive approaches such as hermeneutic review [13] and critical interpretive synthesis [14]. All these approaches share a desire to generate meaning; they favour sense-making and theory-building over methodological scoring systems and checklists.

Search strategy

We sought to identify all studies relating to populations that explored individuals' risk perceptions and/or the psychological, social, cultural and material influences on lifestyle change in pre-diabetes. There is international inconsistency in how to define pre-diabetes with different countries using different parameters and inclusion criteria in prevention programmes. To reflect this, we looked for studies that assessed the impact on health-related behaviours of informing people they were at risk. Such behaviours included attendance for testing, engagement with lifestyle programmes and changes in diet and activity levels. Peer-reviewed qualitative (semi-structured interview, focus group or ethnography) and quantitative (closed-item questionnaire and survey) studies were eligible. Research on populations with established diabetes and studies focusing exclusively on children were excluded.

Study identification was undertaken between May 2016 and August 2017. With guidance from a specialist librarian, searches of Medline, Pre-Medline and Embase were undertaken. The search strategy is shown in Additional file 1. The search terms (medical subject headings and free text) included 'test', 'screening', 'pre-diabetes', 'impaired glucose tolerance', 'impaired fasting glucose', 'gestational diabetes', 'post-partum', 'ethnic groups qualitative research', 'social cultural', 'risk' and 'health related behaviours'. With a view to identifying papers in both biomedical and social science traditions, we undertook further searches of the Cochrane Database, International Bibliography of the Social Sciences and Web of Science. Citations of key papers were followed in Google Scholar to identify other relevant titles. Preliminary searches were performed in May 2016 with repeat searches for papers published in the last 12 months undertaken in June 2017. In addition, citations of all the key papers identified in our 2016 search were followed in Google Scholar in June 2017 to see if any new papers had cited them. A further paper was added to the data set following a recommendation from a peer reviewer. We manually extracted relevant titles from this data set and reviewed abstracts to identify papers for full review.

Data extraction

Given the large number of studies identified in the initial searches, full text papers were assessed initially for relevance and were subject to rapid appraisal using the Critical Appraisal Skills Programme (CASP) checklist [15] (Additional file 2). Papers not meeting basic criteria for CASP (such as relevance to the review title) were excluded from further analysis.

For each study, data were extracted on four key questions for a meta-narrative review [12]: (a) How has the issue been conceptualised by researchers? (b) How has it been theorised (explicitly or implicitly)? (c) What methodological approaches have been used to study it? (d) What were the key findings? Papers that discussed ethical considerations as well as gaining ethical approval gained a point for their CASP score for this question.

Quality assessment

Further assessment of the quality of the papers was undertaken using an adapted CERQual (Confidence in the Evidence from Reviews of Qualitative Research) framework [16], a tool designed to indicate the level of confidence in research findings. It was created in response to the increasing use of qualitative research in health-care institutions and health-care policy. The CERQual tool is not a technical checklist but gives an overall structure to a quality appraisal, leaving room for the reviewer's interpretation of the evidence [16]. The four domains are methodological limitations, relevance, coherence and adequacy of data. The CERQual tool [17] was adapted using published literature on how to assess the methodology and quality of the studies [17]. Questions pertinent to the four domains as well as questions relevant to quantitative research were included in the checklist (for full details, see Additional file 3).

Theoretical approach

It was evident from our data set that the studies identified sought to account for behavioural change through quite different types of explanation, some using psychological theories, some taking more sociologically informed perspectives and some not using any explicit theoretical framework at all.

To combine these different approaches, we selected Amartya Sen's theoretical model, the health capabilities framework, which states that health outcomes in lifestyle-related diseases are the result of interaction between choices (human behaviour) and chances (the socio-cultural contexts that make some choices more feasible and meaningful than others in particular contexts) [18].

Health lifestyle theory [19] builds on these principles, as illustrated in Fig. 1. Key to this theory is an exploration of the influences forming individual life choices and life chances. Central to this is Bourdieu's notion of habitus, that is, the internal dispositions and tendencies

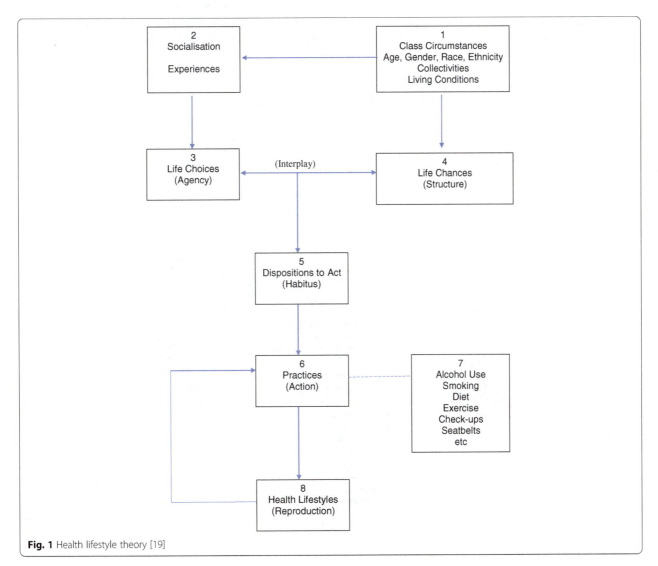

Fig. 1 Health lifestyle theory [19]

that have been generated and shaped by particular socio-cultural experiences. In turn, the way people think and act (including the choices they make) also influences the wider socio-cultural environment and evolves over time [20].

The studies in our data set were mapped diagrammatically onto the healthy lifestyle framework to visualise the approach undertaken by the different studies, identifying which components of the theory the studies focused on.

Synthesising the literature

We took an emergent approach, keeping the initial inclusion criteria broad and selecting papers by relevance to the review question. As the analysis developed, we selected further papers to test emerging theories. Microsoft Excel spreadsheets were used to aid data management. Using the iterative approach recommended for a meta-narrative review, we undertook a critical assessment of the literature, explored contradictory results, challenged authors' interpretations and understanding of problems, and considered the strengths and limitations of the approaches taken. A line of argument incorporating the overarching similarities and differences in the perspectives between different research traditions was developed. These were mapped onto the healthy lifestyle framework.

Results

Search results

The study flowchart is shown in Fig. 2.

A large number of articles were identified through the search databases but the relevance of many of these to the review question was low. Citation-tracking identified a small number of highly relevant articles (50% of the final sample). In total, 35 publications underwent a full paper review and 15 studies were included in the final analysis. The final sample included four quantitative studies (using questionnaires and surveys), one mixed methods study and 10 qualitative studies (including 154 participants from individual interviews and 312 participants from focus groups). Seven studies recruited participants who were currently or previously enrolled in diabetes prevention trials or interventions.

The list of papers included in the study and their methods are shown in Table 1. Different papers addressed

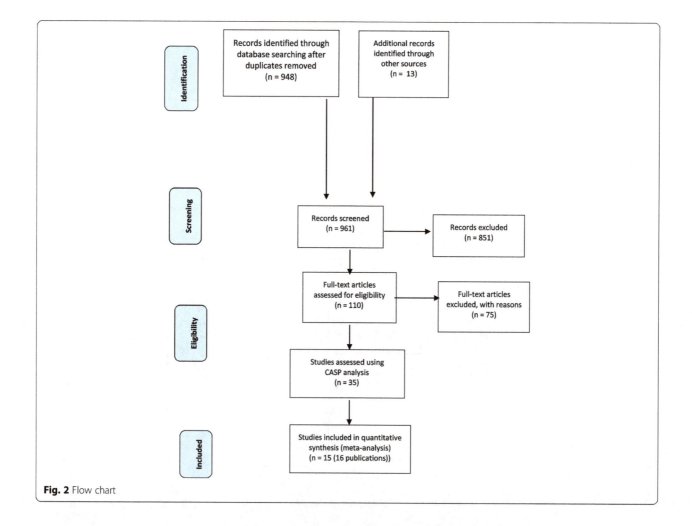

Fig. 2 Flow chart

Table 1 Summary of studies included

Author	Paper no	Research perspective	Study design	Study population	Theory or framework used	CASP score	CERQual score
Hindhede 2014 [29, 30]	1,2	Social realist	In-depth semi-structured interviews	10 individuals participating in intervention; focus groups with 14 clinicians	Bourdieu: habitus Giddens: agency/structure Weber: choices/chances	9	1
Greenhalgh 2015 [31]	3	Social realist	Group storytelling and in-depth narrative interviews	South Asian women with a history of GDM, 17 in focus groups and 28 individual narratives	Glass and McAtee's axis of nested hierarchies influencing behaviours and disease risk Giddens: agency/structure Weber: choices/chances	9	1
Jallinoja 2008 [32]	4	Biomedical	Structured focus groups with pre-defined questions	30 individuals interviewed after a lifestyle intervention.	No explicit theoretical framework, though references to Giddens's reflexivity and individuality and self-determination theory	9	0.5
Walker 2012 [28]	5	Psychological	Structured focus groups	29 people a year after a lifestyle intervention	Health action process approach (Schwarzer)	8	0.5
Troughton 2008 [36]	6	Biomedical	1:1 semi-structured interviews	15 participants, 40% with South Asian ethnicity	Leventhal's self-regulatory model of illness behaviour referred to in discussion but not in analysis	8	0.1
Satterfield 2003 [35]	7	Biomedical	Open-ended focus groups	235 persons from a mixed US population	None	7	0.1
Tang 2015 [38]	8	Psychological	Semi-structured interviews	23 women with a history of GDM within the last year	Health belief model	9	0.5
Vlaar 2014 [27]	9	Psychological	Structured questionnaire (Likert scales)	535 people in a randomised controlled trial on diabetes prevention	Leventhal's self-regulatory model of illness behaviour	9	1
Kim 2007 [24]	10	Psychological	Telephone or written survey	217 women of white ethnicity with a history of GDM	Health belief model	8	0.5
Jones 2011 [25]	11	Psychological	Quantitative survey with semi-structured interview	22 women with a history of GDM within the last 7 years.	Risk perception attitude framework	8	0.5
Morrison 2014 [33]	12	Biomedical	Semi-structured interviews	20 trial participants and four family volunteers	None	9	0.5
Penn 2015 [34]	13	Biomedical	Semi-structured interviews	15 intervention participants from a South Asian ethnic group	None (theoretical domains framework used in structure coding)	8	0.5
Kolb 2015 [26]	14	Psychological	60-item multi-choice survey	54 black or Hispanic women	Trans-theoretical model of stages of change	8	1
Morrison 2010 [39]	15	Biomedical	Cross-sectional analysis of national survey	1381 women with a history of GDM	None	9	1
Penn 2018 [37]	16	Biomedical	Semi-structured interviews and focus group as part of an evaluation	21 people with pre-diabetes undertaking DPP	None	9	1

DPP Diabetes Prevention Programme, *GDM* gestational diabetes

at least one of research questions set out by the review. The maximum CASP score was 10/10 and all papers scored at least 7/10. Reasons for exclusion included lack of relevance to the title of the review [21], participants not meeting our inclusion criteria (e.g. studies undertaken in people who did not have an elevated risk of diabetes or pre-diabetes) [22] and studies that focused exclusively on GDM and the not future risk of diabetes [23]. The CERQual tool was used to assess the quality of the papers included in the review. A score of 1.0 reflects that there were no major methodological flaws in a paper whereas a score of 0.1 signifies that there were several methodological flaws. Full details of the CASP and CERQual assessments can be found in Additional files 2 and 3.

Key research traditions

The studies reviewed revealed a range of assumptions about the nature of reality. Broadly speaking, they fell into three categories, each of which might be considered a meta-narrative [12]. All included studies could be aligned with one of these three meta-narratives, though there was some cross-fertilisation of ideas between traditions (e.g. when a paper in one tradition mentioned a different theoretical perspective in passing in the discussion).

The first category was what we called the biomedical meta-narrative. In this, T2DM was conceptualised in epidemiological terms as resulting from the interplay of antecedent risk factors and environmental causes. From this perspective, the perceptions of participants about how they understood diabetes and their possible actions were themselves analysed as risk factors and causes. These studies did not include theories (either psychological or sociological) as a major element of the analysis and proposed solutions in terms of individual behavioural change as a way of reducing one or more risk factors.

The second category was what we called the psychological meta-narrative. These studies drew on psychological theories to surface and analyse the perceptions of participants. Some of these studies took a cognitive approach (such as focusing on individual perceptions of risk and its relation to behaviour, or stages of change) [24–26]. Others took a social cognitive approach, incorporating participants' perceptions of their social and cultural context within their analysis, such as through Leventhal's self-regulatory model [27] of illness behaviour or the health action process approach [28]. In keeping with a psychological approach, though, these studies focused on the individual within a social context, rather than on the social context itself.

Our third category was what we called the social realist meta-narrative. These studies took a sociological approach, focusing on the social determinants of health, consisting of relevant aspects of the social, cultural and economic environments, which were seen as both shaping and constraining individual predisposition and behaviour. Some of these papers questioned the origins of the category pre-diabetes, viewing it as partly socially constructed and asking whose interests the diagnosis served [29]. These studies used sociological theories to explore the interplay between human behaviour and external social and material influences [29–31]. They framed solutions mainly in terms of addressing the wider social context in which disease (or pre-disease) develops.

Table 2 summaries the key findings from the studies by epistemological perspective. Additional file 4 gives a detailed description of authors' perspectives and findings from individual studies.

In the next section, we describe the three key meta-narratives of pre-diabetes in the research literature before synthesising an overarching account of the condition using health lifestyles theory.

Meta-narrative 1: pre-diabetes as a biomedical condition
The pre-diabetes diagnosis

The studies that took a biomedical perspective accepted pre-diabetes as a medical diagnosis and saw this as a precursor to T2DM. For example, Jallinoja et al. present pre-diabetes as an objective medical condition and summarise empirical evidence of the effectiveness of lifestyle interventions in its prevention [32].

Responses from the participants to the diagnosis of pre-diabetes differed between all the studies. Some described the condition as 'being on the borderline of developing diabetes' [33] and gave a strong incentive to engage in interventions and change lifestyles [34]. Some people welcomed the diagnosis of pre-diabetes and were pleased that it was 'not yet diabetes' [35]. In contrast, a UK community-based qualitative study found participants had 'never heard of this pre-diabetes stuff' [36], rejecting the categorisation with 'I cannot see that I have got, that I am pre-diabetic, because I am not a great sugary lover' [36]. Some revealed confusion on how to prevent diabetes: 'I want to prevent it if I can, and I do not know how. I am up in the air and hoping' [36]. As a consequence of these findings, researchers introduced the term 'non-diabetic hyperglycaemia' as an alternative diagnostic label.

Socio-cultural influences

The biomedical studies focused almost exclusively on the individual to bring about behavioural change with varying degrees of focus on socio-cultural influences. For example, Jallinoja et al. explored how individuals change their lifestyles and to what extent they are autonomous in this [32]. The authors identified key themes of self-regulation, self-control, individualisation and autonomy. They summarised their findings by depicting three contrasting repertoires—hopeless, struggle and self-governing—depending

Table 2 Three meta-narratives of pre-diabetes

Question	Biomedical	Psychological	Social realist
How has the problem been conceptualised by the authors?	Pre-diabetes is a biomedical condition that is a precursor for diabetes. People can reduce their risk by changing their lifestyles in a prescriptive way.	Pre-diabetes is an objective risk state. People require a perception of high risk and knowledge to change their lifestyles and reduce their diabetes risk. Social context has a role to play in changing behaviours within the individual.	Development of type 2 diabetes is a complex process influenced by multiple social, cultural and environmental factors. The term 'pre-diabetes' is (at least in part) a socially constructed and value-laden category that obscures these wider determinants.
How has the problem been theorised?	Chronic disease develops in a linear fashion (genetic predisposition to risk state to established disease).	Psychological models of health-related behaviour (especially Leventhal's self-regulatory model of illness behaviour and the health belief model).	Sociological models of the interaction between agency (individual behaviour and choices) and wider social influences (structure), especially Bourdieu's notion of habitus (internal predispositions shaped by cultural experiences).
What methods have been used to research the problem?	Questionnaires and semi-structured focused interviews.	Semi-structured interview and focus group studies seeking data on psychological factors (attitudes, perceptions, concerns and barriers to change or engagement). Questionnaire studies of attitudes, stage of change, self-reported behaviours, risk assessment and disease knowledge.	Interviews and ethnographic studies seeking a rich picture of how wider social and cultural influences affect individual decision-making and action. Lifestyles are viewed as social practices with cultural meaning and moral worth.
What instruments have been used to measure key variables or influences?	Quantitative scales and questionnaires. Qualitative data from focus groups.	Quantitative scales and questionnaires. Qualitative data from focus groups.	Critical ethnography, analysis of individual narratives (e.g. of family life) and analysis of wider cultural storytelling narratives (e.g. of diaspora or oppression).
What are the main findings?	A diagnosis of pre-diabetes is sometimes (but not always) accepted and seen positively as prompting behavioural change.	People with pre-diabetes do not always perceive themselves at high risk of developing type 2 diabetes, even when they know the risk factors. Social context has an important role to play in changing lifestyles.	Perceptions and actions are socio-culturally framed. Lifestyle change is possible only when (and to the extent that) the individual's social context, culture, and material and economic situation support particular behaviours.
What conclusions are drawn from the findings?	Diabetes prevention can be improved through individual lifestyle education. This should focus on improving knowledge.	Diabetes prevention can be improved through lifestyle change by increasing risk perception and knowledge. However, social context is an important determinant of individual behavioural change.	Diabetes prevention through individual lifestyle education will have limited impact unless wider socio-cultural, environmental and material influences are addressed.

on the individual's perceptions and their ability to self-regulate. For example, participants classified as having a hopeless repertoire exhibited

> 'some motivation to show that one went along with the rest of the group and as the sessions ended the individual became disengaged from lifestyle change pursuit, with fading out of the novel behaviours formed during the programme.'

In turn, these participants felt guilty, blaming themselves for this failure. In contrast, the participants classified as having a self-governing repertoire were able to self-monitor and self-govern and had self-control: 'this is part of this life ... and that you can control it... I now control this system in myself' [32]. There is the implication that these behaviours can to some extent be influenced through education. However, the studies did not consider the social circumstances that might make a person with pre-diabetes feel more or less in control.

Many authors discussed 'the importance of social influences, as well as social role and identity' [34]. Satterfield et al. identified structural elements that have been shown to restrict life choices, such as environmental constraints (not enough parks and green spaces), economic constraints and lack of community support [35]. Others identified enablers to lifestyle change, such as person-centred advice from medical professionals and supportive family and friends [36]. Penn et al. also confirmed a number of influences on lifestyle change, such as embarrassment about size, cost of gym access and the emotional complexity of food intake [34]. Morrison et al. [33] identified cultural barriers and enablers to engaging in lifestyle change that determined the extent participants could adhere to such change. For example, dietary interventions did not resonate with international food preferences, creating barriers to lifestyle change:

> 'Once a week they have children all come so we feel that the food should be much nicer according to the

tradition and also children don't like ordinary vegetables they fancy food like from McDonald's so just to compete with that kind of food we try to make our old Indo-Pakistani dishes.'

Moreover, 'food was described as a cultural representation of warmth'. Penn et al.'s [37] paper evaluating the NHS DPP identified difficulties faced by individuals when changes to behaviours (such as healthy eating) conflicted with social practices:

"When you go to somebody's home and they've invited you in and they've prepared a meal for you, it's very difficult to say, 'I won't eat that. I can't eat that. I shouldn't eat that.'" [37]

In summary, biomedical studies did appreciate the presence of wider social, cultural and economic influences on behavioural change. However, their focus at an individual level meant that these wider influences were documented as individual descriptions. These studies did not further analyse wider structural influences as objects of study using psychological or social theories. As a consequence, future research and policy recommendations focused on individual-level interventions.

Meta-narrative 2: pre-diabetes from a psychological perspective
Pre-diabetes and risk

The psychological studies took an individual approach to studying pre-diabetes. These authors accepted the categorisation of pre-diabetes [28, 38] and did not question its establishment. Four psychological studies examined the effects of the diagnosis by asking participants about their perceived risk of developing T2DM. They calculated mathematical estimates of people's risk perception, with regression analyses to see which risk factors (such as physical activity, weight, ethnicity, diet or family history) were associated with a perception of higher risk. They found that no individual risk factor was associated with a perception of high diabetes risk at a statistically significant level, although people with a family history of diabetes perceived themselves as having a higher risk of developing diabetes [25]. These studies reported that participants were able to identify risk factors associated with diabetes. For example, >90% of participants recognised that GDM was a risk factor for diabetes development [24, 25].

The ability to identify risk factors for diabetes did not always result in participants identifying themselves as being at high risk. Kim et al. [24] reported that over 90% of participants with a history of GDM were aware of the lifestyle changes required to prevent diabetes but only 16% thought they were at high risk of developing diabetes. In Vlaar et al.'s study of people with pre-diabetes,

72.5% identified South Asian ethnicity and 88.9% identified family history as risk factors for diabetes development [27]. Despite this, only 44% of respondents thought they were at high risk of developing diabetes. The participants in this study who attended a lifestyle intervention had a higher risk perception score and more knowledge of diabetes risk factors, compared to those who did not attend the intervention. However, this was not statistically significantly associated with attendance of the lifestyle intervention (odds ratio 1·76; 95% confidence interval 1·01–3·07) [27]. The studies that identified the disparity between understanding the high risk factors and a perception of low risk drew on Weinstein's theory of unrealistic optimism, which suggests that people believe they are healthier than others because they focus on protective actions in their own case, but on risks when it comes to others [24, 27, 39].

Kolb et al.'s [26] study of American pre-diabetics also identified a high level of knowledge of diabetes risk factors and prevention strategies among the participants. This study reported that the participants felt it was their responsibility to change their behaviours and reported high motivation for changing their lifestyles. They identified the importance of social support in enabling lifestyle change but did not explore the role of wider contexts. Rather, this study used the trans theoretical model to analyse stages of behavioural change and was, thus, focused at the individual level.

Socio-cultural influences

Three of the psychological studies examined how socio-cultural contexts influence behavioural change within the individual and used social cognitive psychological theories to explain how these interacted with the individual.

Jones et al. used both questionnaires and semi-structured interviews of Indian American women with a previous history of GDM. They identified a discrepancy between the self-efficacy reported in questionnaires (which found that participants reported a high level of personal control in efforts to prevent diabetes) and the self-efficacy reported in semi-structured interviews. These women reported that they did not feel they could control their diabetes risk due to 'American Indian cultures' [25]. For example, one said:

'Trying to actually practice it [behavioural change] in my home, yeah, it's somewhat difficult, you know, because we're all used to this lifestyle. And it's a major change'. [25].

Food was identified as central to socialising within the American Indian community:

'Everything revolves around food, and a lot of native peoples, that's their highlight of any kind of social gathering is that you've got to have food to celebrate'.

Further to this:

'Cooking like most of all Indians do; we fry everything, deep fry everything. Fry bread, fried potatoes, and we love it. That's what was our meal; that's what we were raised on.' [25]

Many women in this study reported low confidence in preventing diabetes due to their family history of diabetes or ethnicity:

'You know when you grow up and you just hear about those things, you know 'Indians get diabetes.' ... It's pounded in my head growing up.' [25]

This study used a risk perception attitude framework in the analysis of the qualitative interviews, but this framework did not integrate an analysis of the wider social factors identified by participants.

Tang et al. [38] also explored how individual risk perception influenced engagement in behavioural change. Using qualitative interviews of women with a history of GDM, they found that the majority of participants perceived they had a high risk of developing diabetes. However, this did not act as a motivator for reducing their risk of diabetes and changing lifestyles. Children acted as a positive influence on behavioural change (women wanted to be healthy for them) but also were a barrier for change. Women reported difficulties accepting or accessing social support for childcare assistance, which meant they were unable to partake in lifestyle change such as exercise:

'I don't leave the children alone with non-family members and so that is difficult because if I am not exercising with them, with me, then I feel I have really leaned on my mother a lot for sitting so I don't want to overdo it.' [38]

Walker et al. [28], whilst focusing on the individual, explored how social support and community influences were critical in determining the success of lifestyle change strategies. Social support from partners and roles within the family unit were key in helping people change their lifestyles:

'It's difficult to change your own lifestyle if your partner and family don't want to change theirs.' [28]

In addition, life circumstances and community or group support were key in increasing physical activity. However, there were also community barriers such as hospitality and social acceptability of meals:

'Households needed supplies of biscuits and cakes for visitors, while savoury scones or biscuits and cheese were healthy alternatives to cake for morning tea'. [28]

Social context and acceptability of lifestyle choices were seen as some of the greatest threats to sustained behavioural change. Walker et al. [28] analysed their results using the health action process approach model, which embeds the individual processes and stages of behavioural change within external contextual influences, such as family and community support. These were linked to the quantitative targets of the lifestyle intervention.

The psychological studies found that knowledge of diabetes risk factors and risk perception did not themselves lead to behavioural change. Qualitative psychological studies identified a number of structural barriers to lifestyle change and used psychological theories to explore how these were considered by individuals. Recommendations for further research and policy focused on individual-level interventions.

Meta-narrative 3: pre-diabetes as a social realist construct
The pre-diabetes diagnosis
The two social realist papers framed their studies very differently. Whilst the individually focused studies implicitly assumed that individuals should be responsible for behavioural change, Hindhede et al.'s paper is a critique of how the medical diagnosis of pre-diabetes puts the full responsibility for behavioural change on the individual, thereby downplaying the importance of social and material circumstances in the development of T2DM [29]. Pre-diabetes is described as a 'statistically constructed risk object' [29], and linking risk to lifestyle leads to a portrayal of the individual being the greatest risk to their own health. Hindhede et al. report that this is a strategy for disciplinary power to monitor and govern individuals to achieve behavioural change [29]. Participants in their qualitative study interpreted the pre-diabetes diagnosis as an individual failing that needed a response through self-regulation. Fear of developing diabetes and the threat of medication by health-care professionals were all motivating influences in encouraging behavioural change. The Hindhede study also explored the views of health professionals who welcomed this categorisation. They saw pre-diabetes as a way to identify those in need of education, surveillance, self-management and behavioural change [29].

Greenhalgh et al. did not use the phrase 'pre-diabetes' because they deliberately adopted the words used by the study participants to describe their condition. Their study included participants who described themselves as having abnormal blood sugar levels following diabetes that came on in pregnancy [31]. Participants were anxious about the implications for subsequent pregnancies and the need for annual testing for diabetes. The participants' fear of diabetes stemmed from the negative physical and emotional symptoms experienced in pregnancy alongside feelings of lack of control. This study found that health-related behavioural changes during pregnancy were performed primarily for the health of the unborn baby. These ante-natal efforts diminished after birth because the mother's attentions were focused on the new baby and not themselves:

'Right now, I'm just like whatever. It is just me. I am not worrying about another human being in my womb. It makes a big difference. Right now, I just need to get energy to take care of this guy right here.' [31]

This study collected and analysed a number of narrative accounts identifying socio-cultural enablers and constraints influencing an individual's risk perception and ability to act. This allowed the authors to undertake an in-depth exploration of the complexity behind diabetes development.

Socio-cultural influences

The social-orientated studies demonstrate how social and cultural factors have significant influences on lifestyle change. The Hindhede study included middle-class participants of white ethnicity and exhibited how social influences, such as identity, social capital, material circumstances, economic circumstances and self-regulation, acted as positive influences on lifestyle change [29]. The behavioural changes participants were being asked to adopt were not far removed from their existing lifestyles and could be readily incorporated into their existing routines. For example,

'I liked it the minute I entered [the fitness club] ... I cannot run on the treadmill, I only walk for like 10 min at a brisk trot.' [29]

Another participant reported:

'I have already exercised away much of the fat. I wake up every morning and cycle 11 km... I love it. It has become my way of life.' [29]

In sum, these educated white European participants were able to incorporate a fitness identity within their existing lives and used this to enable their behavioural change.

This study also identified the importance of social capital as an enabler to lifestyle change, such as a supportive spouse: 'I can ride a bike and that's what we've been doing' (pointing at his wife) [29]. However, social influences can also be negative:

'There is peer pressure involved, you know…. When we are with friends, they do not accept a 'no', so you end up drinking that beer. It's hard to lose weight'. [29]

A further influence identified in this study is the medicalisation of lifestyles through self-regulation (similar to the self-control group in the paper by Jallinoja et al. [32]). Participants use medical language and numerical values to monitor their progress and provide a source of motivation:

'I didn't like to look at myself in the mirror; it didn't look good with that stomach. And twice a week, I measure my circumference and my weight. I write it down in my book here.' [29]

Drawing on Bourdieu's theory of habitus, Hindhede illustrates that lifestyle change is possible if the interventions being suggested are within material and economic reach of a participant and familiar to their existing social world.

In contrast, the study by Greenhalgh et al., which focused exclusively on South Asian women living in a deprived part of London, found that socio-cultural influences made health-related lifestyle change difficult [31]. Issues of identity, social capital, social context and material poverty were all important inhibitors of health-related lifestyle change. Deeply held cultural beliefs and practices (notably the heavy expectations of women's domestic role) meant that women rejected exercise and fitness identities to keep their identity within traditional female roles. In this study, the same lifestyle changes that were accommodated readily by middle-class white Europeans (in the Hindhede paper) were depicted by these South Asian participants as unfamiliar, devoid of social meaning and lacking moral resonance.

In this study, friends and family depicted the kind of lifestyle changes recommended by doctors for people with pre-diabetes (dietary restriction and increased exercise levels) as unusual, inappropriate and even as a risk to their health. In the context of a group discussion on weight gain in pregnancy, for example, one woman said: 'A lot of people advised me to eat this or eat that... so I followed their orders rather than just the doctors' [31]. This, alongside the lack of social support, made it very difficult for these women to challenge peer advice and change their lifestyles. There were a number of constraints described by the cohort including scarcity of affordable healthy food, housing insecurity, cramped living conditions, high crime area and low walkability of the inner-city environment [31]. Participants reported that medical professionals presented unrealistic lifestyle strategies that were effectively impossible under the participants' current socio-cultural and material constraints.

Whereas Hindhede's middle-class white European participants sought to control their risk of developing diabetes through self-regulation, British South Asian participants in the Greenhalgh paper perceived their GDM to be out of control, and their accounts after the pregnancy reveal what a psychologist might describe as an external locus of control responsible for diabetes development (due to their perception that constraints on their lifestyle were insurmountable). As a consequence, these women tended to seek medication rather than lifestyle interventions to reduce their risk of T2DM.

Hindhede et al. and Greenhalgh et al. explored the dynamic interplay between agency and structure and how these interrelate to create the individual's habitus and subsequent actions or inactions to change lifestyle. For example, the quote above about 'following orders' of family members and close friends illustrates that the social structure of peer pressure was often more influential than medical advice.

Greenhalgh et al. adapted Glass and McAtee's axis of nested hierarchies, depicted by Fig. 3 [31]. It shows how medium- and longer-term socio-cultural influences alongside individual considerations influence behaviour and disease risk. The perpetual cycle of these influences accumulates over time to restrict the life chances of the individual and their family. This shows how wider social processes interrelate to shape lifestyles and the health-related behaviours of women and their families.

Health lifestyle theory

Health lifestyle theory proved a good fit to the data and helped synthesise and map the approach taken by the studies included in this review [19]. Figure 4 is a depiction of this with each number corresponding to a study in Table 1. Added to the theory is an overriding box that recognises that there is a political context within which socialisation processes are created and structural disparities, such as class circumstances, are constructed. Again this was explored by Hindhede and Greenhalgh et al. [29–31] in their discussions and no other papers explored these influences. Figure 4 shows that the individually focused literature focuses on socialisation experiences and the life choices of individuals, reflecting the overriding emphasis for the individual to act. As we can see, all papers identify life choices as the area to target in diabetes prevention. Over half of the papers were able to identify socio-cultural structural factors that influenced lifestyle change. However, only two papers identify these as structural influences to be targeted in population-level diabetes-prevention strategies. Further to this, only two studies [29–31] using a social realist perspective looked at the interaction between agency and structure. They used the sociological theories of

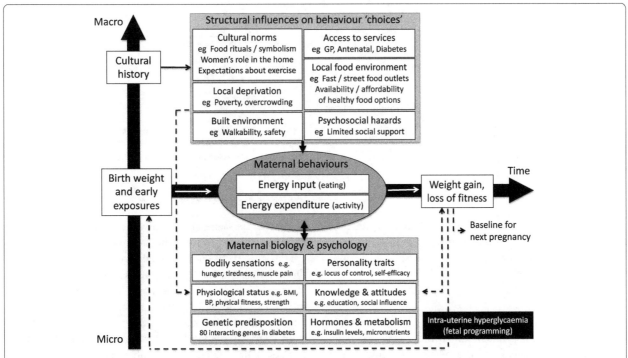

Fig. 3 Schematic diagram adapted from Glass and McAttee showing the hierarchy of influences on diabetes risk, reproduced with permission from Greenhalgh et al. [31]

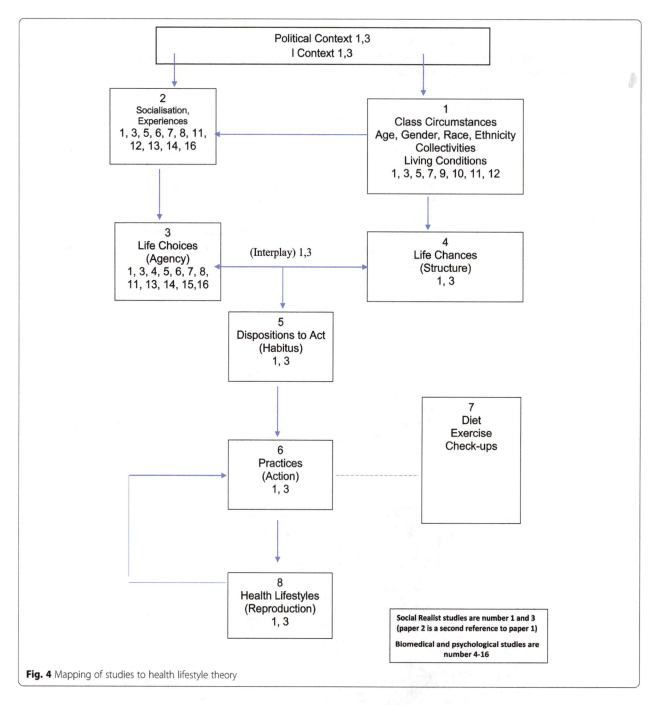

Fig. 4 Mapping of studies to health lifestyle theory

Bourdieu, Weber and Giddens [29–31] to interpret their findings and explain the practices and lifestyles depicted by their participants' narratives.

Discussion
Principal findings
This meta-narrative systematic review explored how socio-cultural influences and risk perception contribute to health-related behaviours. The studies fell on an epistemological continuum from strong interpretivist to strong positivist approaches. For clarity, three main research traditions were identified from the literature.

The studies taking a biomedical perspective accepted the pre-diabetes categorisation. An implicit assumption in this labelling is that the participants will act linearly to reduce their risk of diabetes. This places the emphasis on the individual to act and assumes that people are free from everyday demands and constraints and can rationally adapt their lives. Social realists critique the biomedical use of risk as being void of context and reductionist [40]. Some studies outlined the importance of personal and social structural influences on behavioural change. However, none of these explored the complexity of the condition or how structural influences are incorporated into the individual as part of the decision-making process. This draws attention away from population-level strategies and as a consequence, the authors' discussions focus on individual life choices with the emphasis on the individual's agency to reduce their own risk of diabetes.

Psychological studies also took an individual-level approach to exploring knowledge on diabetes risk factors, risk perception and whether these led to behavioural change. Risk perception was not associated with behavioural change and this was explored using cognitive psychological theories. Qualitative studies identified a number of social barriers to lifestyle change, such as peer, family and community support. The social cognitive psychological theories used in these papers analysed how these contextual influences affect the individual regarding behavioural change and intervention behaviour targets. However, none of the psychology studies discussed the contextual barriers as objects of study or as intervention targets in further research [34, 35].

Social realist studies, in contrast, challenged the pre-diabetes risk diagnosis as a construct that could be applied unproblematically to individuals. They used social theory to explore how agency and structure interrelate to create dispositions to act and lifestyle decisions. One study, of middle-class white Europeans with high social capital, contrasted with another, of deprived South Asians with low social capital. The main themes influencing lifestyle change in these studies included cultural obligations, identity, self-control, self-surveillance, social capital, and economic and material circumstances. Lifestyle interventions were more likely to be successful if aligned to existing reality and if an individual has the personal and material resources to support change. However, for many, overwhelming structural influences will restrict their life chances, preventing any dispositions to act.

However, the social realist papers did not measure or theorise about individual psychological constructs such as self-efficacy and empowerment or draw on psychological theories in their analysis of the thoughts and actions of individuals. Had they done so, they may have identified psychological factors that help to overcome the structural influences for their choices. Hindhede [29] does not mention any psychological influences within the sociological paradigm. Greenhalgh's [31] study references an 'external locus of control' in which individuals feel that diabetes development is out of their control, but did not draw on relevant psychological theory to situate that construct. It is presumed that this is due to overwhelming socio-cultural influences. A social realist analysis could be enhanced by the use of formal psychological frameworks to consider issues as self-efficacy and locus of control.

Mapping the studies onto the health lifestyle framework shows that the vast majority of studies focus on individual life choices as a way to change health-related behaviours. Neglecting the rest of the pathways means that current diabetes prevention interventions are unlikely to reduce the overall burden of disease. The mapping of the studies onto the health lifestyle framework shows that the majority of studies funded take an individual-level perspective. As a consequence, this limits the evidence available for policy use, perpetuating individual-level solutions to diabetes prevention.

Comparison to other systematic reviews

Three qualitative literature reviews explore the experiences of those with pre-diabetes. The first was a review undertaken by O'Reilly et al. that focused on T2DM prevention in those with a history of GDM. This review identified international inconsistencies in diabetes prevention guidelines and explored qualitative work that identified many structural barriers to engagement with screening, interventions and breastfeeding. This team concluded that the solutions lie in individual-level interventions based on educating participants [41].

Shaw et al. undertook a systematic review of studies exploring patient experience of cardiovascular and diabetes prevention initiatives, such as NHS Health Checks [42]. The theoretical domains framework was used in the analysis of the qualitative literature, focusing on psychological behaviour models, which place the emphasis on the individual to act. However, the authors also add themes of context and social influence into their analysis, recognising the importance of upstream entry points for action. They conclude that national population-level policy is needed to support individual interventions.

Youngs et al. explore the impact of the pre-diabetes diagnosis on behavioural change [43]. They undertook a descriptive review of qualitative studies, quantitative studies and analysis reports. Many of the studies included in our review were also included in their review. However, their review strongly supports a biomedical approach to diabetes prevention, concluding that more work needs to be done to 'innovatively' increase people's knowledge, self-belief and self-efficacy. One interpretation of their findings and conclusions is that if you look only for individual-level influences, you will find only solutions at that level.

This review increases both the breadth and depth of the understanding of how people change or do not change their behaviours following a diagnosis of pre-diabetes. Socio-cultural influences and risk perception play important roles in health-related behavioural change. It has illustrated how the epistemological perspective of authors has a large impact on how research questions are framed, what methodologies and data collection tools are used and how the data are interpreted.

Two epistemological positions were identified in this review: the individual perspective and the social realist perspective. Findings from this review show that individual framings produce individual solutions and interpretivist sociological framings produce upstream solutions that are harder to implement. The social realist papers give further understanding as to why people respond and behave the way they do. Tensions between agency and structure show that even if people do want to change, increasing a participant's knowledge and risk understanding is unlikely to result in health-related behavioural changes if they are subject to overwhelming structural factors. Bourdieu's theory of habitus show that people are able to adapt their behaviours only if the interventions relate to their social environment and are within their material reach.

Meaning and implications for public health and health policy

This systematic review has shown the wealth of knowledge and insight that can be obtained by public health social research. Current diabetes prevention policies focus on trial-based research, which lacks reflexivity and appreciation of the complex social mechanisms underlying the development of diabetes. Qualitative work that explores the construction of socio-cultural influences, how they contribute to the complexity of diabetes pathogenesis and structural barriers to lifestyle change are overlooked by diabetes prevention policies. By using academic work from different epistemological perspectives, we can gain a greater understanding of the complexity within which public health initiatives are exercised and insights into why these are or are not translated in practice. Here we have shown that authors taking an individual-level approach identify structural elements influencing behavioural change but have not made recommendations based on these.

Despite extensive knowledge of the wider influences constraining individual health behaviour, public health research has largely focused on individual statistical, psychological and economic models, which naturally lead to individualist solutions to diabetes prevention [10]. These paradigms are currently informing evidence-based policy with the assumption that what people do is divorced from society [10]. This creates a linear and oversimplified approach to T2DM prevention. Blue et al. [10] have called for a paradigm shift in how we 'define, frame and evaluate behavioural change' using a societal perspective. Swinburn [44] and Cypress [45] have called for greater attention to wider upstream structural factors to increase the life chances of the population. Taking this further, Green [46] and Rutter [47] et al. have called for a complex systems approach to multi-causal problems (such as diabetes), which require more than focusing on single interventions but rather 'multiple elements in many systems' [44]. These may have small effects on individuals, but may create large changes at a population level [44].

Strengths and limitations of the review

This is a comprehensive meta-narrative systematic review of the literature that applied interpretive analytic methods to explore the role of socio-cultural influences and risk perception on health-related behaviours in diabetes prevention. This is the only systematic review to have explored the epistemological perspectives of studies, which it used to analyse the data with a new innovative approach for a mixed study review. We used CASP and an adapted CERQual tool for data extraction and quality assessment. We found these tools to be very helpful and did not think they restricted the interpretative approach of this review.

The use of two paradigms is an oversimplification and in reality, these studies fall on a continuum from a strong interpretivist perspective to a strong positivist perspective. There were also limitations to the primary studies. Seven of the studies recruited participants from trial settings, who are more likely to be motivated to create change and have a higher level of health literacy and fewer co-morbidities, and therefore, they are unlikely to be representative of the wider population [48]. In addition, some of the papers are almost 10 years old and discuss theories that may now be out of date. Additionally, there were no papers undertaken in a population at the time of diagnosis. Studies retrospectively explored how the diagnosis influenced health-related behaviours (e.g. Hindhede, Morrison and Troughton). Thus, there is a gap in the literature.

Recommendations for future research

With the introduction of the NHS DPP in the UK, the first avenue for future work is expanding the qualitative work discussed in this paper. Only two studies took an interpretivist approach, which represents a gap in the literature. An ethnography taking an interpretivist perspective to explore the lived experience of pre-diabetics and whether this influences health-related behaviours may expand the knowledge base of existing studies. Undertaking an ethnography may also allow the mapping of the complex health system within which diabetes develops. Understanding this complexity will allow for interventions targeted at multiple elements within the system, rather than just the individual, which may provide greater scope for interpretivist perspectives within biomedical academic work. Increasing the dialogue between epidemiological, psychological and sociological perspectives to investigate systematic structural approaches and reviewing upstream processes may enrich policy recommendations [49]. A multi-disciplinary primary prevention strategy may enhance the current individualist research paradigm by exploring population-level approaches, and framing behaviours as social practices rather than individual choice [10]. These strategies may help to reduce the burden of many related long-term conditions, such as obesity, diabetes and cardiovascular disease.

Conclusion

Socio-cultural influences and risk perception play important roles in determining whether the individual can adapt their health-related behaviours in response to being told that they have pre-diabetes. For those with structural influences that support behavioural change, such as material resources and positive social support, increasing their risk perception may be successful in leading to health behavioural change. However, those who have overwhelming socio-cultural structural inhibitors, such as poor housing, low material wealth, unsupportive environments and conflicting cultural influences, are unlikely to change their behaviours despite increasing their risk perception. This may explain the high attrition rates in engagement in interventions in deprived, ethnically diverse populations. Therefore, placing the onus entirely on individual agency to act is unlikely to have an impact on diabetes incidence. The development of a multi-faceted approach with emphasis on wider upstream structural influences to increase life chances may be needed to reduce the burden of disease. Wider involvement of interdisciplinary psychological and sociological perspectives in health policy construction may help to provide a greater understanding of the complexity of the conditions they are trying to prevent and improve the understanding of these in real-world settings.

Abbreviations
CASP: Critical Appraisal Skills Programme; CERQual Framework: Confidence in the Evidence from Reviews of Qualitative research Framework; DPP: Diabetes Prevention Programme; GDM: Gestational diabetes; NHS: National Health Service; NIHR: National Institute for Health Research; T2DM: Type 2 diabetes mellitus

Acknowledgements
EB would like to give special thanks to Helen Elwell, a specialist BMA librarian who assisted with the Medline/Embase database searches for this dissertation. She is especially indebted to her MSc supervisor Dr Jolijn Hendriks for her support and guidance throughout the MSc. We would also like to thank the peer reviewers for their constructive feedback, which has helped to strengthen the paper.

Funding
EB was funded by a National Institute for Health Research (NIHR) in-practice fellowship to undertake this MSc alongside her academic work. She also received NHS Research Capacity Funding to write her work up for publication. TG's salary is part funded by the NIHR Biomedical Research Centre, Oxford, UK (grant NIHR- BRC-1215-20008). NF is funded by the NIHR Biomedical Research Centre, Oxford, UK (grant NIHR- BRC-1215-20008).

Authors' contributions
EB conceptualised the review, undertook searches of the data and extracted the data. EB analysed and interpreted the data. This review formed the basis of EB's MSc dissertation. EB wrote drafts of the paper following the submission of her MSc dissertation. TG supervised the project, provided theoretical guidance and reviewed drafts of this publication. NF undertook a secondary analysis of the papers following peer review and co-wrote a revision of the paper and reviewed subsequent drafts. All authors read and approved the final manuscript.

Competing interests
The authors declare that they have no competing interests.

References
1. Diabetes UK. Facts and stats. 2016. https://www.diabetes.org.uk/resources-s3/2017-11/diabetes-key-stats-guidelines-april2014.pdf
2. NHS England. NHS five year forward view; 2014. https://www.england.nhs.uk/wp-content/uploads/2014/10/5yfv-web.pdf
3. National Institute for Health and Care Excellence (NICE). Type 2 diabetes: prevention in people at high risk. NICE Guideline PH 38: NICE; 2012.
4. Public Health England (PHE). A systematic review and meta-analysis assessing the effectiveness of pragmatic lifestyle interventions for the prevention of type 2 diabetes mellitus in routine practice. London; 2015. https://www.gov.uk/government/publications/diabetes-prevention-programmes-evidence-review
5. Diabetes Prevention Program Research Group. 10-year follow-up of diabetes incidence and weight loss in the diabetes prevention program outcomes study. Lancet. 2009;374(9702):1677–86.
6. Bellamy L, Casas J-P, Hingorani AD, Williams D. Type 2 diabetes mellitus after gestational diabetes: a systematic review and meta-analysis. Lancet. 2009;373(9677):1773–9.
7. National Institute for Health Research (NIHR). Let's prevent diabetes through education NIHR2016. Available from. https://www.nihr.ac.uk/news/lets-prevent-diabetes-through-education/4886.
8. Barry E, Roberts S, Finer S, Vijayaraghavan S, Greenhalgh T. Time to question the NHS diabetes prevention programme. BMJ. 2015;351:h4717.
9. Barry E, Roberts S, Oke J, Vijayaraghavan S, Normansell R, Greenhalgh T. Efficacy and effectiveness of screen and treat policies in prevention of type 2 diabetes: systematic review and meta-analysis of screening tests and interventions. BMJ. 2017;356:i6538.
10. Blue S, Shove E, Carmona C, Kelly MP. Theories of practice and public health: understanding (un)healthy practices. Crit Public Health. 2014;26(1):36–50.
11. Pluye P, Gagnon MP, Griffiths F, Johnson-Lafleur J. A scoring system for appraising mixed methods research, and concomitantly appraising qualitative, quantitative and mixed methods primary studies in mixed studies reviews. Int J Nurs Stud. 2009;46(4):529–46.
12. Wong G, Greenhalgh T, Westhorp G, Buckingham J, Pawson R. RAMESES publication standards: realist syntheses. BMC Med. 2013;11:21.
13. Barnett-Page E, Thomas J. Methods for the synthesis of qualitative research: a critical review. BMC Med Res Methodol. 2009;9:59.
14. Dixon-Woods M, Cavers D, Agarwal S, Annandale E, Arthur A, Harvey J, et al. Conducting a critical interpretive synthesis of the literature on access to healthcare by vulnerable groups. BMC Med Res Methodol. 2006;6:35.
15. Critical Appraisal Skills Programme (CASP). CASP CHECKLISTS: CASP UK; 2017 Available from: http://www.casp-uk.net/checklists.
16. Lewin S, Glenton C, Munthe-Kaas H, Carlsen B, Colvin CJ, Gulmezoglu M, et al. Using qualitative evidence in decision making for health and social interventions: an approach to assess confidence in findings from qualitative evidence syntheses (GRADE-CERQual). PLoS Med. 2015;12(10):e1001895.
17. Greenhalgh T. How to read a paper: assessing the methodological quality of published papers. BMJ. 1997;315(7103):305–8.
18. Weaver RR, Lemonde M, Payman N, Goodman WM. Health capabilities and diabetes self-management: the impact of economic, social, and cultural resources. Soc Sci Med. 2014;102:58–68.
19. Cockerham WC. Health lifestyle theory and the convergence of agency and structure. J Health Soc Behav. 2005;46(1):51–67.
20. Lupton D. Sociology and Risk. In: Lupton D, editor. Risk. New York: Routledge; 2013. p. 77–105.
21. Grigsby-Toussaint DS, Jones A, Kubo J, Bradford N. Residential segregation and diabetes risk among latinos. Ethn Dis. 2015;25(4):451–8.
22. Gele AA, Torheim LE, Pettersen KS, Kumar B. Beyond culture and language: access to diabetes preventive health services among Somali women in Norway. J Diabetes Res. 2015;2015:549795.

23. Kaptein S, Evans M, McTavish S, Banerjee AT, Feig DS, Lowe J, et al. The subjective impact of a diagnosis of gestational diabetes among ethnically diverse pregnant women: a qualitative study. Can J Diabetes. 2015;39(2):117–22.
24. Kim C, McEwen LN, Piette JD, Goewey J, Ferrara A, Walker EA. Risk perception for diabetes among women with histories of gestational diabetes mellitus. Diabetes Care. 2007;30(9):2281–6.
25. Jones EJ, Appel SJ, Eaves YD, Moneyham L, Oster RA, Ovalle F. Cardiometabolic risk, knowledge, risk perception, and self-efficacy among American Indian women with previous gestational diabetes. J Obstet Gynecol Neonatal Nurs. 2012;41(2):246–57.
26. Kolb JM, Kitos NR, Ramachandran A, Lin JJ, Mann DM. What do primary care prediabetes patients need? A baseline assessment of patients engaging in a technology-enhanced lifestyle intervention. J Bioinform Diabetes. 2014;1(1):4.
27. Vlaar EM, Nierkens V, Nicolaou M, Middelkoop BJ, Stronks K, van Valkengoed IG. Risk perception is not associated with attendance at a preventive intervention for type 2 diabetes mellitus among south Asians at risk of diabetes. Public Health Nutr. 2015;18(6):1109–18.
28. Walker C, Hernan A, Reddy P, Dunbar JA. Sustaining modified behaviours learnt in a diabetes prevention program in regional Australia: the role of social context. BMC Health Serv Res. 2012;12:460.
29. Hindhede AL. Prediabetic categorisation: the making of a new person. Health, Risk & Society. 2014;16(7–8):600–14.
30. Hindhede AL, Aagaard-Hansen J. Risk, the prediabetes diagnosis and preventive strategies: critical insights from a qualitative study. Crit Public Health. 2014;25(5):569–81.
31. Greenhalgh T, Clinch M, Afsar N, Choudhury Y, Sudra R, Campbell-Richards D, et al. Socio-cultural influences on the behaviour of south Asian women with diabetes in pregnancy: qualitative study using a multi-level theoretical approach. BMC Med. 2015;13:120.
32. Jallinoja P, Pajari P, Absetz P. Repertoires of lifestyle change and self-responsibility among participants in an intervention to prevent type 2 diabetes. Scand J Caring Sci. 2008;22(3):455–62.
33. Morrison Z, Douglas A, Bhopal R, Sheikh A, Trial I. Understanding experiences of participating in a weight loss lifestyle intervention trial: a qualitative evaluation of south Asians at high risk of diabetes. BMJ Open. 2014;4(6):e004736.
34. Penn L, Dombrowski SU, Sniehotta FF, White M. Perspectives of UK Pakistani women on their behaviour change to prevent type 2 diabetes: qualitative study using the theory domain framework. BMJ Open. 2014;4(7):e004530.
35. Satterfield DL, May T, Bowman JE, Alfaro-Correa BA, Benjamin A, Stankus C, Learning M. From listening: common concerns and perceptions about diabetes prevention among diverse American populations. J Public Health Manag Pract. 2003:S56–63.
36. Troughton J, Jarvis J, Skinner C, Robertson N, Khunti K, Davies M. Waiting for diabetes: perceptions of people with pre-diabetes: a qualitative study. Patient Educ Couns. 2008;72(1):88–93.
37. Penn L, Rodrigues A, Haste A, Marques MM, Budig K, Sainsbury K, et al. NHS diabetes prevention Programme in England: formative evaluation of the programme in early phase implementation. BMJ Open. 2018;8(2):e019467.
38. Tang JW, Foster KE, Pumarino J, Ackermann RT, Peaceman AM, Cameron KA. Perspectives on prevention of type 2 diabetes after gestational diabetes: a qualitative study of Hispanic, African-American and white women. Matern Child Health J. 2015;19(7):1526–34.
39. Morrison MK, Lowe JM, Collins CE. Perceived risk of type 2 diabetes in Australian women with a recent history of gestational diabetes mellitus. Diabet Med. 2010;27(8):882–6.
40. Nettleton S. The emergence of e-scaped medicine? Sociology. 2004;38(4):661–79.
41. O'Reilly SL. Prevention of diabetes after gestational diabetes: better translation of nutrition and lifestyle messages needed. Healthcare (Basel). 2014;2(4):468–91.
42. Shaw RL, Holland C, Pattison HM, Cooke R. Patients' perceptions and experiences of cardiovascular disease and diabetes prevention programmes: a systematic review and framework synthesis using the theoretical domains framework. Soc Sci Med. 2016;156:192–203.
43. Youngs W, Gillibrand WP, Phillips S. The impact of pre-diabetes diagnosis on behaviour change: an integrative literature review. Pract Diabetes. 2016;33(5):171–5.
44. Swinburn BA, Sacks G, Hall KD, McPherson K, Finegood DT, Moodie ML, et al. The global obesity pandemic: shaped by global drivers and local environments. Lancet. 2011;378(9793):804–14.
45. Cypress M. Looking upstream. Diabetes Spectr. 2004;17(4):249–53.
46. Salway S, Green J. Towards a critical complex systems approach to public health. Crit Public Health. 2017;27(5):523–4.
47. Rutter H, Savona N, Glonti K, Bibby J, Cummins S, Finegood DT, et al. The need for a complex systems model of evidence for public health. Lancet. 2017;390(10112):2602–04.
48. Kennedy-Martin T, Curtis S, Faries D, Robinson S, Johnston J. A literature review on the representativeness of randomized controlled trial samples and implications for the external validity of trial results. Trials. 2015;16:495.
49. Nichter M. Representations that frame health and development policy. In: Nichter M, editor. Global Health: why cultural perceptions, social representations and biopolitics matter. Tuscon: University of Arizona Press; 2008. p. 107–18.

Trends in, and factors associated with, HIV infection amongst tuberculosis patients in the era of anti-retroviral therapy: a retrospective study in England, Wales and Northern Ireland

Joanne R. Winter[1*], Helen R. Stagg[1], Colette J. Smith[1], Maeve K. Lalor[1,2], Jennifer A. Davidson[2], Alison E. Brown[2], James Brown[3], Dominik Zenner[1,2], Marc Lipman[3,4], Anton Pozniak[5], Ibrahim Abubakar[1†] and Valerie Delpech[2†]

Abstract

Background: HIV increases the progression of latent tuberculosis (TB) infection to active disease and contributed to increased TB in the UK until 2004. We describe temporal trends in HIV infection amongst patients with TB and identify factors associated with HIV infection.

Methods: We used national surveillance data of all TB cases reported in England, Wales and Northern Ireland from 2000 to 2014 and determined HIV status through record linkage to national HIV surveillance. We used logistic regression to identify associations between HIV and demographic, clinical and social factors.

Results: There were 106,829 cases of TB in adults (≥ 15 years) reported from 2000 to 2014. The number and proportion of TB patients infected with HIV decreased from 543/6782 (8.0%) in 2004 to 205/6461 (3.2%) in 2014. The proportion of patients diagnosed with HIV > 91 days prior to their TB diagnosis increased from 33.5% in 2000 to 60.2% in 2013. HIV infection was highest in people of black African ethnicity from countries with high HIV prevalence (32.3%), patients who misused drugs (8.1%) and patients with miliary or meningeal TB (17.2%).

Conclusions: There has been an overall decrease in TB-HIV co-infection and a decline in the proportion of patients diagnosed simultaneously with both infections. However, high rates of HIV remain in some sub-populations of patients with TB, particularly black Africans born in countries with high HIV prevalence and people with a history of drug misuse. Whilst the current policy of testing all patients diagnosed with TB for HIV infection is important in ensuring appropriate management of TB patients, many of these TB cases would be preventable if HIV could be diagnosed before TB develops. Improving screening for both latent TB and HIV and ensuring early treatment of HIV in these populations could help prevent these TB cases. British HIV Association guidelines on latent TB testing for people with HIV from sub-Saharan Africa remain relevant, and latent TB screening for people with HIV with a history of drug misuse, homelessness or imprisonment should also be considered.

Keywords: HIV, Tuberculosis, Epidemiology, Trends, Latent tuberculosis, Drug misuse

---

* Correspondence: joanne.winter.14@ucl.ac.uk
†Ibrahim Abubakar and Valerie Delpech contributed equally to this work.
[1]Institute for Global Health, University College London, 30 Guildford Street, London WC1N 1EH, UK
Full list of author information is available at the end of the article

Background

Tuberculosis (TB) cases reported in England and Wales increased from 2000 to 2011, peaking at 8280 cases (15.6/100,000 population), but then declined by a third between 2011 and 2015 [1]. Nevertheless, these rates remain amongst the highest in western Europe.

The number of people living with HIV (PLHIV) in the UK increased by 10% from 2010 to more than 100,000 in 2015, although new diagnoses have remained relatively constant [2]. HIV co-infection contributed substantially to the rise in TB from 1999 to 2003; 31% of the increase in TB was in people with HIV, and by 2003 the prevalence of HIV was 8.3% [3]. However, HIV prevalence amongst patients with TB decreased to 3.2% by 2014 [1]. Between 2002 and 2010, more than 50% of TB-HIV co-infections in heterosexual PLHIV were diagnosed simultaneously (within 91 days) [4]. The epidemiology of both TB and HIV in the UK have changed over the last decade; migration from sub-Saharan Africa has decreased since the mid-2000s, whilst migration from Asia and eastern Europe has increased [5, 6], leading to fewer new HIV infections in individuals of black African ethnicity [4] and more TB in patients from the Indian sub-continent and eastern Europe [1]. However, trends in TB-HIV epidemiology have not been recently described.

Social risk factors are also a concern in TB-HIV epidemiology. The proportion of TB patients in England with such risk factors (particularly drug misuse, homelessness and imprisonment) rose from 9.8% in 2010 to 12% in 2015, although the numbers remained relatively constant [1]. Tackling TB in under-served populations is one of the key areas for action in the 2015–2020 Collaborative tuberculosis strategy for England [7]. A study from the Netherlands also found substantially higher HIV prevalence amongst TB patients who misused drugs or were homeless [8]. HIV acquisition by injecting drug use is a known risk factor for developing TB [9, 10]; however, the interactions between different social risk factors and HIV infection amongst patients with TB have not been investigated in the UK.

In the UK, HIV testing is universally recommended in sexual health clinics, antenatal services, drug dependency programmes and healthcare services for people diagnosed with TB, hepatitis B and C, or lymphoma. It is also recommended as part of routine practice where the HIV prevalence in the local population exceeds 2 per 1000 and for patients with risk factors for HIV such as other sexually transmitted infections or high-risk sexual behaviour [11]. Understanding factors currently associated with TB-HIV allows us to target screening for both HIV and latent tuberculosis infection (LTBI) to patients most at risk of developing TB disease. In this study we describe temporal trends in HIV infection of TB patients and identify characteristics of TB patients associated with HIV, focussing on social risk factors (drug and alcohol misuse, homelessness and imprisonment) to determine whether current British HIV Association (BHIVA) guidelines on testing for HIV and LTBI remain appropriate.

Methods

Study population

Statutory notifications of TB cases are reported to Public Health England (PHE)'s Enhanced TB Surveillance (ETS) system by clinicians, along with data on the clinical and sociodemographic characteristics of each TB case. We conducted a retrospective study of all adult (≥ 15 years) patients with TB in England, Wales and Northern Ireland, notified to ETS from 2000 to 2014.

Outcome: HIV status

The national HIV and AIDS Reporting System (HARS) comprises reports of all new HIV/AIDS diagnoses and deaths from the HIV and AIDS New Diagnoses Database; annual reporting on all people accessing HIV care at National Health Service (NHS) sites from the Survey of Prevalent HIV Infections Diagnosed; and death reports from the Office for National Statistics [12, 13]. As HARS does not collect unique personal identifiers, ETS and HARS data were linked to determine the HIV status of TB patients using a probabilistic matching algorithm (adapted from [14]), with supplementary deterministic matching to accept/reject borderline matches [15].

Exposure variables

We included sociodemographic (sex, ethnicity, HIV prevalence in country of birth, index of multiple deprivation [IMD] decile and history of drug misuse, alcohol misuse, homelessness or imprisonment) and clinical (site(s) of disease, year of TB notification, age at TB notification) exposure variables.

IMD score deciles represent relative levels of deprivation of income, employment, health, education, housing and services, crime and living environment for small areas in England and Wales, where 1 = most deprived and 10 = least deprived [16, 17]. Data on social risk factors (IMD decile, current alcohol misuse, current or previous drug misuse, imprisonment or homelessness) were only available from 2010 onwards.

Composite variables were created combining ethnicity and country of birth due to known interactions. As a proxy for HIV exposure, countries of birth were grouped by HIV prevalence; 'high prevalence' was defined as > 1% in the adult population living with HIV, as per World Health Organization (WHO) estimates [18]. Site of TB disease was categorised into three discrete groups: miliary or meningeal TB (with or without pulmonary disease), pulmonary disease with or without other extra-pulmonary disease (excluding miliary or meningeal TB) and other extra-pulmonary disease only. Patients with miliary and meningeal TB have low rates of treatment completion and high rates of death; therefore, we treated this as a separate category.

Statistical analysis

Data were analysed in Stata version 13.1. Descriptive analyses of the study population were undertaken, examining the proportion of people with TB who were infected with HIV and trends over the study period. Diagnoses were considered 'simultaneous' when HIV and TB diagnoses were made within 91 days of each other.

To investigate factors associated with HIV infection, we calculated the proportion of cases with HIV stratified by exposure variable and estimated odds ratios (ORs) using univariable logistic regression models. Two multivariable models were then built, a 'whole-population' model including all cases, and a model including only cases from 2010 to 2014. Year of TB notification, age at TB notification, sex, ethnicity and country of birth were included in both models; data on social risk factors were only available for 2010 to 2014. Site of TB disease was not included in the regression models, as it may be an outcome of HIV co-infection rather than a risk factor. Linearity (of age group, year and IMD decile) was assessed using likelihood-ratio tests, and variables were treated as categorical if $P > 0.05$. We excluded patients missing data on one or more variables. To assess the impact of missing data, we compared the distributions of all demographic factors for cases with missing vs. complete data. Sensitivity analyses investigated the impact of excluding weaker matches between ETS and HARS and the impact of excluding year of TB notification, as it may have confounded the relationship between ethnicity/country of birth and HIV status as the demographics of TB cases in the UK changed over the study period due to changing migration patterns.

Results

Descriptive epidemiology

There were 106,829 cases of TB in adults (≥ 15 years) reported to ETS in England, Wales and Northern Ireland for the period 2000–2014. Overall, 5792 patients (5.4%) were identified as having HIV through record linkage. There were no substantial differences in HIV prevalence amongst those with missing data for any variable (Table 1).

The proportion of TB patients with HIV peaked in 2004 (543/6782, 8.0%, Table 1), although the number was higher in 2005 (555/7489). This decreased to 205/6461 (3.2%) in 2014 (Fig. 1). The number of co-infected patients diagnosed with HIV first rose substantially from 33.5% in 2000 to 57.1% in 2014 (Fig. 2), whilst the number of cases diagnosed with TB first fell from 22.8% to 4.4%. The number of simultaneous diagnoses peaked at 54.9% in 2004, but has since decreased to 38.5%. This was largely due to a decline in simultaneous HIV and TB diagnoses amongst black African people who acquired HIV through heterosexual sex (Additional file 1: Figure S1 and Additional file 2: Figure S2). HIV testing at the time of TB diagnosis increased across all ethnic groups from 2011 to 2014, with the greatest increase occurring in populations with a low prevalence of HIV (Additional file 3: Table S1).

During the study period, HIV infection was more frequent in women (2935/46,696, 6.3%) than in men (2846/59,931, 4.7%); however, the decline was larger in women (Fig. 3). There were also declines in HIV infection in TB patients aged 15–44, but not in patients aged 45 or older (Fig. 4).

HIV infection was most frequent in TB patients of black African ethnicity born in countries with a high HIV prevalence (3537/10,956, 32.3%), compared to 477/18,947 (2.5%) in white TB patients born in countries with low HIV prevalence. Temporal changes in the ethnicity of patients with TB (Fig. 5) correlate with overall trends in the number and percentage of people with TB and HIV; TB in people of black African ethnicity peaked in 2006 and has since been decreasing, whereas the number of Asian patients with TB was increasing until 2011.

Factors associated with HIV infection

Factors associated with HIV infection were consistent between the univariable and multivariable results (Table 2). Year and age were included as categorical variables (tests for linearity both $P < 0.001$).

Sensitivity analyses investigating the impact of excluding weaker matches between ETS and HARS, and the impact of excluding year of TB notification from the multivariable models, showed results consistent with the main models (Additional file 3: Tables S2 and S3).

Social risk factors associated with HIV infection

From 2010 to 2014, 37,162 TB cases were notified, and 1393 (3.8%) were infected with HIV. Complete data on social risk factors (drug and alcohol misuse, homelessness, imprisonment and IMD decile) were available for 30,105 patients (81%).

Compared to TB patients without social risk factors, HIV was more frequent in people with current or previous drug misuse (8.1%), homelessness (8.9%), imprisonment (6.0%) or alcohol misuse (4.6%) (Table 1). There was no substantial difference in the year of notification, age or site of disease for patients with completed social

Table 1 The number and percentage of notified tuberculosis cases with and without HIV infection in England, Wales and Northern Ireland, 2000–2014

	Number of TB cases (whole population)		
	HIV–	HIV+ (%)	Total
Total	101,037	5792 (5.4%)	106,829
Year			
2000	5701	224 (3.8%)	5925
2001	5697	279 (4.7%)	5976
2002	6057	440 (6.8%)	6497
2003	6003	511 (7.8%)	6514
2004	6239	543 (8.0%)	6782
2005	6934	555 (7.4%)	7489
2006	7027	527 (7.0%)	7554
2007	6926	454 (6.2%)	7380
2008	7102	473 (6.2%)	7575
2009	7582	393 (4.9%)	7975
2010	7168	364 (4.8%)	7532
2011	7769	316 (3.9%)	8085
2012	7631	277 (3.5%)	7908
2013	6945	231 (3.2%)	7176
2014	6256	205 (3.2%)	6461
Sex			
Female	43,761	2935 (6.3%)	46,696
Male	57,085	2846 (4.7%)	59,931
Missing	191	11 (5.4%)	202
Age group (years)			
15–24	16,628	320 (1.9%)	16,948
25–34	28,658	1969 (6.4%)	30,627
35–44	17,521	2281 (11.5%)	19,802
45–54	12,347	872 (6.6%)	13,219
55–64	9283	255 (2.7%)	9538
65+	16,576	94 (0.6%)	16,670
Missing	24	1 (4.0%)	25
Ethnicity/country of birth			
White, low HIV prevalence	18,470	477 (2.5%)	18,947
Black African, low HIV prevalence	7672	249 (3.1%)	7921
Indian sub-continent, low HIV prevalence	38,745	179 (0.5%)	38,924
Other/unknown, low HIV prevalence	8692	197 (2.2%)	8889
White, high HIV prevalence	232	20 (7.9%)	252
Black African, high HIV prevalence	7419	3537 (32.3%)	10,956
Indian sub-continent, high HIV prevalence	1325	29 (2.1%)	1354
Other/unknown, high HIV prevalence	1673	254 (13.2%)	1927
Country of birth unknown	16,809	850 (4.8%)	17,659
Site of TB disease			
Pulmonary, +/–extra-pulmonary[a]	52,770	3227 (5.8%)	55,997
Miliary/meningeal TB	3747	780 (17.2%)	4527

Table 1 The number and percentage of notified tuberculosis cases with and without HIV infection in England, Wales and Northern Ireland, 2000–2014 (Continued)

	Number of TB cases (whole population)		
	HIV–	HIV+ (%)	Total
Extra-pulmonary only	44,218	1761 (3.8%)	45,979
Missing	302	24 (7.4%)	326
Homelessness[b]			
No	32,129	1136 (3.4%)	33,265
Yes	947	92 (8.9%)	1039
Missing	2693	165 (5.8%)	2858
Imprisonment[b]			
No	31,092	1102 (3.4%)	32,194
Yes	958	61 (6.0%)	1019
Missing	3719	230 (5.8%)	3949
Drug misuse[b]			
No	31,823	1125 (3.4%)	32,948
Yes	980	86 (8.1%)	1066
Missing	2966	182 (5.8%)	3148
Alcohol misuse[b]			
No	31,297	1098 (3.4%)	32,395
Yes	1134	55 (4.6%)	1189
Missing	3338	240 (6.7%)	3578
IMD decile[b]			
1	7547	350 (4.4%)	7897
2	6836	287 (4.0%)	7123
3	5531	218 (3.8%)	5749
4	4207	134 (3.1%)	4341
5	3050	112 (3.5%)	3162
6	2294	89 (3.7%)	2383
7	1669	61 (3.5%)	1730
8	1408	48 (3.3%)	1456
9	1228	45 (3.5%)	1273
10	994	19 (1.9%)	1013
Missing	1005	30 (2.9%)	1035

[a]Excluding miliary and meningeal tuberculosis
[b]2010–2014 only
IMD index of multiple deprivation, TB tuberculosis

risk factor data and patients missing data on one or more social risk factors. However, patients with missing social risk factor data were more likely to be women and/or from the Indian sub-continent.

Table 3 shows the percentage of TB patients with combinations of different risk factors, and the proportion with HIV. There was substantial correlation between different social risk factors amongst patients with TB. HIV infection was most frequent amongst TB patients with a history of drug misuse and homelessness (11.5% infected). HIV prevalence amongst TB patients with no history of drug misuse, homelessness or imprisonment was 3.2%.

In univariable analyses we found positive associations with HIV infection for homelessness (OR 2.75 [2.20–3.43]), imprisonment (OR 1.80 [1.38–2.34]), drug misuse (OR 2.48 [1.98–3.12]) and alcohol misuse (OR 1.38 [1.05–1.82]). The associations for other explanatory variables were consistent with the whole-population model. IMD decile was retained as a linear variable (test for linearity $P = 0.14$). In a multivariable model adjusted for all variables shown in Table 1, the only social risk factor

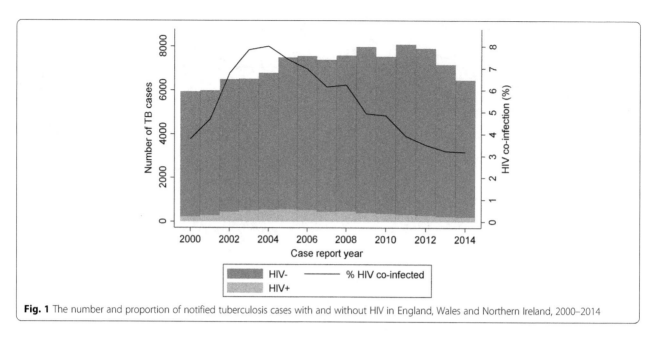

Fig. 1 The number and proportion of notified tuberculosis cases with and without HIV in England, Wales and Northern Ireland, 2000–2014

with strong statistical evidence for an association with HIV infection was drug misuse (OR 2.70 [1.90–3.84], $P < 0.001$). There was no evidence for statistical interactions between the social risk factors in the regression model ($P > 0.25$ for all combinations).

Discussion

In this retrospective study of notified TB cases in England, Wales and Northern Ireland, we report a substantial decline in both the number and proportion of TB cases with HIV since 2005 and 2004 respectively, particularly in women. HIV infection was most frequent amongst people of black African ethnicity born in countries with a high HIV prevalence. Drug misuse was the only social risk factor independently associated with HIV infection.

Implications of our findings

The proportion of TB cases diagnosed > 91 days after an HIV diagnosis rose during the study period, whilst the proportion diagnosed before HIV diagnosis decreased. This is probably the result of increased HIV testing, earlier HIV diagnoses and a healthier population of PLHIV due to initiation of anti-retroviral therapy (ART) [19].

The BHIVA and the National Institute of Health and Care Excellence (NICE) have recommended HIV testing

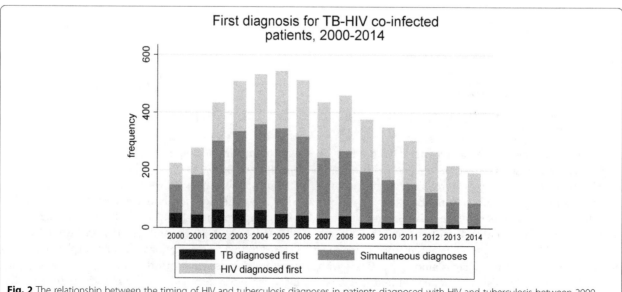

Fig. 2 The relationship between the timing of HIV and tuberculosis diagnoses in patients diagnosed with HIV and tuberculosis between 2000 and 2014

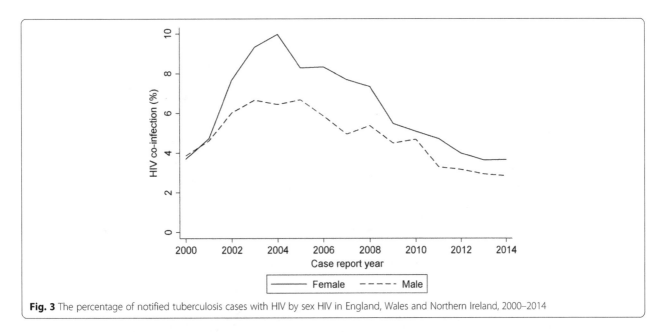

Fig. 3 The percentage of notified tuberculosis cases with HIV by sex HIV in England, Wales and Northern Ireland, 2000–2014

for all patients diagnosed with TB since 2011 [11, 20]. Between 2011 and 2015 more than 90% of TB patients with previously unknown HIV status were tested for HIV [1]. However, a substantial proportion of patients (38.5% in 2014) were diagnosed simultaneously with TB and HIV. Routine testing of new TB patients for HIV provides no opportunity to prevent TB disease, and these TB cases may have been preventable if HIV had been diagnosed earlier and patients had initiated ART sooner or been treated for LTBI. In 2008, BHIVA introduced specific guidelines recommending more HIV testing in populations at high risk of infection, and increased the CD4 count threshold at which they recommend PLHIV start ART. This is reflected in the rise in median CD4 count representing a healthier population of PLHIV [19], contributing to the observed decline in infections. Since 2015, BHIVA guidelines recommend ART for all PLHIV regardless of their CD4 count, which should further decrease TB incidence in PLHIV. More community HIV testing in populations at risk for TB is necessary to diagnose HIV sooner, to enable previously undiagnosed PLHIV to begin ART and prevent progression of LTBI to active disease.

The majority of TB-HIV now occurs in people who were already known to have HIV and subsequently developed TB. This has important implications for TB prevention strategies. Focussing on HIV testing and ART initiation is insufficient to prevent TB in PLHIV, and

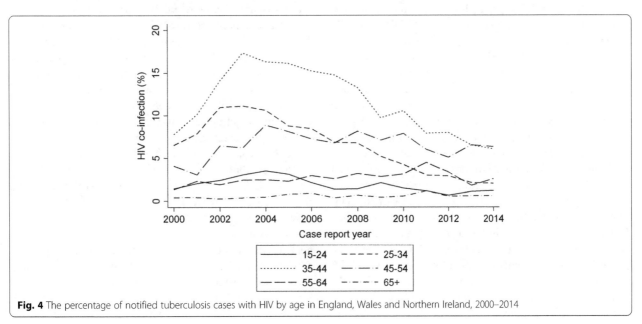

Fig. 4 The percentage of notified tuberculosis cases with HIV by age in England, Wales and Northern Ireland, 2000–2014

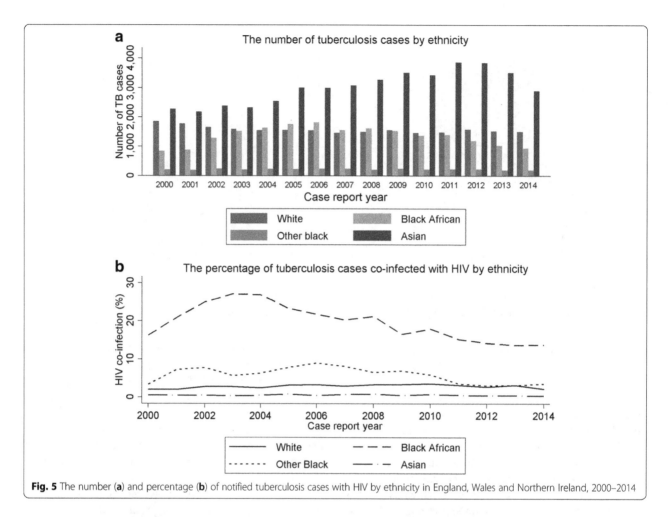

Fig. 5 The number (**a**) and percentage (**b**) of notified tuberculosis cases with HIV by ethnicity in England, Wales and Northern Ireland, 2000–2014

increasing testing and treatment of LTBI may further reduce TB-HIV. Our data indicate that people of black African ethnicity still have high rates of HIV-associated TB, and that the BHIVA guidelines recommending LTBI screening in this population of PLHIV remain appropriate.

Part of the decline in HIV infection can be attributed to changing migration patterns, resulting in less TB in black African individuals from countries with a high HIV prevalence and more amongst individuals from Asian countries with low HIV prevalence [5]. Whilst the largest decreases in HIV infection were in black African TB patients, they remain the most at-risk population. HIV infection was greater amongst women with TB than men. This reflects the gender ratio of heterosexual PLHIV in the UK, where there are more women diagnosed with HIV than men, particularly amongst black Africans [2]. This is likely because of higher diagnostic rates in women [2] due to antenatal HIV testing; thus, the decline reflects both the changes in ethnicity of TB patients and the healthier cohort of women with HIV. HIV infection declined in patients with TB aged 15–44, but not in older people. This may be due to the ageing cohort of PLHIV and the higher rates of late HIV diagnosis in older patients, increasing the risk of TB [2].

HIV infection was more frequent in TB patients with any social risk factor (drug and alcohol misuse, imprisonment and homelessness) than in those without, and overall even more frequent amongst TB patients with multiple social risk factors. However, after adjusting for other social risk factors in the multivariable model, only drug misuse remained associated with greater odds of HIV infection; this is probably the result of HIV acquisition from injecting drug use. As TB incidence amongst PLHIV who inject drugs is comparable to that amongst black Africans from countries with high TB burden [10], we suggest that LTBI screening and preventive TB therapy for PLHIV with social risk factors, particularly drug misuse, could decrease TB in this population.

We found a much greater proportion of HIV co-infection amongst patients with miliary and meningeal TB than pulmonary TB, and a lower proportion amongst patients with other extra-pulmonary disease. This was consistent over the study period and with previous work [21], probably because extra-pulmonary TB is common in patients with TB from the Indian

Table 2 Results from univariable and two multivariable logistic regression models of factors associated with HIV infection in notified tuberculosis cases in England, Wales and Northern Ireland, for the periods 2000–2014 and 2010–2014

	Univariable results (whole population)		Multivariable results (whole population)		Multivariable results (2010–2014)	
	OR (95% CI)	P value	OR (95% CI)	P value	OR (95% CI)	P value
Year						
2000	1.00	< 0.001	1.00	< 0.001	–	
2001	1.25 (1.04–1.49)		1.22 (1.00–1.48)		–	
2002	1.85 (1.57–2.18)		1.45 (1.20–1.74)		–	
2003	2.17 (1.84–2.55)		1.51 (1.26–1.80)		–	
2004	2.22 (1.89–2.60)		1.56 (1.31–1.87)		–	
2005	2.04 (1.74–2.39)		1.40 (1.17–1.67)		–	
2006	1.91 (1.63–2.24)		1.36 (1.14–1.62)		–	
2007	1.67 (1.42–1.97)		1.22 (1.01–1.46)		–	
2008	1.70 (1.44–1.99)		1.25 (1.04–1.50)		–	
2009	1.32 (1.12–1.56)		1.04 (0.86–1.25)		–	
2010	1.29 (1.09–1.53)		1.06 (0.87–1.28)		1.00	< 0.001
2011	1.04 (0.87–1.23)		0.83 (0.68–1.01)		0.76 (0.61–0.93)	
2012	0.92 (0.77–1.11)		0.82 (0.67–1.00)		0.81 (0.65–0.99)	
2013	0.85 (0.70–1.02)		0.76 (0.62–0.94)		0.66 (0.53–0.83)	
2014	0.83 (0.69–1.01)		0.72 (0.58–0.89)		0.68 (0.54–0.85)	
Sex						
Female	1.00	< 0.001	1.00	< 0.001	1.00	0.03
Male	0.74 (0.70–0.78)		0.84 (0.79–0.90)		0.85 (0.74–0.98)	
Age group (years)						
15–24	0.28 (0.25–0.32)	< 0.001	0.28 (0.24–0.32)	< 0.001	0.31 (0.22–0.44)	< 0.001
25–34	1.00		1.00		1.00	
35–44	1.89 (1.78–2.02)		1.97 (1.83–2.13)		2.16 (1.79–2.59)	
45–54	1.03 (0.95–1.12)		1.33 (1.21–1.47)		1.97 (1.60–2.44)	
55–64	0.40 (0.35–0.46)		0.62 (0.54–0.72)		1.35 (1.02–1.78)	
65+	0.08 (0.07–0.10)		0.16 (0.13–0.19)		0.31 (0.20–0.49)	
Ethnicity/country of birth						
White, low HIV prevalence	1.00	< 0.001	1.00	< 0.001	1.00	< 0.001
Black African, low HIV prevalence	1.26 (1.08–1.47)		1.07 (0.91–1.26)		1.07 (0.74–1.55)	
Indian sub-continent, low HIV prevalence	0.18 (0.15–0.21)		0.16 (0.14–0.20)		0.20 (0.14–0.28)	
Other/unknown, low HIV prevalence	0.88 (0.74–1.04)		0.73 (0.62–0.87)		0.67 (0.46–0.96)	
White, high HIV prevalence	3.34 (2.10–5.32)		2.43 (1.51–3.91)		3.85 (1.45–10.23)	
Black African, high HIV prevalence	18.46 (16.71–20.39)		13.02 (11.69–14.50)		10.39 (8.13–13.29)	
Indian sub-continent, high HIV prevalence	0.85 (0.58–1.24)		0.69 (0.47–1.01)		0.51 (0.20–1.26)	
Other/unknown, high HIV prevalence	5.88 (5.01–6.90)		4.56 (3.85–5.39)		4.07 (2.79–5.94)	
Country of birth unknown	1.96 (1.75–2.19)		1.62 (1.44–1.82)		1.51 (1.14–2.00)	
Site of TB disease						
Pulmonary, +/−extra-pulmonary[a]	1.00	< 0.001	1.00	< 0.001	1.00	< 0.001
Miliary/meningeal TB	3.40 (3.13–3.71)		3.30 (2.96–3.68)		3.81 (3.02–4.80)	
Extra-pulmonary only	0.65 (0.61–0.69)		0.70 (0.65–0.75)		0.73 (0.63–0.86)	

Table 2 Results from univariable and two multivariable logistic regression models of factors associated with HIV infection in notified tuberculosis cases in England, Wales and Northern Ireland, for the periods 2000–2014 and 2010–2014 *(Continued)*

	Univariable results (whole population)		Multivariable results (whole population)		Multivariable results (2010–2014)	
	OR (95% CI)	P value	OR (95% CI)	P value	OR (95% CI)	P value
Homelessness						
No	1.00	< 0.001	–		1.00	0.26
Yes	2.75 (2.20–3.43)		–		1.22 (0.87–1.72)	
Imprisonment						
No	1.00	< 0.001	–		1.00	0.19
Yes	1.80 (1.38–2.34)		–		0.77 (0.52–1.15)	
Drug misuse						
No	1.00	< 0.001	–		1.00	< 0.001
Yes	2.48 (1.98–3.12)		–		2.70 (1.90–3.84)	
Alcohol misuse						
No	1.00	0.03	–		1.00	0.73
Yes	1.38 (1.05–1.82)		–		0.93 (0.64–1.37)	
IMD decile						
(for each unit increase)	0.95 (0.93–0.97)	< 0.001	–		0.99 (0.96–1.02)	0.47

[a]Excluding miliary and meningeal TB. *CI* confidence interval, *IMD* index of multiple deprivation, *OR* odds ratio, *TB* tuberculosis
The whole-population model excluded 226 (0.2%) TB cases missing data on sex ($n = 202$) and/or age ($n = 25$), and was adjusted for year of TB notification, age, sex and ethnicity and HIV prevalence in country of birth. The 2010–2014 model excluded 7098 (19%) TB cases missing data on sex ($n = 60$), homelessness ($n = 2693$), imprisonment ($n = 3719$), drug misuse ($n = 2966$), alcohol misuse ($n = 3338$) and/or IMD decile ($n = 1035$) and adjusted for all variables in the table

sub-continent [21] where HIV prevalence is low. Our results were consistent with other studies reporting higher prevalence of HIV co-infection amongst cases of miliary [22] and meningeal [23] TB, and lower HIV prevalence amongst other forms of extra-pulmonary TB. Recent work in the UK showed that patients with severe extra-pulmonary TB have worse outcomes than those with pulmonary TB, whilst patients with other extra-pulmonary TB generally have better outcomes [1]. It is unclear whether this is solely because of severe disease presentation or whether these patients could be influenced by higher rates of HIV co-infection (and corresponding clinical complexity). Regardless, as diagnosis of extra-pulmonary TB is often difficult, increasing awareness of extra-pulmonary TB symptoms amongst PLHIV and populations with high rates of undiagnosed HIV might allow earlier diagnosis of extra-pulmonary TB.

Strengths and limitations

This study benefits from 15 years of case notifications to robust national surveillance programmes, representing comprehensive coverage of TB cases in England, Wales and Northern Ireland. However, there are some limitations. The HIV surveillance dataset does not contain

Table 3 The number of notified tuberculosis cases with and without a history of drug misuse, homelessness or imprisonment, and the HIV prevalence in each of these groups in England, Wales and Northern Ireland, 2000–2014

		Drug misuse		Total
		No	Yes	
Total (homeless and not homeless, number)	No prison	30,711 (3.2% [3.1–3.4])	506 (8.3% [5.9–10.7])	31,217 (3.3% [3.1–3.5])
(% with HIV [95% CI])	Prison	480 (4.4% [2.5–6.2])	365 (6.8% [4.3–9.4])	845 (5.4% [3.9–7.0])
	Total	31,191 (3.3% [3.1–3.5])	871 (7.7% [5.9–9.5])	32,062 (3.4% [3.2–3.6])
Homeless (number)	No prison	465 (7.1% [4.8–9.4])	86 (14.0% [6.6–21.3])	551 (8.2% [5.9–10.5])
(% with HIV [95% CI])	Prison	99 (3.0% [0.4–6.4])	149 (10.1% [5.2–14.9])	248 (7.3% [4.0–10.5])
	Total	564 (6.4% [4.4–8.4])	235 (11.5% [7.4–15.6])	799 (7.9% [6.0–9.8])
Not homeless (number)	No prison	30,246 (3.2% [3.0–3.4])	420 (7.1% [4.7–9.6])	30,666 (3.2% [3.0–3.4])
(% with HIV [95% CI])	Prison	381 (4.7% [2.6–6.9])	216 (4.6% [1.8–7.4])	597 (4.7% [3.0–6.4])
	Total	30,627 (3.2% [3.0–3.4])	636 (6.3% [4.4–8.2])	31,263 (3.3% [3.1–3.5])

Excluding 5899 (16%) cases missing data on homelessness ($n = 2693$), imprisonment ($n = 3719$) and/or drug misuse ($n = 2966$)
CI confidence interval

personally identifiable information (PII), meaning that record linkage to the TB data was necessary. The probabilistic algorithm we adapted has very high sensitivity (97.1%) and specificity (100.0%), even when PII such as NHS numbers and addresses are not available [14]. To reduce bias, we adapted the algorithm, removing the need for subjective manual review of borderline matches by replacing this step with deterministic record linkage [15]. The record linkage algorithm used ethnicity, year and country of birth to link cases, and although the completeness of these variables was high (Table 1), cases missing these variables (in either dataset) were less likely to be linked. It is therefore possible that we underestimated the prevalence of TB-HIV if we could not link some records due to missing data. We conducted sensitivity analyses, excluding weaker matches between TB and HIV records to assess whether risk factors differed for patients about whose HIV status we were less certain. These provided consistent results, suggesting that the matching algorithm did not affect our conclusions. Robust, high-quality national disease surveillance databases are essential for monitoring progress towards the WHO's sustainable development goals. Both the TB and HIV surveillance systems in the UK are of very high quality, but the inclusion of HIV status in the TB surveillance system, or the ability to link the two datasets using unique patient identifiers, would be beneficial for future research.

Most variables had little missing data; however, 19% of patients from 2010 to 2014 were missing some social risk factor data. These patients were more likely to be women or from the Indian sub-continent; both groups had low levels of social risk factors [1]. Consequently, any bias in our results will be towards the null, underestimating the association between TB and social risk factors.

We were only able to identify infected individuals with diagnosed HIV, and an estimated 13% of HIV infections were undiagnosed in 2015 [2]. However, 94% of people diagnosed with TB in 2015 received HIV testing or were already aware of their HIV status [1], and therefore we would expect very low prevalence of undiagnosed HIV in this population. There may be more undiagnosed HIV amongst patients prior to 2011, when testing TB patients for HIV became routine; however, most of these patients would have since presented to care and been linked in our dataset. As this was a retrospective, observational study of TB cases, we could not establish causality between HIV infection and TB disease, but it is likely that HIV infection precedes TB disease. Our study demonstrates a continuing risk of infection with HIV amongst patients with TB, supporting the guidance for universal HIV testing for all patients diagnosed with TB and highlighting the groups that should be prioritised for interventions that improve testing uptake.

Conclusions

TB-HIV infection has substantially decreased over the past decade in England, Wales and Northern Ireland, as has the proportion of patients diagnosed simultaneously with both infections. However, sub-populations of patients with high rates of infection remain. Whilst the current policy of testing all patients diagnosed with TB for HIV infection is important in ensuring appropriate management of TB patients, many of these TB cases would be preventable if HIV could be diagnosed before TB develops. Increasing HIV testing and ensuring early treatment of HIV infection in black African populations (particularly people born in countries with high HIV prevalence) and people with a history of drug misuse could help prevent these TB cases. The BHIVA guidelines on LTBI testing for PLHIV from sub-Saharan Africa remain relevant, and LTBI screening for PLHIV with a history of drug misuse, homelessness or imprisonment should also be considered.

Additional files

> **Additional file 1 Figure S1** The relationship between the timing of HIV and tuberculosis diagnoses in people diagnosed with HIV and tuberculosis between 2000 and 2014, by ethnicity.
>
> **Additional file 2 Figure S2** The relationship between the timing of HIV and tuberculosis diagnoses in people diagnosed with HIV and tuberculosis between 2000 and 2014, by route of HIV transmission.
>
> **Additional file 3 Table S1** HIV testing amongst TB cases, stratified by ethnicity and year, in England, Wales and Northern Ireland from 2011 to 2014. **Table S2** Results from univariable and two multivariable logistic regression models of factors associated with HIV infection, excluding year, in notified tuberculosis cases in England, Wales and Northern Ireland, for the periods 2000–2014 and 2010–2014. **Table S3** Sensitivity analyses, excluding TB cases with HIV co-infection where the match between the HIV and tuberculosis datasets was weak, for two multivariable logistic regression models of factors associated with HIV co-infection in notified tuberculosis cases in England, Wales and Northern Ireland, in 2000–2014 and 2010–2014.

Abbreviations
ART: Anti-retroviral therapy; BHIVA: British HIV Association; ETS: Enhanced Tuberculosis Surveillance; HARS: HIV and AIDS Reporting System; HIV: Human immunodeficiency virus; NHS: National Health Service; NICE: National Institute of Health and Care Excellence; OR: Odds ratio; PHE: Public Health England; PII: Personally identifying information; PLHIV: People living with HIV; TB: Tuberculosis; WHO: World Health Organization

Funding
JRW was funded by a University College London (UCL) IMPACT studentship. This report is the result of independent research supported by the National Institute for Health Research (NIHR, Post Doctoral Fellowship, HRS, PDF-2014-07-008). IA is supported by the NIHR (SRF-2011-04-001, NF-SI-0616-10037), the Medical Research Council, the UK Department of Health and the Wellcome Trust. The views expressed in this publication are those of the authors and not necessarily those of the NHS, the NIHR or the Department of Health. The funding source had no involvement in the study design; the collection, analysis and interpretation of the data; the writing of the report; or the decision to submit the paper for publication.

Authors' contributions

JRW designed the study, linked the TB and HIV surveillance datasets, conducted the analysis, interpreted the results and drafted the paper. HRS, CJS, ML, AP, IA and VD designed the study, interpreted the data and critically revised the paper. MKL, JAD, AEB, JB and DZ gave input on the study design, collected, linked and interpreted the data and revised the paper. All authors approved the final version of the paper for publication.

Competing interests

HRS reports grants from the National Institute of Health Research, outside the submitted work. CJS reports personal fees from Gilead and Janssen, outside the submitted work. AP is chair of the BHIVA guidelines committee. All other authors declare that they have no competing interests.

Author details

[1]Institute for Global Health, University College London, 30 Guildford Street, London WC1N 1EH, UK. [2]National Infections Service, Public Health England, 61 Colindale Avenue, London NW9 5EQ, UK. [3]Royal Free London National Health Service Foundation Trust, Royal Free Hospital, Pond Street, London NW3 2QG, UK. [4]UCL Respiratory, Division of Medicine, University College London, Royal Free Campus, Pond Street, London NW3 2PF, UK. [5]Chelsea and Westminster Hospital, 369 Fulham Road, London SW10 9NH, UK.

References

1. Public Health England. Tuberculosis in England: 2016 report. London: Public Health England; 2016.
2. Kirwan PD, et al. HIV in the UK — 2016 report. London: Public Health England; 2016.
3. Ahmed AB, et al. The growing impact of HIV infection on the epidemiology of tuberculosis in England and Wales: 1999-2003. Thorax. 2007;62(8):672–6.
4. Rice B, et al. Decreasing incidence of tuberculosis among heterosexuals living with diagnosed HIV in England and Wales. AIDS. 2013;27(7):1151–7.
5. Public Health England. Tuberculosis in England: 2015 report. London: Public Health England; 2015.
6. Public Health England. Tuberculosis in the UK: 2014 report. London: Public Health England; 2014.
7. Public Health England. Tuberculosis (TB): collaborative strategy for England. 2015; https://www.gov.uk/government/publications/collaborative-tuberculosis-strategy-for-england. Accessed 11 July 2017.
8. Haar CH, et al. HIV prevalence among tuberculosis patients in The Netherlands, 1993-2001: trends and risk factors. Int J Tuberc Lung Dis. 2006; 10(7):768–74.
9. Gupta RK, et al. Does antiretroviral therapy reduce HIV-associated tuberculosis incidence to background rates? A national observational cohort study from England, Wales, and Northern Ireland. Lancet HIV. 2015;2(6): e243–51.
10. Winter JR, et al. Injecting drug use predicts active tuberculosis in a national cohort of people living with HIV. AIDS. 2017;31(17):2403–13.
11. British HIV Association (BHIVA). UK National Guidelines for HIV Testing. London: BHIVA; 2008.
12. Gupta RK, et al. CD4+ cell count responses to antiretroviral therapy are not impaired in HIV-infected individuals with tuberculosis co-infection. AIDS. 2015;29(11):1363–8.
13. Zenner D, et al. Impact of TB on the survival of people living with HIV infection in England, Wales and Northern Ireland. Thorax. 2015;70(6):566–73.
14. Aldridge RW, et al. Accuracy of probabilistic linkage using the enhanced matching system for public health and epidemiological studies. PLoS One. 2015;10(8):e0136179.
15. Winter JR, et al. Linkage of UK HIV and tuberculosis data using probabilistic and deterministic methods. Conference on Retroviruses and Opportunistic Infections. Boston; 2016.
16. Department for Communities and Local Government. English Indices of Deprivation. 2015; https://www.gov.uk/government/collections/english-indices-of-deprivation. Accessed 20 May 2016.
17. Welsh Govenment. Welsh Index of Multiple Deprivation (WIMD). 2015; http://gov.wales/statistics-and-research/welsh-index-multiple-deprivation/?lang=en. 20 May 2016.
18. WHO Global Health Observatory. Prevalence of HIV among adults aged 15 to 49. Estimates by country (2000-2014). 2016; http://apps.who.int/gho/data/view.main.22500?lang=en. Accessed 28 Sept 2016.
19. Public Health England. National HIV surveillance data tables. 2016; https://www.gov.uk/government/statistics/hiv-annual-data-tables. Accessed 21 June 2017.
20. NICE, HIV testing: increasing uptake among people who may have undiagnosed HIV. 2011.
21. Kruijshaar, Abubakar I. Increase in extrapulmonary tuberculosis in England and Wales 1999-2006. Thorax. 2009;64(12):1090–5.
22. Fortun J, et al. Extra-pulmonary tuberculosis: differential aspects and role of 16S-rRNA in urine. Int J Tuberc Lung Dis. 2014;18(4):478–85.
23. Namme LH, et al. Extrapulmonary tuberculosis and HIV coinfection in patients treated for tuberculosis at the Douala General Hospital in Cameroon. Ann Trop Med Public Health. 2013;6(1):100–4.

Participatory design of an improvement intervention for the primary care management of possible sepsis using the Functional Resonance Analysis Method

Duncan McNab[1,2,3*], John Freestone[2], Chris Black[1,2], Andrew Carson-Stevens[4,5,6] and Paul Bowie[1,3]

Abstract

Background: Ensuring effective identification and management of sepsis is a healthcare priority in many countries. Recommendations for sepsis management in primary care have been produced, but in complex healthcare systems, an in-depth understanding of current system interactions and functioning is often essential before improvement interventions can be successfully designed and implemented. A structured participatory design approach to model a primary care system was employed to hypothesise gaps between work as intended and work delivered to inform improvement and implementation priorities for sepsis management.

Methods: In a Scottish regional health authority, multiple stakeholders were interviewed and the records of patients admitted from primary care to hospital with possible sepsis analysed. This identified the key work functions required to manage these patients successfully, the influence of system conditions (such as resource availability) and the resulting variability of function output. This information was used to model the system using the Functional Resonance Analysis Method (FRAM). The multiple stakeholder interviews also explored perspectives on system improvement needs which were subsequently themed. The FRAM model directed an expert group to reconcile improvement suggestions with current work systems and design an intervention to improve clinical management of sepsis.

Results: Fourteen key system functions were identified, and a FRAM model was created. Variability was found in the output of all functions. The overall system purpose and improvement priorities were agreed. Improvement interventions were reconciled with the FRAM model of current work to understand how best to implement change, and a multi-component improvement intervention was designed.

Conclusions: Traditional improvement approaches often focus on individual performance or a specific care process, rather than seeking to understand and improve overall performance in a complex system. The construction of the FRAM model facilitated an understanding of the complexity of interactions within the current system, how system conditions influence everyday sepsis management and how proposed interventions would work within the context of the current system.
This directed the design of a multi-component improvement intervention that organisations could locally adapt and implement with the aim of improving overall system functioning and performance to improve sepsis management.

Keywords: Quality improvement, Complexity, Functional resonance analysis method, Sepsis, Primary care

---

* Correspondence: Duncan.mcnab@nes.scot.nhs.uk
[1]NHS Education for Scotland, 2 Central Quay, Glasgow, Scotland G3 8BW, UK
[2]NHS Ayrshire and Arran, Ayr, UK
Full list of author information is available at the end of the article

Background

Sepsis is a life-threatening condition where tissue damage, organ failure and death may result due to the body's own response to infection [1, 2]. It is thought to cause at least six million deaths per annum worldwide, many of which are thought to be preventable with early recognition and treatment [1, 2]. There is international expert consensus that increased awareness, earlier presentation and detection, rapid administration of antibiotics and treatment according to locally developed guidelines can significantly reduce sepsis-related deaths [3, 4]. In secondary care, compliance with care protocols for patients with signs suggestive of sepsis is believed critical to improving outcomes and minimising sepsis-related deaths [5]. However, the implementation of sepsis management interventions has been problematic with only 10–20% of patients receiving care that is fully compliant with intervention recommendations [6, 7].

While a significant amount has been reported about work undertaken within the hospital setting to improve sepsis management, work in primary care is at a much earlier stage but has become a national priority in Scotland [8–11]. Presentations with infective conditions in this setting are exceedingly common, with only a very small proportion developing sepsis, while initial symptoms of sepsis can be vague—making early, accurate identification of patients who have sepsis or may develop it a challenge [12]. In several high-profile cases, primary care management of patients who had sepsis was thought to be inadequate [13, 14]. Guidelines to aid the identification of acutely ill patients who may have sepsis in primary care have been published that recommend the use of a structured set of clinical observations to stratify the risk of sepsis including pulse, temperature, blood pressure, respiratory rate, peripheral oxygen saturation and consciousness level [10].

Quality improvement (QI) as both a philosophy and suite of methods [15] has underpinned the design of major national preventive efforts to tackle sepsis internationally [16–18]. Recent perspectives on QI argue that in complex healthcare systems the design of improvement interventions risks being flawed if there is limited focus beforehand to gain a deep insight into how the system under study actually functions when things go right and wrong [19–26].

Primary healthcare has been described as a complex socio-technical system [28, 30]. Such systems consist of many dynamic and interacting components (e.g. clinicians, patients, tasks, information technology, protocols, equipment and culture) and are affected by rapid changes in conditions (such as patient deterioration, reduced staff capacity, increased patient demand, limited information and availability of resources) [28–31]. Often, different parts of systems can be closely coupled resulting in changes in one area affecting other areas in a non-linear, unpredictable manner. Rather than being purposively designed, systems of work often emerge and evolve over time due to the interactions between different components. People employ workarounds (for example, when information is not available) and trade-offs (such as when staff have to prioritise task efficiency over thoroughness) to achieve safe care [31–34]. "Work-as-done" (WAD), including performance adjustments, represents everyday work and is often different from "work-as-imagined" (WAI) as encapsulated in clinical guidelines and protocols and imagined by those in other parts of the system such as senior managers and policymakers.

Healthcare improvement projects to implement recommendations or clinical guidelines are often complex interventions that include multiple interacting and interdependent components; for example, education, new care protocols, new staff roles and new ways of accessing services [19, 20]. There is a growing awareness of the importance of understanding the complexity of current work and considering interactions between proposed interventions and the existing system in the planning and design stages of improvement projects to inform potential success [24–26].

The rationale for this study was to explore and better understand how acutely ill patients who may have sepsis are currently identified and managed in the community, obtain multiple perspectives on potential improvement interventions and determine how best these suggestions can inform the design of a system-centred improvement intervention.

Methods

The methods and results of this project have been reported in keeping with current, best practice guidelines advised by Tong et al. [35]. A COREQ checklist (Additional file 1) is included as Table 6 in Appendix 1.

Clinical setting

The study was conducted in a primary care setting within a single, Scottish, regional health board, NHS (National Health Service) Ayrshire and Arran (NHSAA). The identification and management of sepsis is a priority patient safety improvement focus for NHSAA but the best way to design and implement a related intervention in community settings was not clear to local clinical leaders, management and improvement advisors. To access appropriate treatment including antibiotics and fluid management, patients may self-present at the hospital Emergency Department (ED) either by themselves or through telephoning for an ambulance. Alternatively, they may be assessed in the community by a general practitioner (GP) or advanced nurse practitioner (ANP). During normal working hours (8:00 am to 6:00 pm Monday to Friday), clinical assessment is arranged by GP reception staff, while at other times it is arranged by NHS24 (a special national health board within NHS

Scotland that provides health information and facilitates patient access to primary care out-of-hours services provided regionally by Ayrshire Doctors On Call (ADOC)). Other healthcare professionals, such as nurses who work in the community and in nursing care homes, can arrange out-of-hours clinical review directly using the single point of contact (SPOC—a non-clinical administrative member of staff who arranges ADOC appointments directly based on the instruction from the healthcare professionals). If, after clinical assessment, it is thought that admission is required, clinicians discuss secondary care assessment with colleagues in the Combined Medical Assessment Unit (CMAU) and then forward documentation summarising their findings and presumed diagnosis and arrange transport.

Study design

A mixed methods approach, including semi-structured interviews, group interviews and documentary analysis, was used to identify system functions and their interactions and output variability to inform a contextually grounded design of a Functional Resonance Analysis Method (FRAM) model [36, 37]. Multiple clinical, management and administrative perspectives on potential system improvements were identified and themed. A participatory design approach [38] using a key stakeholder workshop was then used to reflect on FRAM findings and improvement suggestions and identify and agree improvement interventions based on a systems approach to this issue.

Functional Resonance Analysis Method (FRAM)

The Functional Resonance Analysis Method (FRAM) is one way to begin to model and understand non-trivial, complex, socio-technical systems [36]. The FRAM involves exploring "work-as-done" with frontline workers to identify the "functions" that are being performed. A function is defined as "the activities—or set of activities—that are required to produce a certain outcome" [36]. Identified system functions are entered into the FRAM Model Visualiser software (FMV). FRAM studies the relationships within a system by exploring potential interactions between functions to identify coupling between different parts of the system. To achieve this, links are created between functions by identifying six specific aspects of each function: input, output, preconditions, resources, controls and time factors (Table 1). For example, the output of a function <book appointment> is <appointment booked> which is a precondition of the function <perform clinical assessment>. A key component of the FRAM is to study and record the variability of the output of each function. Functional resonance refers to how variability of different functions can combine to produce amplified and unpredicted effects (both wanted and unwanted).

Table 1 Aspects of FRAM functions

Aspect	Description	Example for function <perform clinical assessment>
Input (I)	What the function acts on or changes and starts the function	Patient arriving at the consulting room
Output (O)	What emerges from the function—this can be an outcome or a state change	Clinical assessment complete
Precondition (P)	Some condition that must be met before the function can start	Appointment booked
Resources (R)	Anything (people, information, materials) needed to carry out the function or anything that is used up by the function	Thermometer, stethoscope
Control (C)	Anything that controls or monitors the function	Protocol or guidelines
Time (T)	Time constraint that may influence the function	10-min consultation

The FRAM is one method to facilitate the adoption of a complex systems approach. Exploring and building a model of work-as-done allows consideration of how people adapt to deal with unexpected clinical presentations, system conditions (such as availability of information or time) and competing goals (such as efficiency and thoroughness). Exploring how these adaptations combine with variability elsewhere in the system encourages a shift from considering systems as linear, where event A causes outcome B in a predictable manner, to adopting a complex systems approach to focus on the relationships between components and how outcomes emerge from these interactions. FRAM has previously been used in healthcare to explore the complexity of the system for taking blood prior to blood transfusion [39] and to guide implementation of guidelines [40] by exploring current work systems with health care professionals to ensure proposed changes were compatible with current ways of working. It is used regularly in parts of Denmark to explore complex systems in order to plan improvements [41].

Real linkages can only be found by looking at the system with a specified set of conditions, such as an event that has occurred or by predicting how a particular event may occur—these are called instantiations. The linkages present in any given instantiation are a subset of all the potential linkages in the FRAM model and can be used to understand how historical events occurred, consider how the system may perform in varying conditions or how system performance may be altered by change to one function. The FRAM also describes variability of function output. This variability, or functional resonance, reflects the normal, everyday variability of function output caused by altering system conditions and the adaptations people employ to continue successful operations in these conditions. Rather than being quantified, variability is recorded as present or not within a function and can be described as too early, on time, too late, not at all, precise, acceptable and imprecise. Resonance (or variability) in one function can combine with resonance in other functions and lead to unpredicted outcomes both positive and negative.

Study participants
A pragmatic, purposive sampling strategy was employed to identify appropriate healthcare professionals working in primary, secondary and interface care settings with experience and knowledge of their part of the NHSAA Sepsis identification and management system who were then invited to participate in semi-structured interviews. Twenty-two healthcare professionals and administrators were contacted by email and all agreed to participate. Fifteen interviews were completed (Table 2).

To assess variability of functions, ADOC were asked to provide relevant out-of-hours data and a pragmatic, convenience sample of NHSAA general practices was approached to provide in-hours data (Table 3). Twenty (of 55 NHSAA) general practices were asked to provide data on recent admissions of which eight practices returned requested data (40%).

Data collection and analysis
The following data collection, interpretation and analytical methods were applied to enable construction of a preliminary FRAM Model, identify and theme improvement suggestions and design an improvement intervention.

Semi-structured interviews
Fifteen semi-structured, face-to-face, individual ($n = 11$) and group ($n = 4$) interviews were conducted at the

Table 2 List of interviews

Professional role	Number of interviewees	Individual or group interview
General practitioners with both in-hours and out-of-hours roles	4	Individual
GP specialty trainee—who work both in and out-of-hours	1	Individual
In-hours ANPs	2	Group
Out-of-hours advanced nurse practitioners	1	Individual
NHS 24 nursing staff	5	Group
ADOC administrative staff (single point of contact and reception staff)	2	Individual
Combined assessment unit (secondary care) senior nurse	1	Individual
Accident and emergency senior nurse	1	Individual
Accident and emergency consultant	1	Individual
General practice receptionist	2	Group
Community nurses	2	Group

Table 3 Data extracted from ADOC electronic records

Date and time seen
Age
Case summary (consultation text and values)
Diagnostic codes applied
Priority assigned by NHS24 (to be seen within 1, 2 or 4 h)
The use of a specific sepsis template (yes/no)

participants' place of work by DM. Only DM, who is a GP in the area and an experienced qualitative researcher, and the participants were present during interviews, and no repeat interviews were conducted. The duration of interviews was from 22 to 54 min. Study aims were explained and a definition of sepsis was provided to participants. Interviews were informed by an inductive approach [42] and structured in design to ensure data collection identified functions and their aspects to construct the FRAM model and suggestions for system improvement.

GP in-hours data
Participating GP practices ($n = 8$) provided data on their last ten admissions for adults with a presumed infective cause (chest infection, urine infection, cellulitis or other presumed infective cause based on the recorded consultation). A worksheet was completed by either a GP within the practice or the practice manager to record if the following were explicitly stated in the admission letter: patient's pulse, temperature, oxygen saturations, blood pressure, a comment on level of consciousness and if a working diagnosis of sepsis or possible sepsis was noted.

GP out-of-hours data
Anonymised data for all acute hospital admissions was extracted from the ADOC computer system for a full calendar month in 2016 and downloaded to MS Excel Software [Microsoft Corporation, version 12.0 / 2007] for analysis (Table 3). Patients aged 16 or over admitted with a suspected infective cause were identified and selected by the lead author (DM). The Microsoft Excel random number generator was used to select 50 patient cases, which the research team agreed should be sufficient to provide evidence of variability within this part of the system.

Identification of system functions and aspects
All individual and group interviews with participants were audio-recorded and transcribed with consent. A systematic and iterative approach to analysis of the interview data based on the constant comparative method was adopted [43]. Transcription text was read and re-read by DM to facilitate a deep understanding of the data. Functions required in the current system for the identification and management of sepsis were identified and treated as themes. Responses were coded within QDA Miner [Provalis Research, Montreal, Canada,

Table 4 Functions from the Functional Resonance Analysis Method (FRAM) model

Function	Description of influence of system conditions on function and output variability Data from audit in bold Quotes from interviews in italics
a) Process request for clinical assessment NHS24	• Capacity/demand mismatches (more requests from patients to speak to staff than number of staff available to meet this demand) may delay commencement of this function. • Staff reported deviating from the algorithm (which may be considered a control) when necessary in an attempt to achieve success ○ *We have got the algorithm but quickly you learn that it's only a guide. I mean, when I was new I used to stick to it but now I do not refer to it. I mean I know it in my head anyway, but I ask other things and get them to hold the phone next to them to hear the breathing, ask them if they feel warm and ask them about confusion. I think that is more helpful.* NHS24 • Variability of assigned triage times was observed with no association between triage time and the likelihood of a patient subsequently being admitted with suspected sepsis. **NHS24 triage time, n (%), when admitted with infective cause from out-of-hours** ○ 1 h = 12 (24) ○ 2 h = 18 (36) ○ 4 h = 20 (40) **NHS24 triage time, n (%), when sepsis suspected at out of hours** ○ 1 h = 7 (24) ○ 2 h = 10 (34) ○ 4 h = 12 (41)
b) Process request for clinical assessment GP surgery	• There was a difference between work-as-done by administrative staff and work-as-imagined by the GPs. ○ *In general… our staff are good at saying this person doesn't sound well and they are concerned and they don't call often and they let us know so they will put it onto the emergency doctor.* GP3 ○ *I don't know if I would necessarily recognise it in a patient coming in because a lot of it is like fever and sickness - it could be anything. Training or a checklist may help.* Receptionist 2 ○ *I think it is easy for us to recognise someone that comes in with chest pains rather than someone who comes in with sepsis.* Receptionist 1 • Capacity/demand issues influenced function output resulting in staff taking less time to assess potential urgency of the medical condition at busy periods. ○ *It can be quite hard on a Monday morning when you have got lots of patients waiting for an on-the-day appointment and we just get a sea of people it would be quite hard to say then could you give me indication of the problem.* Receptionist 2 • Resources such as training, experience and knowledge of the patient were also thought to influence function output. • There were no guidelines or protocols in place for staff. These may act as potentially beneficial controls that help staff to decide actions such as the urgency of speaking to a GP—when to interrupt and when to wait. ○ *I think it's difficult I don't think they have had adequate training on it I don't think years of practice or as a Health Board have addressed training for admin reception type staff.* GP3
c) Process request for clinical assessment by an out-of-hours clinician via the single point of contact	• Output was based on the information given by community healthcare workers and was thought to be variable. • There was no guidance to direct the required urgency of clinical assessment.
d) Perform clinical assessment	• Resource availability to aid clinical assessment was thought to be adequate in both in-hours and out-of-hours care. • In-hours electronic templates were thought to be more useful. ○ *In the surgery we have a template we use that is easy and helpful.* GPANP ○ *The out-of-hours template makes it more difficult – you see it when you are back in the car writing up the case after you have made your decision – it's too late. I think if it was quick, easy and straightforward you might get better recording (of observations).* GP2 • Clinicians stated that patients with possible sepsis would take more time to assess and manage. This was not thought to influence actions with these patients, but would cause increased time pressure when consulting with subsequent patients. ○ *Time is a major factor although when you are dealing it is not a factor because you blank everything else out and you deal with it - you have to suck it up after.* GPANP ○ *I think often these patients are unwell so you take the time anyway.* GPANP • It was felt that the lack of information available through the Key Information Summary (KIS), an electronic summary of important clinical and social information created by the patient's GP practice and available to out-of-hours GPs and secondary care, could influence clinical assessment as usual physiological parameters were not available

Table 4 Functions from the Functional Resonance Analysis Method (FRAM) model (Continued)

Function	Description of influence of system conditions on function and output variability Data from audit in bold Quotes from interviews in italics

e) Create and maintain KIS	• The information contained in KIS was noted to be variable by GPs and by hospital teams. This was thought to reflect both a lack of guidance on completion and lack of time to perform this task properly by in-hours clinical teams.
	  ○ *I think it is variable sometimes it is excellent (the KIS) and it makes such a difference - and then other times it is not - and I think that is probably one of the reasons why it is not being accessed strategically because it is not the easiest or quickest thing to get into and it is almost like a lottery if you get one that is going to help you or not.* AE cons
	  ○ *I know it is hard to find the time during the day to complete these (KIS) but in OOH the most important things I have is background observation and base line observations.* GP
	  ○ *In out of hours and you have a confused buddy you don't have any background information. You have no carer to tell you why, there is no relative it is very tricky there is a good chance you are going to miss something. Then as you don't know if they are confused normally - you don't know anything - so that makes it tricky.* GP2

f) Record patient observations in clinical record	• In May 2016, there were a total of 731 admissions via ADOC, of which 592 were patients aged 16 or over (Table 5). Of these, 270 were for a presumed infective cause (66.2%).
	Out-of-hours
	All physiological parameters present to calculate NEWS score.
	• **Those with infective cause: 32 of 50 (64%)**
	• **Those with presumed sepsis: 10 of 29 (34%)**
	• **NEWS score never calculated**
	• **Electronic template used in 5 patients (10%)**
	In-hours
	All physiological parameters present to calculate NEWS score.
	• **Those with infective cause: 11 of 76 (14.5%)**
	• **Those with presumed sepsis: 2 of 11 (18.2%)**
	• Recording of observations in out-of-hours was higher than in-hours and varied between practices. Despite the out-of-hours templates being described as a less usable resource, clinicians described feeling more vulnerable in an out-of-hours setting and were more likely to record all values. Most clinicians discussed measuring and recording physiological parameters to aid diagnosis and to defend themselves if something went wrong, but were not aware if secondary care colleagues found this information useful.
	  ○ *I feel in out of hours you don't know the patient so well so I am very precise in out of hours of recording observations and I think it would be a good idea if more people did that.* GP
	• All physiological parameters were recorded less frequently for patients admitted with presumed sepsis, as opposed to an infective cause where sepsis was not suspected. One GP reported that once the decision to admit a patient had been made, further observations were not made. This was felt to be a beneficial trade-off to deal with the competing goals of efficiency versus thoroughness.
	  ○ *I saw this man on a visit and from the moment I walked in I knew I was admitting him. We had the information that he was getting chemo and was a bit shaky, I did his temp and pulse and thought – right you are going in – so I did not do the other values.* GP2

g) Decide to admit patient	• This function was thought to vary dependent on the clinical picture and also clinician experience.
	  ○ *I think it is variable I think it is probably clinician dependant. Experience dependant. Possibly patient dependant or practice dependant.* GP1
	• The lack of time to observe the trajectory of the patient condition was reported.
	  ○ *The fact so many other things could be going on and the rapidly changing clinical picture cause you have only 10-15 maybe 20 mins, if you are lucky, with the patients.* GP1
	• Some clinicians used early warning scoring systems to aid decision making. These involve assigning a value to each physiological value and calculating a composite score to stratify risk. Others felt such scores were not helpful as routinely recording early warning scores would make normal work more difficult to do (through extra time to calculate and record scores).
	  ○ *I do observations - I probably do a version of NEWS …. and I make the clinical decision based on that.* GP2
	• The overall clinical picture was felt to be a more important indicator of the severity of illness.
	  ○ *You have got to put it together with other observations and clinical picture and the history it gives you more weight, it is all about picking up things that help you make your decision.* GP4
	• When a patient comes through SPOC we do not get KIS access – surely this could be changed. GP1
	  ○ *It would be good to have access to previous notes to help decision making.* GP1

Table 4 Functions from the Functional Resonance Analysis Method (FRAM) model (Continued)

Function	Description of influence of system conditions on function and output variability Data from audit in bold Quotes from interviews in italics
h) Transfer patient to secondary care	• One GP reported that specialty trainees, who he supervised, usually ordered an immediate ambulance if sepsis was considered whereas, if the patient was relatively stable, he may order an ambulance that would transfer the patient to hospital within one hour. Variability in this area was thought to relate to a lack of guidance on transfer urgency. ◦ *I dunno...I suppose we should get a blue light ambulance.. yeah that's what the trainees I supervise do. Sometimes I have arranged a 1 h though... I mean not if they are like very ill but if some of their obs are off but they are still well enough.* GP2

i) Communicate with secondary care	• Variability was seen in the output of this function. Secondary care clinicians reported that the number of physiological parameters communicated during admission was variable. In addition, the use of the word sepsis to alert secondary care colleagues that the patient being admitted may require immediate clinical assessment was variable.
	   ◦ *In OOH there is a variation of what information we get a lot of times em so the girls manning the phone will still ask the same questions it just that information isn't always to hand it is person dependent.* CAU
	• So, the most important thing for us is the more warning we have - and clear communication comes is really helpful - because as soon as the word sepsis is used it will precipitate a certain response amongst our team. AE
	   ◦ *I don't think I have ever used the word sepsis I am admitting this patient with sepsis.* GPANP
	   ◦ *I would describe the situation rather than say sepsis maybe I should say sepsis.* GP2

j) Assess in secondary care	• It was felt that the variability of information received in admission communication and in the KIS had the potential to influence this function and result in delayed assessment, treatment and possible poorer patient outcomes.
	   ◦ *Right we know this patient is coming we are expecting him as soon as that ambulance arrives they are straight into our resus bay where the team are waiting.* CAU
	   ◦ *I think if there has been abnormal physiology it is useful to have that documented.* AE

k) Perform assessment of patient by community healthcare staff	• The output of this function was influenced by lack of available resources (thermometers, oxygen saturation monitors) and absence of controls - guidance on how to assess patients, what information should be communicated to clinical colleagues and to guide urgency of clinical review. ◦ *I know that the chemo folk need admitted and we are able to call the surgery to get a GP to see them. At the weekend, we can use the SPOC [single point of contact] to directly request a GP visit but I am not sure how quickly that [visit] happens.* Community nurse

l) Make guidelines available to clinical staff	• NHS24 had electronic versions of guidelines and two GPs reported having and using an electronic smart phone application for sepsis management. Others were not aware of new guidance or did not know where it could be accessed.
	   ◦ *I have not seen the new guidelines.* GP4
	   ◦ *I mean if there were some guidelines - get guidelines out.* GP2
	   ◦ *I do carry the [sepsis] app.* GP1

m) Educate clinicians on sepsis management	• Educational meetings were considered valuable in raising awareness of guidelines for sepsis management by those that attended them, but many had not attended any local learning events. Other forms of delivering targeted education were suggested. ◦ *Education sessions trying to get people to engage – different people like different things and meetings are not suitable for everyone so not everyone has attended before.* GP2

n) Maintain and stock equipment	• Variable access to resources such as thermometers and saturation monitors was reported by community nurses. For both in-hours and out-of-ours GPs and ANPs, this was thought to be adequate.
	   ◦ *Most of the time in ADOC you have the thermometer and stuff and have spare batteries - I have never had a problem with that.* GP1
	   ◦ *In the surgery there is everything you need but I suppose sometimes I have to go and find stuff. I mean like a thermometer or a sats monitor.* GPANP
	   ◦ *We do not carry thermometers or sats monitors.* DNs

Version 1.4.6.0, 2002] based on these themes. The data for each theme was analysed to identify aspects of each function. All data were cross checked with other authors with any disagreements resolved by discussion until consensus was achieved. Finally, system functions and aspects were uploaded to FMV software [Zerprize, New Zealand, Version 0.4.1, 2016].

Assessment of variability of function output

Variability of function output was assessed through analysis of interview data for reported variability in function output. In addition, out-of-hours and in-hours admission data was analysed to determine the number and percentage of patients with each physiological parameter recorded, the number and percentage with all parameters recorded and the median number of physiological parameters recorded per patient. The median was calculated as it was thought that some practices may have either very high or very low levels of recording physiological parameters [44]. For out-of-hours admissions, the use of an electronic template for recording observations and priority (1, 2 or 4 h) assigned by NHS24 was recorded. This was determined for all patients and separately for those with a presumed diagnosis of sepsis. Variability of function output was entered into the FMV software.

Design of improvement intervention

A separate thematic analysis identified suggested areas for system improvement. Suggestions from interviewees were coded in QDA Miner by DM and arranged into themes through discussion of codes by authors (DM, JF and CB). A workshop was held for key local stakeholders with primary care management, leadership and frontline clinical roles ($n = 6$) to both validate the FRAM model and gain consensus on improvement priorities and strategies. Through discussion, the FRAM model was used to reconcile improvement suggestions with work-as-done and consensus was sought on the design of an improvement intervention. A Driver Diagram was constructed to link the overall aim of the project with the major improvement drivers identified enabling a multi-component improvement intervention strategy to be designed [45]. Consensus was deemed to have been reached when full agreement was achieved by all attendees.

Results
FRAM model

Fourteen foreground system functions were identified with description of the function and output variability outlined in Tables 4 and 5 (Fig. 1). Seventeen background functions were required to complete the FRAM model of which the key stakeholder group felt ten were relevant to discussions on improvement intervention design. For example, the function <Create guidance on KIS completion> was not the focus of the FRAM; therefore, its aspects were not explored, meaning it only had an output and was thus a background function. It was considered relevant in the design of the improvement intervention as change to this function may influence the function <Create and maintain KIS>. In contrast, it was thought that an intervention would be unlikely to influence the background function <Manage staff capacity> and so this was not included in the FRAM model that was discussed.

Co-design of improvement intervention

Six improvement intervention themes were identified comprising of (1) feedback to facilitate reflective learning, (2) improving communication pathways, (3) use of early warning scores, (4) improving electronic template for

Table 5 Recording of physiological parameters admissions data

Data set	Mean age	Number of physiological parameters recorded per patient (max 6) median (interquartile range)	Temp, n (%)	Pulse, n (%)	BP, n (%)	Saturations, n (%)	Resp rate, n (%)	Consciousness level, n (%)	All physiological parameters present to calculate NEWS score, n (%)
Out-of-hours admissions diagnosed as possible infection ($n = 50$)	66.2	5 (1)	50 (100)	50 (100)	48 (96)	45 (90)	31 (62)	38 (76)	32 (64)
Out-of-hours admissions diagnosed as sepsis or possible sepsis ($n = 29$)	66.1	5 (1)	29 (100)	28 (97)	20 (69)	26 (90)	18 (62)	22 (76)	10 (34)
In hours patients diagnosed with possible infection ($n = 76$)	Not recorded	4 (2)	53 (69.7)	66 (86.8)	40 (52.6)	53 (69.7)	42 (55.2)	37 (48.7)	11 (14.5)
In-hours patients where sepsis considered diagnosis ($n = 11$)	Not recorded	4 (1)	10 (90.9)	10 (90.9)	6 (54.5)	7 (63.6)	6 (54.5)	6 (54.5)	2 (18.2)

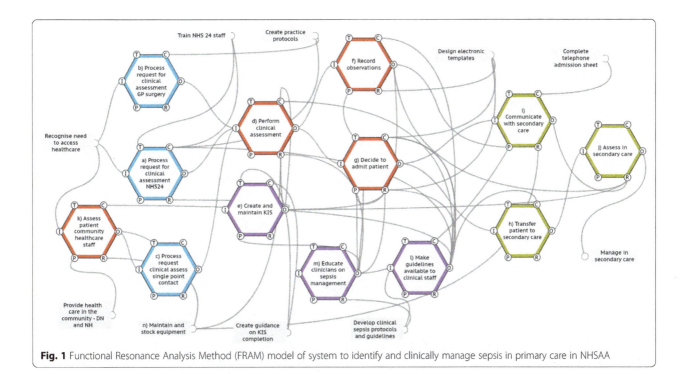

Fig. 1 Functional Resonance Analysis Method (FRAM) model of system to identify and clinically manage sepsis in primary care in NHSAA

recording physiological parameters, (5) provision of sepsis education and (6) improving KIS completion.

1) Feedback to facilitate reflective learning

Many of the professionals interviewed stated that they wanted feedback on their own practice to facilitate learning but this was rarely given. A system-based reflective tool was developed to direct practice teams to reflect on their current systems. This could be used to investigate events when patients were diagnosed with sepsis or to prospectively examine their systems and share learning within teams on how they manage difficult system conditions. The tool provided data from the FRAM to encourage individual and team reflection on their role in the overall system and how this influences other parts of the system. This included how work-as-imagined and work-as-done differ in areas such as arranging clinical review, assessing patients and communication across interfaces.

For example, practice teams were encouraged to analyse their own recording of physiological parameters and compare this to the data collected when constructing the FRAM. It was felt that recording, interpreting and communicating the individual physiological parameters was essential to successfully recognise and manage patients who may be at risk of sepsis. This is demonstrated in the FRAM model which shows that the function <record observations> links to four other functions (<decide to admit patient>, <communicate with secondary care>, <transfer patient to secondary care> and <assess in secondary care>). Variability in this function could influence all of these functions (Fig. 2).

Clinicians were much more likely to record physiological parameters in an out-of-hours setting than an in-hours setting. This was due to feeling that out-of-hours work was riskier as they did not know the patients as well as those seen in their own practices during normal in-hours working.

> I feel in out of hours you don't know the patient so well so I am very precise in out of hours of recording observations and I think it would be a good idea if more people did that. GP1

When patients were admitted and the diagnosis was thought to be sepsis, it was less likely that all physiological parameters were recorded. Clinicians recognised that this was due to employing an efficiency thoroughness trade off based on making a rapid decision to quickly admit patients who appeared acutely ill and so did not record all parameters.

> I saw this man on a visit and from the moment I walked in I knew I was admitting him. We had the information that he was getting chemo and was a bit shaky. I did his temp and pulse and thought – right you're going in – so I didn't do the other values. GP2

Although this is an effective trade-off from the GP perspective, this physiological information is considered extremely important when the patient is assessed in secondary care which was not fully appreciated by those in the community.

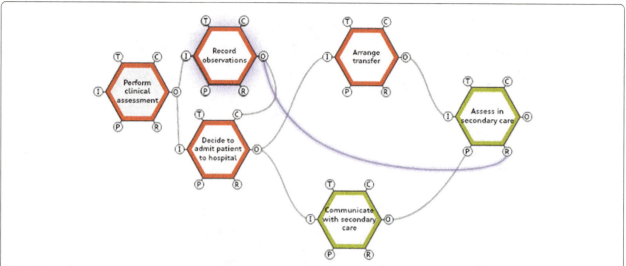

Fig. 2 Extract from Functional Resonance Analysis Method (FRAM) model demonstrating importance of recording observations to other functions in the system

I think if there has been abnormal physiology it is useful to have that documented. AE

Teams were asked to reflect on their own data and the presented data to consider if changes to local systems were required. Trade-offs and performance variability are needed in complex healthcare systems, but it is essential that we understand the potential effects at a local and wider system level through exploring and understanding the system [34, 46].

2) Communication pathways

Physiological parameter values were important when the patient is assessed in hospital (Fig. 2). The results of this project fed into existing work-streams on communication between primary and secondary care. During telephone admission calls to the secondary care combined assessment unit, all physiological parameters will routinely be requested by receiving staff. This allows a degree of flexibility for community staff while still encouraging communication of all parameters.

3) Use of early warning scores

Although early warning scores have been endorsed as a way to detect acute illness due to sepsis, there were mixed opinions on the use of early warning score.

There is much more of a push to do observations which I think gives you more of an objective measurement which might push someone towards a potential sepsis rather than just an unwell diagnosis and make you act a bit more promptly. GPST3

I think [a score] gives you more weight to make the decision that this person is unwell - Even young people for example could be septic and still look alright you know. GP4

I don't think it would change what I do much it would just be more to stimulate me to remember more things. GP2

Yeah and I think a lot of the times when you have this scoring system we are taking away people's common sense it is just a scoring system, it's just a helpful tool it shouldn't replace your clinical judgement. CAU senior nurse

There is less evidence for the use of a "one off" early warning score in the community to identify patients with possible sepsis as opposed to repeatedly recording early warning scores to identify clinical deterioration of a patient. It was felt that the use of an early warning score did not fit with the way that GPs currently worked as they were more likely to consider the whole clinical situation. They felt that the interpretation of parameters and the communication of concern between health professionals were more important than the calculation of the score which also increased workload.

You have got to put it together with other observations and clinical picture and the history it gives you more weight, it is all about picking up things that help you make your decision. GP4

There was concern by some clinicians that if early warning scores were used as part of a QI intervention, compliance would be rigidly monitored reducing scope for clinicians to adapt their behaviour to suit the patient in front of them and the work conditions experienced. Instead, a less rigid approach was recommended focussing on the social aspects of communicating across interfaces and providing opportunity for feedback to encourage reflection on when and why to record physiological parameters.

> But people want every box ticked. Because someone will audit it, someone will look at it and then they will come round and go like we have had a complaint from a patient who had a sore throat turned out two days later he had quinsy you don't seem to have recorded saturations on him. GP1

Despite this, it was agreed that the early warning score may be useful to communicate with professionals in other parts of the system, for example, ambulance services or community nurses. To test this, a pilot project was planned involving community nurses using early warning scores to assess patients and communicate with clinicians in an out of hours setting. Study of the FRAM allowed anticipation of potential problems when implementing these changes by identifying functions that would be influenced by the intervention (Fig. 3). Systems need to be in place to ensure availability of resources such as thermometers and oxygen saturation monitors for community nurses. The output of community nurse assessment will direct the priority of clinical review required. Communication and escalation policies will be required to direct this process for the single point of contact and clinicians.

4) Electronic template for recording physiological parameters

The existing electronic templates were non-intuitive and did not fit with the way work was currently done. Because of this mismatch, clinicians used workarounds such as hand-writing values or typing them into the electronic record as free text. The template available on the in-hours system was considered more useful as it provided information to aid interpretation of results but it often still took time to find and open. Some practices had created shortcuts to allow its use within the consultation—a code, that when typed, automatically opened the template. The

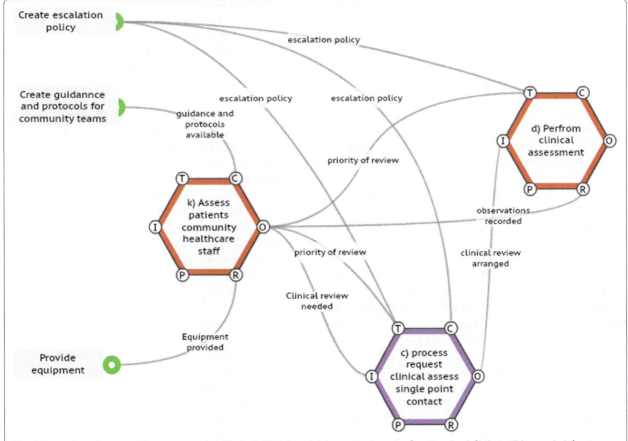

Fig. 3 Extract from Functional Resonance Analysis Method (FRAM) model demonstrating extra functions (on left) that will be needed if system is changed

out-of-hours template was rarely used as values had to be entered after the clinician had left the patient and so any guidance from the template came too late.

> The out-of-hours template makes it more difficult – you see it when you are back in the car writing up the case after you have made your decision – it's too late. I think if it was quick, easy and straightforward you might get better recording (of observations). GP2

The stakeholder group recommended the design of an electronic template that fits with the current work to make its use as simple as hand written notes or free text entries. Work is underway to develop a template to alert clinicians in real time to abnormal physiological parameters that may prompt recording of all relevant parameters with automatic calculation of an early warning score.

5) Provision of sepsis training

By exploring multiple perspectives, the FRAM helped identify the conditions of work that result in divergence of work-as-imagined by clinicians and work-as-done by administrative staff. Clinicians generally thought that their administrative staff could accurately identify patients who may need early assessment and knew how to arrange this. However, administrative staff felt that they had no training or guidance on how to identify patients who may be at risk of sepsis and often had no clear advice on how to arrange rapid review.

> In general, our staff are good at saying this person doesn't sound well and they are concerned and they don't call often and they let us know so they will put it onto the emergency doctor. GP3

> I don't know if I would necessarily recognise it in a patient coming in because a lot of it is like fever and sickness - it could be anything. Training or a checklist may help. Receptionist 2

System conditions affected the output of the function describing staff arranging clinical review and so, even with training, staff may not be able to successfully identify and deal with patients who may have sepsis. This information was used to design educational materials that accompany the system-based reflective tool. The aim is to allow teams to consider how the sepsis education material can be applied in their own setting to improve care. For example, if staff are more aware of the vague symptoms that may indicate risk of sepsis (such as confusion) they need a way to raise their concerns with clinical staff and the clinical staff need a way to respond flexibility dependent on the situation (such as knowledge of patient and competing priorities).

> It can be quite hard on a Monday morning when you have got lots of patients waiting for an on-the-day appointment and we just get a sea of people it would be quite hard to say then could you give me indication of the problem. Receptionist 2

> I think it is easy for us to recognise someone that comes in with chest pains rather than someone who comes in with sepsis. Receptionist 1

> I need to be able to go to someone comfortably and say I am just raising this. To make you aware as I am concerned. Receptionist 2

6) KIS completion

The importance of the Key Information Summary became clear when interviewing professionals in different parts of the system and was demonstrated within the FRAM model (Fig. 4). Work was already underway locally to improve KIS completion in terms of identifying patients appropriate for KIS completion and recording relevant details such as usual oxygen level, pulse, blood pressure, level of confusion and wishes regarding ceilings of care. The FRAM model was used to inform further work in this work-stream as well as providing evidence in the system-based reflective tool of the importance of this task elsewhere in the system.

> I think it is variable sometimes it is excellent (the KIS) and it makes such a difference - and then other times it isn't - and I think that is probably one of the reasons why it is not being accessed strategically because it is not the easiest or quickest thing to get into and it is almost like it is a bit like a lottery if you get one that is going to help you or not. AE consultant

> I know it is hard to find the time during the day to complete these (KIS) but in OOH the most important things I have is background observation and base line observations. GP

It was also identified that the KIS was not available when the SPOC was used to refer patients to primary care out-of-hours clinicians. Information Technology systems were altered to solve this problem.

Following consideration of each improvement theme, consensus was reached on the design of a Driver Diagram and multi-component improvement intervention (Figure 5, Appendices 1 and 2). It was agreed that the overall purpose of the system was the identification and management of sepsis in the community. The boundary of the system

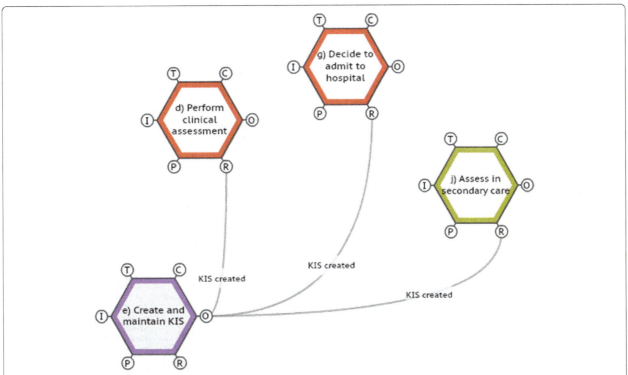

Fig. 4 Extract from Functional Resonance Analysis Method (FRAM) model demonstrating the importance of the Key Information Summary (KIS) to several functions in the system

for improvement excluded NHS24 as this was a national organisation over which we would have little influence.

Discussion

In this paper, we described how a FRAM model of the complex system to identify and manage sepsis in primary care was constructed to understand how conditions of work and system interactions influenced everyday work in a regional NHS Board. This information directly allowed reconciliation between improvement suggestions from frontline staff and current works systems and informed the design of a multi-component improvement intervention to improve overall system functioning.

Despite the complex systems that exist in healthcare, many improvement projects fail to take a "systems approach", or misunderstand and misapply this concept. Many seek to introduce new procedures in a top-down manner or implement change and improvement at the level of individual performance through, for example, audit and feedback strategies [24, 47]. As a result, the focus of many interventions has been on single-system components such as performing a clinical assessment more reliably or effectively [48–51]. Improvement interventions often target the person through education and training, protocol dissemination or recommend the use of a tool or technology, such as an IT template or early warning scores [49–51]. Educational interventions alone are considered weak as they depend on memory of training whereas introducing tools or technology to aid recall is considered to be of intermediate strength as an improvement intervention [52]. Evaluation of such interventions involves measuring compliance (of the component targeted) with the proposed change. It is thought that this attempt to reduce process variation will improve health outcomes [53]. However, the evidence frequently demonstrates that these types of interventions often fail to have the sustainable impact anticipated leading to missed opportunities to improve system performance and reduce avoidable patient harm [28].

Rather than persisting with linear, cause and effect approaches, the use of a complex system lens may help to maximise the impact of improvement interventions [26, 27]. One way to do this is to engage the people in the system who are expert at doing the work to both understand the system and identify potential improvements [26]. In this way, improvement strategies can be co-designed that consider important contextual factors when implementing change and include strategies to support local adaptation to cope with the conditions faced [34, 54]. In this study, the interventions did not over specify work by mandating and measuring the use of early warning scores but encouraged recording and communication of physiological parameters while allowing clinicians to adapt if needed based on the conditions they experience. The edges of systems are blurry and interact with other systems [26]. As such, treating sepsis

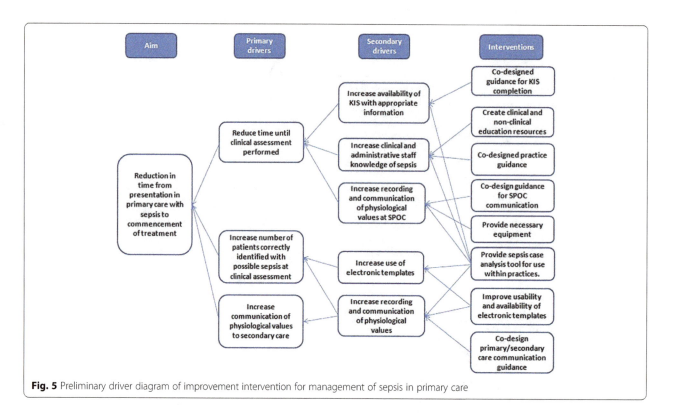

Fig. 5 Preliminary driver diagram of improvement intervention for management of sepsis in primary care

identification as a standalone system, and educating administrative staff on its identification, is unlikely to be effective unless consideration is given to the other task they are doing and the other systems with which they are interacting. We believe that the method described in this study is one way to involve multiple perspectives in the co-design of change and will add value to existing quality improvement methods.

It may be argued that simply discussing implementation of the improvement suggestions with a multidisciplinary team would yield similar results. The benefit of using the FRAM is that it allowed the qualitative and quantitative data to be synthesised and the whole system to be conceptualised. By identifying the conditions and interactions that influence work and cause variable function output, we believe it helped support clinical teams to consider where improvement efforts should be targeted. Constructing the FRAM model is a trade-off between showing all related functions and ensuring that it is useable and understandable. It may be argued that the FRAM could describe many other background functions (such as <manage staff capacity>) and links to other systems (such as <patient obtain access to laboratory results>). FRAM models can be constructed with different levels of resolution. For example, if the function <process request for clinical assessment – GP surgery> was the main object of improvement, this could be broken down to include all the functions needed to complete this task, such as <answer the telephone>. This has potential to increase the complexity of the FRAM model by identifying more interrelated functions. The level of detail required is dependent on the data collected and validated by those doing the work. If links to other systems significantly influence work in the system under study, then they should be included, and if variability in a specific task within a function (such as how the telephone is answered) is important, then it should be included as a separate function [36].

Consensus already exists on how improvement interventions should be described and reported [55, 56] and recent recommendations to improve the design of improvement interventions in complex systems have been published [23]. These include rigorously defining the problem, co-designing improvement interventions, use of a programme theory and considering the interaction between the social and the technical aspects of change. We have described one way to rigorously explore and understand the system to identify potential problems by exploring local work-as-done by frontline staff—for example, expected actions of administrative staff when patients present with possible sepsis and the lack of community nursing equipment. Improvement ideas were generated and interventions co-designed with frontline staff. The reflective sepsis tool promoted co-design of specific practice level interventions. It may be argued that this will produce a new work-as-imagined from which people will have to vary when conditions change in an unexpected way. However, the tool encourages repeated team reflection on performance to understand different perspectives on how the system functions and will support further adaptation to guidance to bring work-as-imagined and work-as-done closer.

The FRAM explored how the system worked and how interactions, resources, controls and time influence output. This allowed us to develop a programme theory, presented in the Driver Diagram (Fig. 2), that defines how interventions may lead to overall system improvement and how each intervention could be evaluated [57]. This will be used by local teams to learn about and adapt local processes to maximise success and is currently being piloted. As recently recommended for improvement interventions in complex systems, we have agreed a measurement of the final outcome of interest allowing for local adaptation of processes to create success [46].

The participatory approach we adopted helped us to explore the social and technical aspects of change. Increasingly, the use of risk stratification and early warning scores are being promoted in primary care but there is little evidence of their benefit as part of a one-off pre-hospital clinical assessment [9, 10]. The key stakeholder group felt that the social "processes" that lead to the interpretation and communication of the output of these tools (the actual physiological parameters and an indication of clinical condition) are what will ultimately influence the quality and safety of care [58].

Many factors that should be considered to maximise implementation and sustainability of improvement interventions within complex system have been described [59]. These include how the intervention fits with current work, demonstrating the benefits of the intervention and the ability to adapt it to local conditions [59]. Considering these factors can help understand why measuring the use of early warning scores as a quality improvement process measure was rejected by the key stakeholder group. The current electronic templates are not simple to use and do not fit with the way work is currently done. The benefits were not obvious to community clinicians—although there may be benefits in other parts of the system. There was also concern that if they were used as part of a QI intervention, compliance would be rigidly monitored reducing scope for clinicians to adapt their behaviour to suit the patient in front of them and the work conditions experienced. Instead, a less rigid approach was recommended focussing on the social aspects of communicating across interfaces and providing opportunity for feedback to encourage reflection on when and why to record physiological parameters.

This study has several limitations. First, several key stakeholders were not involved—most notably patients, home care teams and the Scottish Ambulance Service. We did not know if this approach would work and wished to initially test it with healthcare professionals. Better integrated patient participation will be sought to develop the improvement intervention design. The study included small numbers of participants in each professional group. This did not present a problem in the construction of the FRAM model and it appeared that data saturation was achieved for improvement suggestions. However, with more participants, it is possible other ideas for change may have been generated. The FRAM model was constructed based on work-as-disclosed by participants and observation of actual work may have revealed other ways of working. Interviewees may have been guarded in their description of how they completed work as they were speaking to a local GP; however, this made access to participants' easier and improved understanding of contextual factors such as the limitations of existing electronic templates. Transcripts were not returned to participants for checking. Data from NHS24 only included patients who received an out-of-hours clinician review, and did not include how often an emergency ambulance was called. It may be that NHS24 identify most patients with sepsis and arrange ambulance transport. Nevertheless, it allowed assessment of the variability of output of the function of arranging clinical review that may delay transfer to hospital. Similarly, the low rate of GP practice participation in data collection may mean levels of recording are not representative but they do demonstrate variability which was the main objective. The stakeholder meeting held to agree the improvement intervention did not include representation from all staff groups but their perspective was considered through the discussion of the suggested improvement interventions. The methods used to explore and understand the system require considerable experience and time investment that will not be available in all improvement projects. FRAM model construction through facilitated group discussion is successfully used elsewhere and this may be a more time efficient method to allow wider application and inclusion of more participants from each professional group [40, 41]. This method has only been used to design the intervention, and future evaluation of the intervention is required. Similarly, the method has only been tested in a single regional health board and further evaluation of its application in different settings is required. A full evaluation of the impact of this approach is planned and further research on the application of this method in different healthcare areas is required.

Conclusion

We have demonstrated the use of FRAM in a complex system to aid the design of a quality improvement intervention for identifying and managing sepsis in a single regional NHS board. This allowed an exploration of how conditions and interactions influence performance and output and how improvement suggestions from frontline staff could be reconciled with current work systems.

Appendix 1

Table 6 System improvement intervention informed by SEIPS 2.0 model [60]

Part of work system	Improvement aim	How will this be done?	Anticipated outcomes	Evaluation
Person	1. Increase administrative staff knowledge on sepsis. 2. Increase clinical staff knowledge on the identification and management of sepsis in the community.	1. Development of sepsis case analysis tool for use within practices. 2. Education session for receptionist staff, production of learning pack deliverable in practices. 3. Clinical educational sessions and production of accessible educational material (e.g. webinar, online module, dissemination of learning pack) Containing summary of guidelines, systems approach, recommendations and their rationale for standardising communication to increase recording of physiological parameters. 4. Training for adult community nurses on sepsis management and measuring and interpreting physiological values.	1. Reception staff aware of how sepsis will present and possible red flags—prompting them to arrange sooner clinical review. 2. Increased knowledge of guidelines, available tools (IT templates and NEWS), appreciation by clinical staff of reasons for recording and communicating values and how this can be achieved. 3. Earlier recognition by community adult nurses of septic patients and more effective communication of concern resulting in sooner clinical review by GP.	1. Evaluate satisfaction with training and other educational materials. 2. Evaluate change in attitude and knowledge following training.
Tools and Technology	1. Provide adult community nurses with required resources—thermometers and saturation monitors. 2. Facilitate recording of physiological values.	1. Resources provided through health board funding. 2. Improved IT systems that are a useful resource, available when needed that may help positively constrain behaviour. 3. Dissemination of existing in-hours IT templates to practice managers with instructions on how to use short cuts to open—work with frontline staff to improve out-of-hours IT systems	1. All necessary equipment available. 2. Easier to record physiological values. 3. Awareness of guideline that supports everyday work (positive control). Patients who are potentially septic are identified earlier.	1. Assess via survey—satisfaction with created protocols and templates. 2. Survey staff to determine if protocols and templates are a beneficial control and represent work-as-done. 3. Measure use of templates.
Tasks	1. Increase recording and communication of physiological parameters 2. Improve the ability of practice administrative staff to identify patients who may have sepsis. 3. Improve completion of Key Information Summary to include—the recording of risk factors for sepsis and normal physiological parameters	1. Development of sepsis case analysis tool for use within practices. 2. Through educational events that describe importance of recording values in other parts of the system. 3. Co-design guidance with community nurses following education on sepsis—potentially positive control. 4. Co-design protocol for communication between primary/secondary care. 5. Co-design guidance with practice administrative staff following educational sessions—potentially positive control. 6. Improvement in KIS completion will be achieved through existing programme of work—sepsis work will feed into this.	1. Increase recording and communication of physiological parameters. 2. More accurate and useful information contained in KIS—allows interpretation of physiology to facilitate accurate diagnosis in out-of-hours and secondary care.	1. Measure use of protocols and templates to determine if they represent work-as-done. 2. Evaluate information contained in KIS—through existing GP cluster and locality work. 3. Evaluate patients admitted with sepsis to determine if all parameters recorded—results to be used for reflection and not as a performance indicator.
Internal Environment	1. Develop practice culture where receptionists can interrupt clinicians if needed. 2. Improve culture within out-of-hours to reduce concern regarding auditing of data.	1. Development of sepsis case analysis tool for use within practices. 2. Co-design of protocols with clinical and administrative staff in practices following reception and GP training. 3. Regular reinforcement of use of data and incident investigation for learning—recording of	1. Receptionists know when to adapt behaviour—when to seek early review and have confidence to implement—supports staff wellbeing and improves performance. 2. Feedback from incident investigation and data used for learning—supports staff wellbeing.	1. Survey of perceptions of culture.

Table 6 System improvement intervention informed by SEIPS 2.0 model [60] (Continued)

Part of work system	Improvement aim	How will this be done?	Anticipated outcomes	Evaluation
		observations or early warning scores should not be used as a performance indicator without appreciation of the context within which the patient was assessed.		
Organisation	1. KIS available when SPOC used—resource provision. 2. Improve communication when out-of-hours community healthcare staff use the single point of contact. 3. Improve communication between primary/secondary care	1. Change system to ensure KIS available—arranged with out-of-hours leaders. 2. Following education sessions with adult community nurses and out-of-hours administrative staff—co-design guidance for communication including communication of physiological values. Potentially positive behaviour control. 3. The sepsis work would feed into existing cross interface programme boards—co-design protocol for communication between primary/secondary care.	1. Normal values available for out-of-hours and secondary care clinicians to facilitate early diagnosis and treatment. 2. Awareness of guideline that helps work (positive control). Patients who are potentially septic are identified earlier.	1. Evaluation as above.
External Influences	1. Sepsis management prioritised by Health board. 2. Nice Guidelines widely distributed 3. Reflection on management of sepsis patients with other GP practices	1. Report sent to health board for discussion and approval at Primary Care Leadership committee. 2. Dissemination guidelines and sepsis app as part of educational intervention—potentially positive behaviour control.	1. Resources available to implement and evaluate changes. 2. More patients managed following guidance.	1. Use of guidance can be evaluated following educational events using a survey.
Processes	1. Increased rates of provision of relevant physiological values when admission arranged by primary care clinicians. 2. Increased rates of provision of relevant physiological values when community healthcare staff contacts out-of-hours services.	1. Work with secondary care sepsis leads—for all admissions receiving team will request all physiological parameters—GP expected to provide values when relevant—educational sessions detail when it is relevant. This will include all admissions with infective, cardiac or respiratory cause. Efficiency thoroughness trade-offs may lead to performance variability and this should be recognised. 2. SPOC will use a template and ask for all physiological parameters.	1. Improved communication of physiological values so secondary care aware of admissions and have values from community for comparison. Results in quicker assessment and initiation of appropriate treatment. 2. Out-of-hours staff will be aware of severity of illness of patient and, if necessary see sooner and ensure treatment initiated sooner, resulting in improved healthcare outcomes.	1. Measure rates of communication of relevant values when SPOC used and at admission. 2. Survey—perceptions of clinical staff in acute care hub to new system for adult community nurses.
Outcomes	1. Reduce time from contacting health services to receiving antibiotics for ten patients with a confirmed admission diagnosis of sepsis per month.	1. Long term outcome of all above measures	1. Improved mortality and morbidity outcomes for patients presenting to primary care with sepsis.	1. Measure for ten patients per month and feedback to all GPs and ANPs. Once baseline measure obtained specific target will be set.

Appendix 2

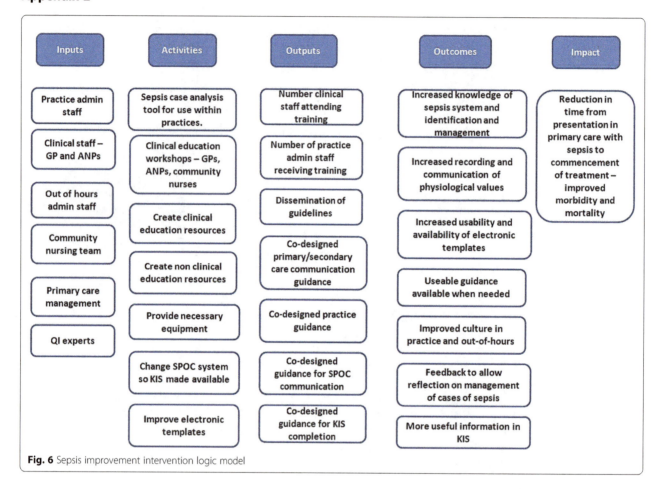

Fig. 6 Sepsis improvement intervention logic model

Abbreviations
ADOC: Ayrshire Doctors on Call; ANP: Advanced nurse practitioner; CMAU: Combined Medical Assessment Unit; COREQ: Consolidated criteria for reporting qualitative research; ED: Emergency department; FMV: FRAM Model Visualiser; FRAM: Functional Resonance Analysis Method; GP: General practitioner; GPST3: General Practitioner Specialty Trainee 3; KIS: Key Information Summary; NHSAA: National Health Service Ayrshire and Arran; QI: Quality improvement; SPOC: Single point of contact; WAD: Work-as-done; WAI: Work-as-imagined

Acknowledgements
The authors would like to thank all those that participated in interviews, the practices that submitted data, the ADOC staff who collected data and the key stakeholder group who designed the intervention and Julie Anderson, Associate Director Scottish Improvement Science Collaborating Centre for feedback on the paper.

Authors' contributions
The project was devised and planned by DM, PB, JF and CB. DM conducted the interviews, coded the data and analysed the quantitative data. DM, JF and CB developed themes from the coded data. All authors contributed equally to develop the improvement intervention. DM produced the first draft of the manuscript and all authors reviewed, edited and revised the manuscript. All authors read and approved the final manuscript.

Competing interests
The authors declare that they have no competing interests.

Author details
[1]NHS Education for Scotland, 2 Central Quay, Glasgow, Scotland G3 8BW, UK. [2]NHS Ayrshire and Arran, Ayr, UK. [3]Institute of Health and Wellbeing, University of Glasgow, Glasgow, UK. [4]Division of Population Medicine, School of Medicine, Cardiff University, Cardiff, UK. [5]Department of Family Practice, University of British Columbia, Vancouver, Canada. [6]Australian Institute of Health Innovation, Macquarie University, Sydney, Australia.

References
1. National Confidential Enquiry into Patient Outcome and Death. Sepsis: just say sepsis! (2015) http://www.ncepod.org.uk/2015sepsis.html. Accessed 11 Sept 2018.
2. Fleischmann C, Scherag A, Adhikari NKJ, et al. Assessment of global incidence and mortality of hospital-treated sepsis: current estimates and limitations. Am J Respir Crit Care Med. 2016;193:259–72.
3. Reinhart K, Daniels R, Kissoon N, Machado FR, Schachter RD, Finfer S. Recognizing sepsis as a global health priority—a WHO resolution. N Engl J Med. 2017;377(5):414–7.
4. Herlitz J, Bang A, Wireklint-Sundstrom B, et al. Suspicion and treatment of severe sepsis. An overview of the prehospital chain of care. Scand J Trauma Resusc Emerg Med. 2012;20:42.
5. Rivers E, Nguyen B, Havstad S, Early Goal-Directed Therapy Collaborative Group, et al. Early goal-directed therapy in the treatment of severe sepsis and septic shock. N Engl J Med. 2001;345:1368–77.
6. Delaney A. Protocolized sepsis care is not helpful for patients. Crit Care Med. 2017;45(3):473–5.
7. Schlapbach LJ, Javouhey E, Jansen NJG. Paediatric sepsis: old wine in new bottles? Intensive Care Med. 2017;43(11):1686–9.

8. The Scottish Patient Safety Programme. Scottish Patient Safety Programme in Primary Care. http://www.scottishpatientsafetyprogramme.scot.nhs.uk/programmes/primary-care. Accessed 11 Sept 2018.
9. Gilham C. Sepsis: the primary care focus. Br J Gen Pract. 2016;66(644):120–1.
10. National Institute for Health and Care Excellence (NICE). Sepsis: recognition, diagnosis and early management. London: National Institute for Health and Care Excellence (NICE); 2016.
11. Esteban A, Frutos-Vivar F, Ferguson ND, et al. Sepsis incidence and outcome: contrasting the intensive care unit with the hospital ward. Crit Care Med. 2007;35(5):1284–9.
12. NHS England Cross Systems Sepsis Prevention Programme Board. In: NHS England, editor. Improving outcomes for patients with sepsis: a cross-system action plan. London: NHS England; 2015.
13. Health Service Ombudsman. Time to act: severe sepsis rapid diagnosis and treatment saves lives. London: Parliamentary and Health Service Ombudsman; 2014.
14. Health Service Ombudsman. An avoidable death of a three year old. London: Parliamentary and Health Service Ombudsman; 2014.
15. Cork N, Rooney KD, Carson-Stevens A. When I say… quality improvement. Med Educ. 2017;51(5):467–8.
16. Gatewood MO, Wemple M, Greco S, et al. A quality improvement project to improve early sepsis care in the emergency department. BMJ Qual Saf. 2015;24:787–95.
17. Levy MM, Dellinger RP, Townsend SR, Linde-Zwirble WT, Marshall JC, Bion J, et al. The surviving sepsis campaign: results of an international guideline-based performance improvement program targeting severe sepsis. Intensive Care Med. 2010;36(2):222–31.
18. Ferrer R, Martin-Loeches I, Phillips G, Osborn TM, Townsend S, Dellinger RP, et al. Empiric antibiotic treatment reduces mortality in severe sepsis and septic shock from the first hour: results from a guideline-based performance improvement program. Crit Care Med. 2014;42(8):1749–55.
19. Craig P, Dieppe P, Macintyre S, Michie S, et al. Developing and evaluating complex interventions: the new Medical Research Council guidance. BMJ. 2008;337:a1655.
20. Campbell NC, Murray E, Darbyshire J, Emery J, Farmer A, Griffiths F, Guthrie B, Lester H, Wilson P, Kinmonth AL. Designing and evaluating complex interventions to improve health care. BMJ. 2007;334:455–9.
21. Kaplan H, Brady P, Dritz M, Hooper D, et al. The influence of context on quality improvement success in health care: a systematic review of the literature. Millbank Q. 2010;88:500–9.
22. Parry GJ, Carson-Stevens A, Luff DF, McPherson ME, Goldmann DA. Recommendations for evaluation of health care improvement initiatives. Acad Pediatr. 2013;31(13 Supple 6):23–30.
23. Marshall M, de Silva D, Cruikshank L, et al. What we know about designing an effective improvement intervention (but too often fail to put into practice). BMJ Qual Saf. 2017;26(7):578–82. https://doi.org/10.1136/bmjqs-2016-006143.
24. Lau R, Stevenson F, Ong BN, et al. Achieving change in primary care—effectiveness of strategies for improving implementation of complex interventions: systematic review of reviews. BMJ Open. 2015;5:e009993. https://doi.org/10.1136/bmjopen-2015-009993.
25. May CR, Johnson M, Finch T. Implementation, context and complexity. Implement Sci. 2016;11:141.
26. Greenhalgh T, Papoutsi C. Studying complexity in health services research: desperately seeking an overdue paradigm shift. BMC Medicine. 2018;16:95 https://doi.org/10.1186/s12916-018-1089-4.
27. Braithewaite J, Chirruca K, Long J, Ellis LA, et al. When complexity science meets implementation science: a theoretical and empirical analysis of systems change. BMC Medicine. 2018;16:63 https://doi.org/10.1186/s12916-018-1057-z.
28. The Health Foundation. Evidence scan: complex adaptive systems. London: The Health Foundation; 2010.
29. Braithwaite J, Clay-Williams R, Nugus P, Plumb J. Health care as a complex adaptive system. In: Hollnagel E, Braithwaite J, Wears R, editors. Resilient health care. Surrey: Ashgate Publishing Limited; 2013.
30. Litaker D, Tomolo A, Liberatone V, Stange K, et al. Using complexity theory to build interventions that improve health care delivery in primary care. J Gen Intern Med. 2006;21(Suppl 2):30–4.
31. Hollnagel E. Safety-I and safety-II the past and future of safety management. Surrey: Ashgate Publishing Limited; 2014.
32. Tucker AL, Spear SJ. Operational failures and interruptions in hospital nursing. Health Serv Res. 2006;41(3part1):643–62.
33. Hollnagel E. The ETTO principle: efficiency-thoroughness trade-off: why things that go right sometimes go wrong. London: Ashgate Publishing Limited; 2009.
34. McNab D, Bowie P, Morrison J, Ross A. Understanding patient safety performance and educational needs using the 'Safety-II' approach for complex systems. Educ Prim Care. 2016;27(6):443–50.
35. Tong A, Sainsbury P, Craig J. Consolidated criteria for reporting qualitative research (COREQ): a 32-item checklist for interviews and focus groups. Int J Qual Health Care. 2007;19(6):349–57.
36. Hollnagel E. FRAM: the functional resonance analysis method. Modelling complex socio-technical systems. Surrey: Ashgate publishing limited; 2012.
37. The Functional Resonance Analysis Method: FRAM Model visualiser. http://functionalresonance.com/FMV/index.html. Accessed 11 Sept 2018.
38. Hignett S, Wilson JR, Morris W. Finding ergonomic solutions—participatory approaches. Occup Med. 2005;55:200–7.
39. Pickup L, Atkinson S, Hollnagel E, Bowie P, et al. Blood sampling—two sides to the story. Appl Ergon. 2017;59(Pt A):234–42.
40. Clay-Williams R, Hounsgaard J, Hollnagel E. Where the rubber meets the road: using FRAM to align work-as-imagined with work-as-done when implementing clinical guidelines. Implement Sci. 2015;10:125. https://doi.org/10.1186/s13012-015-0317-y.
41. Hounsgaard J. Patient safety in everyday work: learning from things that go right. 2016 http://functionalresonance.com/onewebmedia/Hounsgaard%20(2016).pdf. Accessed 11 Sept 2018.
42. Hsieh H-F, Shannon SE. Three approaches to qualitative content analysis. Qual Health Res. 2005;15(9):1277–88.
43. Glaser BG, Strauss AL. The discovery of grounded theory: strategies for qualitative research. Chicago: Aldine; 1967.
44. British Medical Journal. Statistics square one - 1. Data display and summary. http://www.bmj.com/about-bmj/resources-readers/publications/statistics-square-one/1-data-display-and-summary. Accessed 11 Sept 2018.
45. Institute for Healthcare Improvement. Driver Diagram Available at http://www.ihi.org/resources/Pages/Tools/Driver-Diagram.aspx. Accessed 11 Sept 2018.
46. Young RA, Roberts RG, Holden RJ. The challenges of measuring, improving, and reporting quality in primary care. Ann Fam Med. 2017;15(2):175–82.
47. Ivers N, Jamtvedt G, Flottorp S. Audit and feedback: effects on professional practice and healthcare outcomes. Cochrane Database Syst Rev. 2012;6:CD000259.
48. Institute for Healthcare Improvement. Science of Improvement: Establishing measures http://www.ihi.org/resources/Pages/HowtoImprove/ScienceofImprovementEstablishingMeasures.aspx. Accessed 11 Sept 2018.
49. McLaughlin S, Houston N, Winter J. Sepsis in primary care: recognition, response and referral using NEWS. http://www.qihub.scot.nhs.uk/media/969883/stephen%20mclaughlin_25.pdf. Accessed 11 Sept 2018.
50. Byers G. Recognizing severe sepsis in the pre hospital setting improves the timeliness of antibiotic administration. http://www.qihub.scot.nhs.uk/media/618286/geraldine%20byers.pdf. Accessed 11 Sept 2018.
51. Ryan L. Early, safe and reliable detection of sepsis in primary care: moving the front door into the community in NHS borders.http://www.qihub.scot.nhs.uk/media/650720/laura%20ryan.pdf. Accessed 11 Sept 2018.
52. US Department for Veterans Affairs. National Centre for patient safety. Root cause analysis tools. NCPS; 2015. http://www.patientsafety.va.gov/docs/joe/rca_tools_2_15.pdf. Accessed 11 Sept 2018.
53. The Health Foundation. Evidence scan: QI made simple. London: The Health Foundation; 2013.
54. Sujan MA, Huang H, Braithwaite J. Learning from incidents in health care: critique from a Safety-II perspective. Safety Sci. 2017;99:115–21.
55. Hoffmann TC, Glasziou PP, Boutron I, Milne R, Perera R, Moher D, Altman DG, Barbour V, Macdonald H, Johnston M, Lamb SE, et al. Better reporting of interventions: template for intervention description and replication (TIDieR) checklist and guide. BMJ. 2014;348:g1687.
56. Ogrinc G, Mooney SE, Estrada C, et al. The SQUIRE (Standards for QUality Improvement Reporting Excellence) guidelines for quality improvement reporting: explanation and elaboration. BMJ Qual Saf. 2008;17:i13–32.
57. Foy R, Ovretveit J, Shekelle PG, et al. The role of theory in research to develop and evaluate the implementation of patient safety practices. BMJ Qual Saf. 2011;20:453–9.
58. Mitchell B, Cristancho S, Nyhof BB, et al. Mobilising or standing still? A narrative review of surgical safety checklist knowledge as developed in 25 highly cited papers from 2009 to 2016. BMJ Qual Saf. 2017. https://doi.org/10.1136/bmjqs-2016-006218.

Avoidable waste of research related to outcome planning and reporting in clinical trials

Youri Yordanov[1,2,3,4*], Agnes Dechartres[1,4,5,6], Ignacio Atal[1,4], Viet-Thi Tran[1,4], Isabelle Boutron[1,4,5,6], Perrine Crequit[1,4] and Philippe Ravaud[1,4,5,6,7]

Abstract

Background: Inadequate planning, selective reporting, and incomplete reporting of outcomes in randomized controlled trials (RCTs) contribute to the problem of waste of research. We aimed to describe such a waste and to examine to what extent this waste could be avoided.

Methods: This research-on-research study was based on RCTs included in Cochrane reviews with a summary of findings (SoF) table. We considered the outcomes reported in the SoF tables as surrogates for important outcomes for patients and other decision makers. We used a three-step approach. (1) First, in each review, we identified, for each important outcome, RCTs that were excluded from the corresponding meta-analysis. (2) Then, for these RCTs, we systematically searched for registrations and protocols to distinguish between inadequate planning (an important outcome was not reported in registries or protocols), selective reporting (an important outcome was reported in registries or protocols but not in publications), and incomplete reporting (an important outcome was incompletely reported in publications). (3) Finally, we assessed, with the consensus of five experts, the feasibility and cost of measuring the important outcomes that were not planned. We considered inadequately planned or selectively or incompletely reported important outcomes as avoidable waste if the outcome could have been easily measured at no additional cost based on expert evaluation.

Results: Of the 2711 RCTs included in the main comparison of 290 reviews, 2115 (78%) were excluded from at least one meta-analysis of important outcomes. Every trial contributed to 55%, on average, of the meta-analyses of important outcomes. Of the 310 RCTs published in 2010 or later, 156 were registered. Inadequate planning affected 79% of these RCTs, whereas incomplete and selective reporting affected 41% and 15%, respectively. For 63% of RCTs, we found at least one missing important outcome for which the waste was avoidable and for 30%, the waste was avoidable for all important outcomes.

Conclusions: Most of the RCTs included in our sample did not contribute to all the important outcomes in meta-analyses, mostly because of inadequate planning or incomplete reporting. A large part of this waste of research seemed to be avoidable.

Keywords: Randomized controlled trial, Waste of research, Outcome, Selective reporting, Core outcome set

---

* Correspondence: youri.yordanov@aphp.fr
[1]INSERM, U1153, Hôpital Hôtel-Dieus, 1, place du parvis Notre Dame, 75004 Paris, France
[2]Sorbonne Universités, UPMC Paris Univ-06, Paris, France
Full list of author information is available at the end of the article

Background

Clinical trials are only as credible as their outcomes, so to inform decision-making appropriately, randomized controlled trials (RCTs) must evaluate the outcomes that are most important to patients and their caregivers [1–8]. Failure to do so could contribute to the overwhelming problem of waste in research [9–16]. Waste of research related to inadequate outcome planning, selective reporting, and incomplete reporting of outcomes in RCTs prevents patients and their physicians from making well-informed decisions, with potential serious consequences if ineffective or harmful treatments are promoted [9, 12–14, 17, 18].

Therefore, when planning an RCT, researchers are expected to measure all important outcomes [9]. However, previous studies found that less than one-fifth of diabetes RCTs and less than one-quarter of cardiovascular trials considered patient-important outcomes as their primary outcomes [19, 20]. Instead, researchers frequently rely on surrogates as a proxy for final patient-important outcomes because these outcomes allow for smaller, faster, and thus, cheaper clinical trials [21–24]. However, surrogates can be misleading, because they may show exaggerated treatment effect sizes or even an apparent benefit of harmful treatments, as was the case for the use of antiarrhythmic drugs after myocardial infarction, which led to the deaths of several thousand patients decades ago [25–28].

Selective reporting has been repeatedly described as another important issue affecting RCT outcomes [29–32]. Outcome reporting bias arises when outcomes are selectively reported based on the nature and direction of the results [33]. In a recent study, the median proportion of RCTs with discrepancies between registered and published primary outcomes was 31% [34]. Statistically significant outcomes were 2 to 4 times more likely to be reported in publications than non-significant ones, which biases the available body of evidence toward more positive results [30].

Similarly, a median of 31% to 50% of efficacy outcomes were found to be incompletely reported in RCT articles [29, 35, 36]. With incomplete reporting of outcomes, outcomes cannot be included in meta-analyses, which poses a serious threat to the usability of trial results: not including all available results in meta-analyses can lead to a truncated vision of the overall body of evidence.

The purpose of this study was to describe the waste of research related to inadequate planning, selective reporting, or incomplete reporting of outcomes in RCTs and to examine to what extent this waste could be avoided. For this, we addressed the following specific questions: (1) What proportion of RCTs are excluded from meta-analyses due to outcome reasons? (2) Were the exclusions related to inadequate planning, selective reporting, or incomplete reporting? (3) Was it feasible to measure the missing outcomes at the planning stage, and at what cost?

Methods

We performed a research-on-research study based on RCTs included in Cochrane systematic reviews. We used the outcomes reported in the summary of findings (SoF) tables of reviews as surrogates for important outcomes, because Cochrane systematic review SoF tables should include the most important outcomes for patients and other decision makers, whether they are available in RCTs or not [7]. This study used a three-step approach. (1) First, for all important outcomes, we identified the RCTs that were included in the Cochrane reviews but excluded from the corresponding meta-analyses because the important outcome was missing. (2) Then, we systematically searched for trial registrations and protocols to distinguish between the outcomes that were not planned (not included in registries or protocols, i.e., inadequate planning) and outcomes that were planned. For the planned outcomes, we distinguished between those that were adequately reported and those that were incompletely reported (poor reporting) or not reported (selective reporting). (3) Finally, we assessed, via expert consensus, the feasibility and cost of measuring the outcomes that were not planned.

The eligibility criteria at each phase of the study are summarized in Additional file 1.

Identification of RCTs excluded from meta-analyses
Data sources
We obtained data from all Cochrane systematic reviews published between March 2011 and September 2014. They were provided by the Cochrane Collaboration editorial unit as XML files and contained all information reported by the review authors in RevMan, the software developed by the Cochrane Collaboration for preparing and maintaining systematic reviews [37]. Cochrane systematic reviews of interventions are organized by comparisons of two treatment groups. Meta-analyses are then performed for one or more outcomes within each comparison. Cochrane reviewers are encouraged to present an SoF table summarizing information on the quality of evidence and treatment effect magnitude (from the meta-analysis result) for the most important outcomes (see example in the review by Mocellin and colleagues [38]) [7]. According to the Cochrane collaboration, these outcomes should be important to all research end users, that is, patients and other decision makers [7]. These outcomes include a "wide variety of events such as mortality and major morbidity (such as stroke and myocardial infarction); however, they may also represent frequent minor and rare major side effects, symptoms and quality of life, burdens associated with treatment, and resource issues (costs)" [7].

Selection of relevant Cochrane systematic reviews

Using R 3.1.1 and the XML package, one of us (IA) removed from the set of reviews provided by the Cochrane Collaboration withdrawn Cochrane reviews and then identified all reviews of RCTs with an SoF table. We excluded reviews that included observational studies and those including only RCTs published before 2007 because we focused on recent RCTs. From all eligible Cochrane reviews, using a random number generator, we drew a random sample of 300 for an in-depth evaluation but excluded a further 10 reviews because their SoF tables mixed various interventions, which resulted in a final sample of 290 Cochrane reviews.

Identification of important outcomes

We considered outcomes reported in the SoF table as a surrogate for important outcomes. Therefore, we manually identified and extracted all outcomes reported in the SoF tables. Most reviews had a single SoF table, but some had several tables, corresponding to different comparisons. In this case, we focused on the main comparison as acknowledged by the authors. If the main comparison was not reported by the review authors or if various comparisons were reported in the same SoF table, we selected the comparison with the most outcomes and included the largest number of RCTs. If the SoF table reported various interventions (e.g., presented three meta-analyses of different outcomes for three different interventions), the review was excluded.

We classified each outcome as follows: mortality, other clinical event (e.g., myocardial infarction or stroke), therapeutic decision (e.g., transfusion), function (e.g., disability), pain, quality of life, adverse events or side effects (identified as such by the review authors), physiological variable (e.g., blood pressure or weight), biological variable (e.g., cholesterol levels), radiological variable (e.g., measure of joint space), compliance (e.g., discontinuation for any reason), process (e.g., duration of surgical procedure), resource use (hospitalization), cost-effectiveness, and satisfaction with care [39].

Identification of RCTs excluded from meta-analyses

For each review and for each important outcome, we identified all RCTs excluded from the outcome in the corresponding meta-analysis. To do so, by using the reference list of all studies included in the Cochrane review, we first identified all RCTs available for the selected comparison by extracting all RCTs included in any meta-analysis reported for this comparison. Then, for each of these RCTs, we manually evaluated whether they contributed to the meta-analysis of each important outcome by screening RCTs included in the corresponding meta-analysis.

Evaluation of the reason for a missing outcome

We a priori hypothesized that the exclusion of an RCT from a meta-analysis for outcome reasons could be related to inadequate planning (i.e., the outcome was not planned to be measured), selective reporting (i.e., the outcome was planned but not reported in the publication), or incomplete reporting (i.e., the outcome was reported in the publication but not in a way that allowed for pooling of data).

To distinguish among inadequate planning, selective reporting, or incomplete reporting, for each RCT excluded from at least one meta-analysis, we screened the data available in Cochrane reviews and systematically searched for trial registration and/or protocols.

We focused on RCTs published in 2010 or later to maximize the chance of identifying trial registration or protocols.

Search for RCT registration and protocols

For each RCT, we individually assessed all available reports and information. To do that, we extracted the references identified from the "References to studies included in this review" section of the Cochrane reviews. One of us (YY) retrieved all the articles, conference abstracts, reports etc. related to the identified RCT. We screened all articles for any information regarding registration (name of trial registry and/or registration number) and/or protocol availability. When no reference to a trial registration was found, we used the following approach:

1. We searched the full text of the Cochrane review for any information regarding trial registration.
2. If no information was found, we searched the World Health Organization (WHO) International Clinical Trials Registry Platform (ICTRP). Also, according to the author's affiliation, we searched the local registry if not part of the WHO ICTRP. We used the article title, the first and last author's name as author or as investigator, or the author's affiliation as search keywords.
3. If no information was found, we searched Google with the publication title and keywords regarding registration (e.g., registry, registration, NCT etc.).
4. If no information was found, we contacted the corresponding author to ask whether the trial was registered and whether a protocol was available.

Evaluation of the reason for the missing outcome

For each identified RCT, one of us (YY) classified each missing outcome into one of the following five categories:

1. Inadequate planning
    - The outcome was not planned according to the protocol or the registry entry. It was not reported in the available trial reports.

2. Selective reporting
   - The outcome was planned according to the protocol or the registry entry but was not reported in the available trial reports.
3. Incomplete reporting
   - The outcome was planned according to the protocol or the registry entry and was reported in the available trial reports but incompletely or not in a way that allowed for meta-analysis (e.g., mixed model analyses reported, no results per group, missing control group results, difference in means without the standard error, etc.).
   - No protocol or registry entry was found. The outcome was reported in the available trial reports but not in a way that allowed for meta-analysis.
4. Unable to distinguish between selective reporting and inadequate planning
   - No protocol or registry entry was found and the outcome was not reported in the available trial reports.
5. Other situations
   - The outcome was listed in the trial reports, but there was no event (e.g., the outcome was death but no death occurred).
   - The outcome concerned adverse events, but there was no event (e.g., the outcome was "Major Complications—Visceral injury," but no complications were reported).
   - The outcome was reported in the available trial reports in a way that could allow for inclusion in a meta-analysis but was not included in the meta-analysis.

As a quality assessment measure, 10% of the RCTs were classified independently by two reviewers (YY and AD), with no disagreements.

Evaluation of research waste

Feasibility and cost of measuring the missing outcomes that were not planned

To evaluate whether the missing outcomes that were not planned could have been easily measured, we used an expert consensus approach. One of us (YY) presented to an expert panel of five methodologists and trialists (AD, IB, PC, PR, and VT) each RCT for which at least one missing outcome was classified as not planned. After evaluating standardized information on the population, interventions in the experimental and control group, and other outcomes evaluated, the panel of experts were asked to answer the following questions regarding the missing outcomes:

- "According to you, given the other outcomes measured in the trial, and based on your experience, would you consider that measuring the presented outcome would be easy, moderately easy, difficult or impossible in most cases from a trialist's perspective?"
- "According to you, given the other outcomes measured in the trial, and based on your experience, would you consider that measuring the presented outcome would be easy, moderately easy, difficult or impossible in most cases from a patient's perspective?"
- "According to you, given the other outcomes measured in the trial, and based on your experience, what would be the approximate cost of measuring this outcome: no cost defined as ≤ 1% of the total cost of the trial; minor cost, defined as ≤ 5%; moderate cost, 5% to 15%; or major cost, 15% or more". These percentages were indicative.
- "According to you, how important is the missing outcome: major importance; non-major importance?"

One of us (YY) ensured that all experts first gave their opinion and then discussed together, to avoid the opinion of one leading person influencing the others. The final feasibility and cost evaluation of every proposed adjustment was based on the group consensus.

The qualifications and areas of expertise of the experts involved are summarized in Additional file 2.

Avoidable waste of research related to missing outcomes

We defined avoidable waste related to missing outcomes as missing important outcomes related to:

- Selective reporting
- Incomplete reporting
- Inadequate planning, if the outcome was judged by the expert panel as easy to collect from both the trialist and patient perspective, not costly (i.e., no or minor additional cost), and of critical importance

At the trial level, such waste could have been partially avoided if the trial could have been included in the meta-analysis of at least one missing outcome and totally if it could have been included in all meta-analyses of missing outcomes.

Statistical analysis

The analysis was mainly descriptive. Continuous data are presented as median (Q1–Q3) and categorical data as frequencies (%, 95% confidence interval [CI]). All analyses involved use of R 3.0.2 (2013-09-25) (R Foundation for Statistical Computing, Vienna, Austria. http://www.r-project.org/).

Results

Identification of RCTs excluded from meta-analyses

Selection and characteristics of the Cochrane systematic reviews

The complete selection process is described in Fig. 1. Briefly, from the 2796 Cochrane systematic reviews published between March 2011 and September 2014, 820 reviews corresponded to our eligibility criteria. Our selection process resulted in a sample of 290 reviews (5047 RCTs), with a median of 11 RCTs per review (Q1–Q3: 5–21) (Fig. 1). The subset of included reviews appeared comparable to the eligible Cochrane Reviews (Additional file 3). The reviews investigated 47 different health research topics, the most common being airways (7%, $n = 21/290$), menstrual disorders and subfertility (7%, $n = 20/290$), and anesthesia (6%, $n = 18/290$) (Table 1). Experimental interventions were pharmacological in 60% of reviews ($n = 175/290$).

The reviews included a median of 5 outcomes per SoF table for the main comparison (Q1–Q3: 3–7, Min–Max: 1–12), for a total of 1414 outcomes. Mortality represented 10% ($n = 138/1414$) of the outcomes, and other clinical events, 14% ($n = 198/1414$); quality of life, 7% ($n = 98/1414$); function, 27% ($n = 384/1414$); and adverse events, 12% ($n = 174/1414$) (Table 1). Biological variables, process and resource use, and physiological variables accounted for 6% ($n = 89/1414$), 5% ($n = 74/1414$), and 4% ($n = 56/1414$), respectively. The corresponding meta-analyses included a median of 3 RCTs (Q1–Q3: 2–7), maximum 76.

Proportion of RCTs excluded from the meta-analyses due to outcome reasons

The 290 reviews included a total of 2711 RCTs in the main comparison; 596 (22%; 95% CI: 20–24) were included in all meta-analyses of important outcomes, and

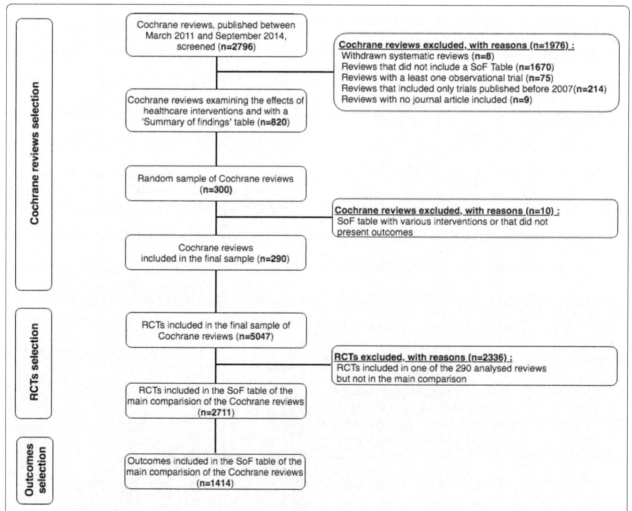

Fig. 1 Flow chart of the selection process. This figure summarizes the selection process for Cochrane reviews, RCTs, and outcomes. The analyzed sample involved 290 Cochrane reviews, which included 2711 RCTs in the SoF table of the main comparison. The SoF tables reported 1414 important outcomes. RCT randomized controlled trial, SoF summary of findings

Table 1 Characteristics of selected systematic reviews and outcomes

Review characteristics	n = 290
	Median (Q1–Q3)
No. of trials per review	11 (5–21)
No. of trials in the main comparison	5 (3–12)
No. of comparisons per review	2 (1–5)
Cochrane review groups	n = 290
	No. (%)
Airways	21 (7)
Menstrual disorders and subfertility	20 (7)
Anesthesia	18 (6)
Oral health	15 (5)
Schizophrenia	15 (5)
Hepato-biliary	12 (4)
Neuromuscular disease	12 (4)
Musculoskeletal	11 (4)
Infectious diseases	10 (3)
Other	156 (54)
Type of assessed intervention	n = 290
	No. (%)
Pharmacological	175 (60)
Non-pharmacological	115 (40)
Outcomes characteristics	n = 141
No. of outcomes per SoF table, median (Q1–Q3)	5 (3–7)
No. of trials per meta-analysis, median (Q1–Q3)	3 (2–7)
Outcome categories	n = 1414
	No. (%)*
Function	384 (27)
Other clinical events	198 (14)
Adverse events; side effects	174 (12)
Mortality	138 (10)
Quality of life	98 (7)
Biological variables	89 (6)
Process, resource use	74 (5)
Pain	71 (5)
Physiological variables	56 (4)
Compliance	45 (3)
Therapeutic decision	33 (2)
Satisfaction with care	24 (2)
Radiological variables	23 (2)
Cost-effectiveness	16 (1)

*The total exceeds 100% because some outcomes were included in more than one category

2115 (78%, 95% CI: 76–80) were excluded from at least one meta-analysis. Every RCT contributed to 55%, on average, of the meta-analyses for important outcomes.

Evaluation of the reason for missing outcomes

Among the 2115 RCTs excluded from at least one meta-analysis of important outcomes, 310 were published in 2010 or later. We further excluded 19 RCTs, because their reports were not accessible (e.g., retracted paper) or were not in English or French (e.g., Chinese), which left 291 RCTs for further evaluation, with a total of 971 missing outcomes. A registration number or a protocol was retrieved for 54% ($n = 156/291$) of these RCTs (corresponding to 461 missing outcomes).

Reasons for missing outcomes were incomplete reporting for 21% of missing outcomes ($n = 204/971$) in 40% of RCTs ($n = 117/291$), and inadequate planning for 29% of missing outcomes ($n = 282/971$) in 42% of RCTs ($n = 123/291$) (Table 2). Confirmed selective reporting represented 4% of missing outcomes ($n = 36/971$) in 9% of RCTs ($n = 25/291$). Nevertheless, 42% of RCTs ($n = 122/291$) had no protocol or registration, so for these, we could not distinguish between selective reporting and inadequate planning.

When restricting our description to registered RCTs ($n = 156$), inadequate planning concerned 61% of missing outcomes ($n = 282/461$) in 79% of RCTs ($n = 123/156$), whereas incomplete reporting accounted for 21% of missing outcomes ($n = 98/461$) in 41% of RCTs ($n = 64/156$), and selective reporting, 7% of missing outcomes ($n = 34/461$) in 15% of RCTs ($n = 23/156$) (Table 2).

Evaluation of research waste
Feasibility of measuring the missing outcomes that were not planned

We submitted the 282 outcomes missing due to inadequate planning from 123 RCTs to our panel of experts. For 78% of outcomes ($n = 221/282$), the experts judged the outcome of critical importance given the context. For these 221 critically important outcomes, they considered that 82% ($n = 182$) could have been easily measured from both the trialist and patient perspective at no cost (Additional file 4).

Avoidable waste of research due to missing important outcomes

For the 291 RCTs published in 2010 or later, taking into account selective or incomplete outcome reporting, waste of research could have been partially avoided for 43% ($n = 126$) and totally (i.e., the trial could have been included in all meta-analyses of important outcomes) for 12% ($n = 34$) (Fig. 2). If we also consider missing outcomes that could have been easily measured from the planning stage at no additional cost as judged by our experts, waste of research could have been partially avoided for 63% of RCTs ($n = 183$) and totally for 30% ($n = 86$) (Fig. 2).

Table 2 Classification of reasons for missing outcomes

	All trials published in 2010 or later			
Reasons for missing outcome	All trials (registered and unregistered)		Registered trials	
	No. of affected outcomes (%) $N = 971$	No. of affected trials (%)* $N = 291$	No. of affected outcomes (%) $N = 461$	No. of affected trials (%)* $N = 156$
Inadequate planning	282 (29)	123 (42)	282 (61)	123 (79)
Selective reporting	36 (4)	25 (9)	34 (7)	23 (15)
Incomplete reporting	204 (21)	117 (40)	98 (21)	64 (41)
Unable to distinguish between selective reporting and lack of planning	363 (39)	122 (42)		
Other situations	86 (9)	63 (24)	47 (10)	41 (26)

*The total exceeds 100% because some outcomes were included in more than one category

Discussion

We evaluated the avoidable waste of research due to outcome-related reasons across a large number of RCTs included in recent Cochrane systematic reviews in a variety of medical fields. Our analysis revealed that 78% of the RCTs were not included in all meta-analyses of important outcomes and that every RCT contributed to 55%, on average, of the meta-analyses of these important outcomes. Among registered RCTs, inadequate planning was the most common reason affecting 79% of RCTs with missing outcomes. Such waste could have been partially avoided for 63% of the RCTs and totally for 30%.

Our findings suggest that many RCTs were not included in all meta-analyses of important outcomes and that every RCT contributed to only half of the meta-analyses, on average. These results seem consistent with the literature. In a recent study of patient-important outcomes, the median proportion of trials included in a meta-analysis for such outcomes was about 60% [39]. Approximately half of the RCTs included in another sample of Cochrane reviews were included in the pooled effect size estimates in the meta-analyses of patient-important outcomes [40], whereas more than one-third of the outcomes prespecified in the review were not reported in the results sections [18, 41].

Although possible reasons for excluding RCTS from meta-analyses have been hypothesized, the respective contribution of inadequate planning and selective reporting or incomplete reporting was unknown. Our results provide major insights into this question, showing that many RCTs do not plan the most important outcomes to evaluate. Inadequate planning represents a missed opportunity within a trial because equipoise remains unchanged after this trial. However, a missed opportunity at the trial level will result in waste of research at the meta-analysis level. Actually, clinical research should be considered a sequential process, with each new trial contributing to the existing body of evidence. If a trial fails to do so because of a missed opportunity, it becomes a source of waste of research and resources at the meta-analysis level because this trial will not contribute to the overall evidence. Cochrane reviewers may select outcomes that differ in importance from those selected by trialists (typically those defined as primary outcomes and used for sample size calculation). Trialists rarely consider adverse events (particularly severe adverse events) as primary outcomes and for sample size calculation. However, these outcomes are crucial to assess and report because they could be included in meta-analyses to increase power and inform decision-making. Identifying important outcomes is challenging, and without a consensus on outcomes, heterogeneity in outcomes evaluated will remain [41].

To overcome these issues, several initiatives have emerged to improve the relevance and consistency of outcomes used in clinical research [4, 42–45]; one is the Core Outcome Measures in Effectiveness Trials (COMET) initiative promoting the development and use of standardized core outcome sets (COSs). COMET offers extremely helpful tools for researchers aiming to develop COSs in their fields. However, although the number of COSs is rapidly increasing, it remains limited [46–48], and searching for specific existing COSs for a given condition is difficult. The COMET website may evolve to present available COSs in a tabular fashion to help trialists identify the outcomes to use and researchers the conditions for which COSs are needed. Another perspective would be to use the outcomes reported in the SoF table of Cochrane reviews to develop COSs, because most of these outcomes seem important to patients.

Incomplete reporting was another common reason for outcomes excluded from meta-analyses. Two main situations can be distinguished. First, the failure to report results adequately (e.g., reporting means without standard deviations) and second, the reporting of an analysis that cannot be included as such in a meta-analysis (e.g., reporting of repeated data analysis). The first situation is clearly related to poor reporting. We previously showed that results were more completely reported at

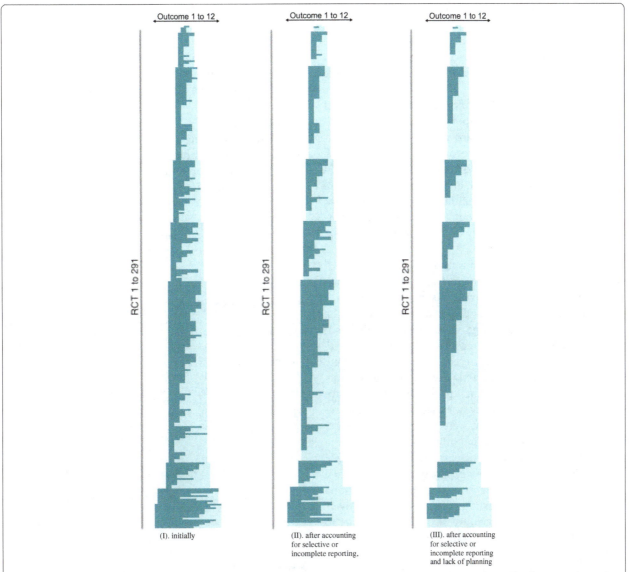

Fig. 2 Avoidable waste of research related to missing outcomes in RCTs published in 2010 or later and not contributing to all meta-analyses of important outcomes (n = 291). This figure summarizes the evolution of the outcomes status of SoF tables (O1 to O12 because SoF tables included from 1 to 12 outcomes per review) for each RCT at the different steps of our study: step I (i.e., information as it was extracted), step II (i.e., after evaluating the reason for the missing outcome) and after considering if there was no selective reporting or incomplete reporting, and finally step III (i.e., evaluation of waste of research) and after accounting for inadequate planning and selective reporting or incomplete reporting (i.e., adequate planning and no selective reporting or incomplete reporting). On the y-axis, each line represents one of the 291 RCTs published in 2010 or later and not contributing to all meta-analyses of the outcomes reported in the SoF table. The x-axis represents the outcomes reported in the SoF table. Each brick represents a single outcome of the SoF table. The color is a visual representation of the presence or absence of the outcome in the RCT. Light blue means that the outcome was present in the corresponding RCT and dark blue that the outcome was absent in the RCT. RCT randomized controlled trial, SoF summary of findings

ClinicalTrials.gov than in publications, probably because of the standardized template used to report results at ClinicalTrials.gov [49]. Such standardized templates may help trialists determine which data should be reported and should be included in reporting guidelines and required by journals to improve the presentation of results. The other situation is more complex because it does not reflect poor reporting, just reporting in a different way. Studies with repeated data are meant to record measurements at numerous time points to inform researchers of changes over time. However, several approaches for meta-analyzing these types of data exist, and they can differ in terms of the data needed for analysis [50]. Therefore, reporting trial results not just for an immediate use but also considering a later inclusion in meta-analyses can be challenging. The Instrument for reporting of Planned Endpoints in Clinical Trials (InsPECT) reporting guidelines (currently under development, https://www.inspect-statement.org/) might help trial authors mitigate the effects of incomplete reporting in RCTs.

Finally, selective reporting of outcomes seems to affect a few trials. It remains an important issue in clinical trials, with, on average, one-third of discrepancies in primary outcomes between protocols and publications [29] or between registry information and publications [31]. In our situation, this concerns only outcomes that were planned and not reported at all in publications. Actually, reviewers consider a given outcome whether this outcome is reported as a primary or a secondary outcome.

Strengths and limitations of the study
In this study, we used an original approach to evaluate the main reasons why a trial was not included in a meta-analysis and the part of this waste that could be avoided. We analyzed a large set of trials included in a vast, unselected, sample of recent Cochrane reviews exploring various health-care research topics. Assembling numerous experts in such a variety of fields to identify the most important outcomes to evaluate would have been challenging. As a proxy, we used the outcomes reported in the SoF tables that were considered by the review authors as the most important to measure for a given comparison in a particular health condition [7]. We used the consensus of an expert panel of recognized methodologists and trialists to assess the feasibility and costs of measuring the missing outcomes. To avoid overestimating waste of research, we also asked the panel to evaluate the importance of outcomes and considered that research was wasted for only those outcomes the panel confirmed to be of critical importance.

Our study has several limitations. First, we focused only on trials included in Cochrane reviews published between 2010 and 2014. However, it has been reported that Cochrane and non-Cochrane reviews have systemic differences, likely reflective of different methodology [51]. Then, we focused on trials included in the reviews but excluded from at least one meta-analysis. We did not consider the number of trials excluded from the reviews for outcome-related reasons. Therefore, we probably underestimated the proportion of trials excluded from meta-analyses for outcome-related reasons. Despite the recommendation of the Cochrane Handbook to determine trial eligibility independently of outcomes measured (studies should not be excluded just because they provide no usable data), some trials may be excluded for this reason [7]. Thus, although, our sample of RCTs was from a large variety of medical fields, the database used (Cochrane reviews published between 2010 and 2014

and with an SoF table), the limited sample size, the language restrictions, or the expertise of our panel of experts may limit the generalizability of our results. Finally, as a quality measure, 10% of the RCTs were classified independently by two reviewers, since this assessment is challenging and implies some subjectivity.

Conclusions
Our study shows that most RCTs included in our sample of Cochrane reviews did not contribute to all meta-analyses of the most important outcomes mainly because of inadequate planning or incomplete reporting. Such waste could have been partially avoided for 63% of the trials and totally for 30%. We need to accelerate the development and dissemination of COSs and reduce poor outcome reporting to avoid this waste.

Additional files

Additional file 1: Summary of the inclusion and exclusion criteria for the different phases of the study.

Additional file 2: Qualifications and areas of expertise of the experts involved in the final step of the study.

Additional file 3: Characteristics of the 820 Cochrane systematic reviews and the analyzed subset of 290 reviews.

Additional file 4: Experts' opinion of the feasibility and costs of measuring the missing outcomes.

Abbreviations
CI: Confidence interval; COMET: Core Outcome Measures in Effectiveness Trials; COS: Core outcome sets; ICTRP: International Clinical Trials Registry Platform; RCT: Randomized controlled trial; SoF: Summary of findings; WHO: World Health Organization

Acknowledgments
We thank Elise Diard for help in designing Fig. 2.

Funding
This study did not receive any specific funding.

Authors' contributions
YY was involved in study conception, selection of trials, data extraction, data analysis, interpretation of results, and drafting the manuscript. AD was involved in study conception, selection of trials, data extraction, data analysis, interpretation of results, and drafting the manuscript. IA was involved in initial data management, interpretation of results, and drafting the manuscript. VT, IB, and PC were involved in the interpretation of results and drafting the manuscript. PR was involved in study conception, interpretation of results, and drafting the manuscript. All authors read and approved the final manuscript.

Competing interests
The authors declare that they have no competing interests. All authors have completed the International Committee of Medical Journal Editors uniform disclosure form at www.icmje.org/coi_disclosure.pdf (available on request from the corresponding author) and declare that they received no support

from any organization for the submitted work, they have no financial relationships with any organizations that might have an interest in the submitted work in the previous 3 years, and they have no other relationships or activities that could appear to have influenced the submitted work.

Author details
[1]INSERM, U1153, Hôpital Hôtel-Dieus, 1, place du parvis Notre Dame, 75004 Paris, France. [2]Sorbonne Universités, UPMC Paris Univ-06, Paris, France. [3]Service des Urgences - Hôpital Saint Antoine, Assistance Publique–Hôpitaux de Paris (APHP), Paris, France. [4]Centre d'Épidémiologie Clinique, Hôpital Hôtel Dieu, Assistance Publique–Hôpitaux de Paris (APHP), Paris, France. [5]Faculté de Médecine, Université Paris Descartes, Sorbonne Paris Cité, Paris, France. [6]Cochrane France, Paris, France. [7]Department of Epidemiology, Columbia University, Mailman School of Public Health, New York, USA.

References
1. Tugwell P, Boers M. OMERACT conference on outcome measures in rheumatoid arthritis clinical trials: introduction. J Rheumatol. 1993;20(3):528–30.
2. Frank L, Basch E, Selby JV. Patient-centered outcomes research I: the PCORI perspective on patient-centered outcomes research. Jama. 2014;312(15):1513–4.
3. Koroshetz W. A core set of trial outcomes for every medical discipline? BMJ. 2015;350:h85.
4. Williamson P, Altman D, Blazeby J, Clarke M, Gargon E. Driving up the quality and relevance of research through the use of agreed core outcomes. J Health Serv Res Policy. 2012;17(1):1–2.
5. Tunis SR, Clarke M, Gorst SL, Gargon E, Blazeby JM, Altman DG, Williamson PR. Improving the relevance and consistency of outcomes in comparative effectiveness research. J Comp Eff Res. 2016;5(2):193-205.
6. Murad MH, Shah ND, Van Houten HK, Ziegenfuss JY, Deming JR, Beebe TJ, Smith SA, Guyatt GH, Montori VM. Individuals with diabetes preferred that future trials use patient-important outcomes and provide pragmatic inferences. J Clin Epidemiol. 2011;64(7):743–8.
7. Higgins JPT, Green S (editors). Cochrane Handbook for Systematic Reviews of Interventions Version 5.1.0 [updated March 2011]. The Cochrane Collaboration, 2011. Available from http://handbook.cochrane.org.
8. Ioannidis JPA. Why most clinical research is not useful. PLoS Med. 2016;13(6):e1002049.
9. Chalmers I, Glasziou P. Avoidable waste in the production and reporting of research evidence. Lancet. 2009;374(9683):86–9.
10. Al-Shahi Salman R, Beller E, Kagan J, Hemminki E, Phillips RS, Savulescu J, Macleod M, Wisely J, Chalmers I. Increasing value and reducing waste in biomedical research regulation and management. Lancet. 2014;383(9912):176–85.
11. Chalmers I, Bracken MB, Djulbegovic B, Garattini S, Grant J, Gulmezoglu AM, Howells DW, Ioannidis JP, Oliver S. How to increase value and reduce waste when research priorities are set. Lancet. 2014;383(9912):156–65.
12. Chan AW, Song F, Vickers A, Jefferson T, Dickersin K, Gotzsche PC, Krumholz HM, Ghersi D, van der Worp HB. Increasing value and reducing waste: addressing inaccessible research. Lancet. 2014;383(9913):257–66.
13. Glasziou P, Altman DG, Bossuyt P, Boutron I, Clarke M, Julious S, Michie S, Moher D, Wager E. Reducing waste from incomplete or unusable reports of biomedical research. Lancet. 2014;383(9913):267–76.
14. Ioannidis JP, Greenland S, Hlatky MA, Khoury MJ, Macleod MR, Moher D, Schulz KF, Tibshirani R. Increasing value and reducing waste in research design, conduct, and analysis. Lancet. 2014;383(9912):166–75.
15. Macleod MR, Michie S, Roberts I, Dirnagl U, Chalmers I, Ioannidis JP, Al-Shahi Salman R, Chan AW, Glasziou P. Biomedical research: increasing value, reducing waste. Lancet. 2014;383(9912):101–4.
16. Moher D, Glasziou P, Chalmers I, Nasser M, Bossuyt PMM, Korevaar DA, Graham ID, Ravaud P, Boutron I. Increasing value and reducing waste in biomedical research: who's listening? Lancet. 2016;387(10027):1573–86.
17. Yordanov Y, Dechartres A, Porcher R, Boutron I, Altman DG, Ravaud P. Avoidable waste of research related to inadequate methods in clinical trials. BMJ. 2015;350:h809.
18. Smith V, Clarke M, Williamson P, Gargon E. Survey of new 2007 and 2011 Cochrane reviews found 37% of prespecified outcomes not reported. J Clin Epidemiol. 2014;68(3):237–45.
19. Gandhi GY, Murad MH, Fujiyoshi A, Mullan RJ, Flynn DN, Elamin MB, Swiglo BA, Isley WL, Guyatt GH, Montori VM. Patient-important outcomes in registered diabetes trials. JAMA. 2008;299(21):2543–9.
20. Rahimi K, Malhotra A, Banning AP, Jenkinson C. Outcome selection and role of patient reported outcomes in contemporary cardiovascular trials: systematic review. BMJ. 2010;341:c5707.
21. Svensson S, Menkes DB, Lexchin J. Surrogate outcomes in clinical trials: a cautionary tale. JAMA Intern Med. 2013;173(8):611–2.
22. Naci H, Ioannidis JP. How good is "evidence" from clinical studies of drug effects and why might such evidence fail in the prediction of the clinical utility of drugs? Annu Rev Pharmacol Toxicol. 2015;55:169–89.
23. Ocana A, Tannock IF. When are "positive" clinical trials in oncology truly positive? J Natl Cancer Inst. 2010;103(1):16–20.
24. Gluud C, Krogsgaard K. Would you trust a surrogate respondent? Lancet. 1997;349(9053):665–6.
25. The Cardiac Arrhythmia Suppression Trial (CAST) Investigators. Preliminary report: effect of encainide and flecainide on mortality in a randomized trial of arrhythmia suppression after myocardial infarction. N Engl J Med. 1989;321(6):406–12.
26. Ciani O, Buyse M, Garside R, Pavey T, Stein K, Sterne JA, Taylor RS. Comparison of treatment effect sizes associated with surrogate and final patient relevant outcomes in randomised controlled trials: meta-epidemiological study. BMJ. 2013;346:f457.
27. Moynihan R. Surrogates under scrutiny: fallible correlations, fatal consequences. BMJ. 2011;343:d5160.
28. Walter SD, Sun X, Heels-Ansdell D, Guyatt G. Treatment effects on patient-important outcomes can be small, even with large effects on surrogate markers. J Clin Epidemiol. 2012;65(9):940–5.
29. Chan AW, Hrobjartsson A, Haahr MT, Gotzsche PC, Altman DG. Empirical evidence for selective reporting of outcomes in randomized trials: comparison of protocols to published articles. JAMA. 2004;291(20):2457–65.
30. Dwan K, Altman DG, Cresswell L, Blundell M, Gamble CL, Williamson PR. Comparison of protocols and registry entries to published reports for randomised controlled trials. Cochrane Database Syst Rev. 2011;1:MR000031.
31. Mathieu S, Boutron I, Moher D, Altman DG, Ravaud P. Comparison of registered and published primary outcomes in randomized controlled trials. JAMA. 2009;302(9):977–84.
32. Williamson PR, Gamble C. Identification and impact of outcome selection bias in meta-analysis. Stat Med. 2005;24(10):1547–61.
33. Kirkham JJ, Dwan KM, Altman DG, Gamble C, Dodd S, Smyth R, Williamson PR. The impact of outcome reporting bias in randomised controlled trials on a cohort of systematic reviews. BMJ. 2010;340:c365.
34. Jones CW, Keil LG, Holland WC, Caughey MC, Platts-Mills TF. Comparison of registered and published outcomes in randomized controlled trials: a systematic review. BMC Med. 2015;13:282.
35. Chan AW, Krleza-Jeric K, Schmid I, Altman DG. Outcome reporting bias in randomized trials funded by the Canadian Institutes of Health Research. CMAJ. 2004;171(7):735–40.
36. Chan A-W, Altman DG. Identifying outcome reporting bias in randomised trials on PubMed: review of publications and survey of authors. BMJ. 2005;330(7494):753.
37. Dechartres A, Ravaud P, Atal I, Riveros C, Boutron I. Association between trial registration and treatment effect estimates: a meta-epidemiological study. BMC Med. 2016;14(1):100.
38. Mocellin S, Lens MB, Pasquali S, Pilati P, Chiarion Sileni V. Interferon alpha for the adjuvant treatment of cutaneous melanoma. Cochrane Database Syst Rev. 2013;6:CD008955.
39. Ameur H, Ravaud P, Fayard F, Riveros C, Dechartres A. Systematic reviews of therapeutic interventions frequently consider patient-important outcomes. J Clin Epidemiol. 2017;84:70–77.
40. Furukawa TA, Watanabe N, Omori IM, Montori VM, Guyatt GH. Association between unreported outcomes and effect size estimates in Cochrane meta-analyses. JAMA. 2007;297(5):468–70.
41. Wuytack F, Smith V, Clarke M, Williamson P, Gargon E. Towards core outcome set (COS) development: a follow-up descriptive survey of outcomes in Cochrane reviews. Syst Rev. 2015;4(1):73.

42. The COMET (Core Outcome Measures in Effectiveness Trials) Initiative [http://www.comet-initiative.org/]. Accessed 11 Apr 2017.
43. Methodology Committee of the Patient-Centered Outcomes Research I. Methodological standards and patient-centeredness in comparative effectiveness research: the PCORI perspective. JAMA. 2012;307(15):1636–40.
44. Selby JV, Beal AC, Frank L. The Patient-Centered Outcomes Research Institute (PCORI) national priorities for research and initial research agenda. JAMA. 2012;307(15):1583–4.
45. Clarke M, Williamson P. Core outcome sets and trial registries. Trials. 2015;16(1):216.
46. Gargon E, Williamson PR, Altman DG, Blazeby JM, Tunis S, Clarke M. The COMET initiative database: progress and activities update (2015). Trials. 2017;18(1):54.
47. Gargon E, Williamson PR, Altman DG, Blazeby JM, Clarke M. The COMET initiative database: progress and activities update (2014). Trials. 2015;16:515.
48. Gargon E, Williamson PR, Altman DG, Blazeby JM, Clarke M. The COMET initiative database: progress and activities from 2011 to 2013. Trials. 2014;15:279.
49. Riveros C, Dechartres A, Perrodeau E, Haneef R, Boutron I, Ravaud P. Timing and completeness of trial results posted at ClinicalTrials.gov and published in journals. PLoS Med. 2013;10(12):e1001566.
50. Peters JL, Mengersen KL. Meta-analysis of repeated measures study designs. J Eval Clin Pract. 2008;14(5):941–50.
51. Useem J, Brennan A, LaValley M, Vickery M, Ameli O, Reinen N, Gill CJ. Systematic differences between Cochrane and non-Cochrane meta-analyses on the same topic: a matched pair analysis. PLoS One. 2015;10(12):e0144980.

Thresholds of socio-economic and environmental conditions necessary to escape from childhood malnutrition: a natural experiment in rural Gambia

Mayya Husseini[1,2], Momodou K Darboe[1], Sophie E Moore[1,3], Helen M Nabwera[4] and Andrew M Prentice[1*]

Abstract

Background: Childhood malnutrition remains highly prevalent in low-income countries, and a 40% reduction in under-5 year stunting is WHO's top Global Target 2025. Disappointingly, meta-analyses of intensive nutrition interventions reveal that they generally have low efficacy at improving growth. Unhygienic environments also contribute to growth failure, but large WASH Benefits and SHINE trials of improved water, sanitation and hygiene (WASH) recently reported no benefits to child growth.

Methods: To explore the thresholds of socio-economic status (SES) and living standards associated with malnutrition, we exploited a natural experiment in which the location of our research centre within a remote rural village created a wide diversity of wealth, education and housing conditions within the same ecological setting and with free health services to all. A composite SES score was generated by grading occupation, education, income, water and sanitation, and housing and families were allocated to 5 groups (SES1 = highest). SES ranged from very poor subsistence-farming villagers to post graduate staff with overseas training. Nutritional status at 24 m was obtained from clinic records for 230 children and expressed relative to WHO Growth Standards.

Results: Height-for-age (HAZ) and weight-for-age (WAZ) Z-scores were strongly predicted by SES group. HAZ varied from − 0.67 to − 2.23 ($P < 0.001$) and WAZ varied from − 0.90 to − 1.64 ($P < 0.001$), from SES1 to SES5, respectively. Weight-for-height (WHZ) showed no gradient. Children in SES1 showed greater dispersion so were further divided in a post hoc analysis. Children resident in Western housing on the research compound (SES1A) had HAZ = + 0.68 and WAZ = + 0.36. The residual gradient between those in SES1B and SES5 spanned only 0.65 Z-score for HAZ (− 1.58 to − 2.23) and was not significant for WAZ or WHZ.

Conclusions: The large difference in growth between children in SES1A living in Western-type housing and SES1B children living in the village, and the very shallow gradient between SES1B and SES5, implies a very high SES threshold before stunting and underweight will be eliminated. This may help to explain the lack of efficacy of the recent WASH interventions and points to the need for what is termed 'Transformative WASH'. Good quality housing, with piped water into the home, may be key to eliminating malnutrition.

Keywords: Child growth, Stunting, Socioeconomic status, Gambia, WASH, Hygiene, Environmental, Enteropathy, Global health

---

* Correspondence: aprentice@mrc.gm
[1]MRC Unit The Gambia at London School of Hygiene and Tropical Medicine, Atlantic Boulevard, Fajara, Banjul, The Gambia
Full list of author information is available at the end of the article

Background

Severe growth faltering leading to stunting and underweight remains highly prevalent in low- and middle-income countries [1] (LMICs) and is estimated to play a role in 45% of under-5 year child deaths [2]. An analysis of data from 54 such countries shows that babies are born small and then follow a remarkably uniform pattern of stunting initiated soon after birth and continuing to a nadir at about 24 months [1]. In Africa and SE Asia average height-for-age Z-scores (HAZ) fall to less than −2 HAZ against the WHO Growth Reference Standard [1]. Weight-for-age Z-scores (WAZ) vary more widely between populations.

Despite many decades of research, the precise aetiology of this growth failure remains obscure. It is ecologically associated with a number of correlates of poverty including generally poor diets of low diversity; food insecurity; poor water supply, sanitation and hygiene; frequent infections and inflammation (including enteric infections that cause a persistent environmental enteropathy that may inhibit nutrient uptake); and constraints on mothers' time combined with poor parental understanding of the principles of childcare. However, amelioration of some of these factors frequently has a disappointing impact on child growth. For instance, during 35 years of intensive clinical and nutritional interventions in rural Gambia, we have reduced child mortality rates over 10-fold [3] and observed a profound decline in diarrhoeal disease [4], yet the prevalence of stunting is still 30% [5]. Others have shown that careful evaluation of nutritional and educational interventions either singly or in combination achieve improvements in HAZ of less than 0.3 Z-scores [6]; representing less than one sixth of the average deficit.

The excellent prenatal and post-natal growth shown by the cohorts of carefully selected children used to derive the INTERGROWTH Fetal Growth [7], and WHO Child Growth Standards [8] demonstrate the potential for excellent growth when the environmental conditions are right. Furthermore, rates of stunting decline quite rapidly as countries pass through the demographic transition. [9]. So why is it so difficult to improve child growth in low-income settings? The current paradigm is that multiple interventions must be introduced simultaneously [10] and numerous trials combining efforts to improve water, sanitation, hygiene (WASH), diet, breast-feeding rates, infant stimulation and parental education are in progress. Notably, the large-scale WASH Benefits trials in Kenya and Bangladesh have recently reported their outcomes with respect to stunting [11, 12]. The intervention arms that promoted infant and young child feeding (IYCF) showed a significant reduction in stunting but with a very modest effect size (0.13–0.16 Z-score for length in Kenya and 0.13–0.25 Z-score in Bangladesh). The SHINE Trial in Zimbabwe has also reported significant but limited success with IYCF (0.16 Z-score for length) [13]. Disappointingly, none of the WASH interventions reduced stunting.

In this study, we exploited a natural experiment to examine thresholds of socio-economic development associated with growth faltering. Our research centre at MRC Keneba is embedded within a rural subsistence-farming Gambian village. The centre employs over 200 indigenous staff ranging from scientists, physicians and senior management, through nurses, laboratory technicians and field-workers to lower grades of support staff such as cleaners many of whom are natives of Keneba or nearby villages. We also studied villagers without any paid employment. These circumstances have created a very wide socio-economic and educational gradient within the same confined ecological setting and allowed us to examine the effects of these gradients on child growth.

Methods

Study location

The UK Medical Research Council has maintained a research presence in the poor rural West Kiang region of The Gambia, since 1948. The field station comprises a self-sufficient 4-acre site with housing, laboratories, clinic and administrative buildings contained within a perimeter fence. All housing is of 'Western' standard with tiled floors, metal roofs and suspended ceilings, fully plumbed kitchens and bathrooms with flushing toilets and hot and cold water to basins and showers, screened and louvered windows, gas cooking, fans and air conditioning. Water and electricity are available constantly and are not charged to staff, thus allowing unlimited usage. The keeping of livestock is strongly discouraged in the compound. Originally sited on the edge of the village, it has now become engulfed by new village compounds as the population has expanded. Most villagers rely for their livelihoods on subsistence farming, occasionally supplemented by some petty trading, and increasingly by remittances from family members who have migrated to urban areas or abroad. The village has a primary and middle school and an Islamic school. Uptake of education has increased in the past two decades, initially male dominated but now more equitable due to universal free education for girls. The MRC compound and the village are both supplied by clean tube-well water. Villagers obtain their water from a series of 30+ standpipes distributed as equitably as possible around the village. Water is potable as it emerges from the taps. Subsequent contamination during collection and storage is possible.

Healthcare

For over 35 years, we have provided an exceptional level of free healthcare for villagers and staff (summarised in Box 1). Thus, availability of healthcare is constant across

> **Box 1: Concordant factors across the population sample**
>
> - Residence within the same 4 km^2
> - Free access to MRC Keneba Clinic providing excellent healthcare (3 qualified medical doctors, diagnostics labs, etc.) 5 days per week. Round-the-clock (24/7) emergency access to on-call staff.
> - Free access to medications with reliable supply. Close to 100% vaccination and vitamin A supplementation rates using full WHO schedule. Guaranteed cold chain. Ready access to oral rehydration fluids.
> - Equal access to 3-monthly growth monitoring. All children called to 3-monthly healthy child clinics.
> - Free referral to secondary and tertiary health care when required. Free transportation provided. Free nutritional rehabilitation according to WHO protocols for any child falling below – 3 WHZ.
> - Universal access to excellent ante-natal and delivery care including provision of blanket FeFol supplementation and malaria prophylaxis in pregnancy.
> - Universal breast-feeding to at least 18 m for village children and similar for staff children. No formula milk available in local markets. Keneba is a Baby Friendly Community supported by the National Nutrition Agency with promotion of exclusive breast-feeding to 6 m.
> - Water supplied from the same borehole and via same storage tank.

all socio-economic and educational levels, and for staff and villagers alike, and uptake is only determined by parental health-seeking behaviours. All women receive regularly scheduled ante-natal care, and their infants have a post-natal check-up and are called to well-baby clinics at 6 week, 3 m and then at 3 m intervals until 2 years of age. All children receive their full schedule of Extended Programme of Immunisation (EPI) vaccines and vitamin A supplementation according to WHO guidelines.

Eligibility and sampling

The greatest variance in SES was associated with MRC employment. Using the Kiang West Demographic Surveillance System (DSS) [14], a list of all children with anthropometric data (length and weight measurements) taken at 24 ± 4 m of age and born between January 1993 and December 2009 was created. The sample size was determined by the number of MRC employees who had children at 24 m within the study window. All MRC employees on the list were approached to participate. This yielded 51 families and 133 children. This list was supplemented with data from 129 village children selected at random from our DSS database and matched by year of measurement. Children with any condition known to affect growth were excluded.

Assessment of parental SES

A total of 98 parents were interviewed during the data collection period. Parental SES was evaluated using a modified version of a 43-item questionnaire originally developed to study the relationship between parental SES and child mortality elsewhere in The Gambia [15]. The questions were grouped according to occupation, income and possessions, education, access to water and sanitation, and housing. In the absence of indications to the contrary, each of these factors was assumed to have an equal impact on child growth; thus, each category was given the same weight of a maximum of 10 points. Each question within each category was then assigned an appropriately weighted score based on information from senior staff at the MRC about the perceived socio-economic value of items in the questionnaire. The aggregate SES score for each set of parents was then determined by adding up the 5 separate scores obtained for each category, giving a total maximum of 50 points. Initially the total parental scores were assigned a priori to 5 SES groups as follows: SES1 = > 25; SES2 = 21–25; SES3 = 17–21; SES4 = 14–17; and SES5 = < 14. It was subsequently noted that SES1 showed a wide dispersion of anthropometric values so this group was further divided as follows: SES1A = > 25 points and resident in Western-style housing within the MRC compound; and SES1B = > 25 points and resident in the village. The headline descriptors of each SES category are listed in Table 1.

Anthropometry

In this population, anthropometric status declines rapidly in the first and second years of life and then remains somewhat stable before recovering slightly in later childhood [16]. We therefore obtained clinic records for heights and weights at 24 ± 4 m. Weight (in minimal clothing) and recumbent length (height) were recorded by trained anthropometrists using standard techniques and regularly calibrated apparatus. Appropriate weight data was found for 262 children, but there were 32 missing heights. The data were then restricted to those that had full anthropometric values available; yielding a final sample size of 230. HAZ, WAZ and WHZ were calculated using WHO Anthro software (version 3.2.2) based on the 2006 WHO Child Growth Standards [8]. Within the narrow age range selected for this study, there was no influence of age on any of the anthropometric measures. There was an influence of sex, so this has been

Table 1 Typical SES characteristics of the five pre hoc determined groups and subsequent post hoc division of group 1

Pre hoc assignment	1A	1B	2	3	4	5
N	8	11	46	72	65	28
Occupation	One or both parents with senior MRC jobs; (e.g. scientific officer and admin staff)	One parent with middle grade job at MRC (e.g. field worker); Mother likely to be housewife	One farmer parent, other with lower grade job at MRC (e.g. cleaner)	Farmer parents	Farmer parents; father likely to be retired
Education	Both parents have > 10 years at English school. Most families have one parent with university qualifications and/or post graduate diplomas from abroad	Fathers have > 10 years at Arabic and English school; Mother likely to have approx. 5 years at English school	One parent with approx. 5 years in English school	Approx. 10 years for father and 5 years for mother in Arabic school	Approx. 5 years in Arabic school for father only
Income	Main income from MRC employment	Main income from MRC employment	Main income from MRC employment, remittances and minor produce sales	Dependent on minor produce sales and remittances	Dependent on remittances
Water and sanitation	Plumbed hot and cold water to kitchens and bathrooms, indoor flushing toilets, modern cooking facilities	Public tap for water, pit latrine exclusive to household, cook with firewood	Public tap for water, pit latrine exclusive to household, cook with firewood	Public tap for water, pit latrine exclusive to household, cook with firewood	Public tap for water, pit latrine exclusive to household, cook with firewood	Public tap for water, pit latrine shared with other households, cook with firewood
Housing	European grade cement housing with ceramic tile flooring, screened windows, fans and air conditioning, located on MRC compound	Local housing, cement as main material. Corrugated iron roofing. Occasional solar electricity. Unscreened windows, located in the village	Local housing, cement as main material. Corrugated iron roofing. Occasional solar electricity. Unscreened windows, located in the village	Local housing, cement as main material. Corrugated iron roofing. Occasional solar electricity. Unscreened windows, located in the village	Local housing, cement as main material. Corrugated iron roofing. Occasional solar electricity. Unscreened windows, located in the village	Basic housing; mud as main material. Corrugated iron or thatched roofing

included in the analysis model. Stunting was defined as HAZ < – 2, underweight as WAZ < – 2 and wasting as WHZ < – 2. Parental heights were obtained from our DHSS database. There were 2 missing maternal heights.

Data analysis

Multi-level linear analysis was performed on anthropometric attainment at 24 m according to the 5 (later 6) SES groups with adjustment for parental heights and with intra-household clustering accounted for by including mother's ID on the basis that children of this age live with their mothers. Date of measurement was included in the model to test for any secular drift but was not significant so was not included in the final analysis. All analyses were performed using the 'Linear Models' function in DataDesk version 7.0.2 (Data description Inc., Ithaca, NY).

Results

On average fathers had 2 wives (range 1–4) and 12 children (range 1–33). Mothers averaged 6 children (range 1–12) and household size averaged 13 (range 4–27). Fathers averaged 3.5 years of formal education (range 0–18 years) and 8.0 years of Arabic/Islamic studies (range 0–24). Mothers averaged 2.0 years of formal education (range 0–16 years) and 4.4 years of Arabic/Islamic studies (range 0–13). Reported incomes ranged from less than US$50 to over US$20,000 per annum. Eight percent of families owned a car, 12% a motorcycle and 55% a bicycle. Seventeen percent had a refrigerator, 32% had a television and 19% had electricity at home. Housing ranged from very basic mud block huts to Western-style housing with hot and cold running water, showers, flushing toilets, gas cooking, refrigerators, mosquito screens, fans and air conditioning.

The mean anthropometric statistics for the whole sample were HAZ (% stunted), boys = – 1.94 (40%), girls = – 1.55 (35%) ($p = 0.018$ for sex); WAZ (% underweight) boys = – 1.46 (31%), girls = – 1.32 (21%) ($p = 0.052$ for sex); and WHZ (% wasted) boys = – 0.64 (5%), girls = – 0.68 (6%) (NS for sex). Notably, The Gambian children's heights and weights at 2 years of age were very similar to the average heights and weights of WHO reference children at 1 year of age.

Table 2 details the mean anthropometric Z-scores according to the 5 pre-determined SES groupings

Table 2 Mean anthropometric scores at 24 m according to the 5 pre hoc SES categories

Variable	Mean per SES category					P value for trend
	1 upper	2 upper-middle	3 middle	4 lower-middle	5 lower	
N	19	46	72	65	28	
HAZ score	− 0.67 [3,4,5]	− 1.58	− 1.69 [1]	− 2.16 [1]	− 2.23 [1]	< 0.001
% stunted	26	37	44	54	54	
WAZ score	− 0.90	− 1.20	− 1.35	− 1.67	− 1.64	< 0.001
% underweight	31	17	19	34	43	
WHZ score	− 0.63	− 0.56	− 0.63	− 0.77	− 0.68	0.255
% wasted	10	4	4	9	4	
Mothers' heights	159.6	162.0	164.0	161.3	161.9	0.014
Fathers' heights	173.5 [4]	171.3 [4]	170.6	167.8 [1,2]	170.4	< 0.001

Superscripts indicate the SES groups against which values are significantly different at $P < 0.01$ by Scheffé's post hoc test. For the children's anthropometry, their parents' heights were included in the model. Child sex was also included in the model

(see Fig. 1 for the interquartile ranges). HAZ varied strongly with SES with a range from − 0.67 in SES1 to − 2.23 in SES5 ($P < 0.001$); the proportions of stunted children were 26 and 54% respectively. Surprisingly, the trend between SES2, defined as upper-middle SES, and the lowest category of SES5 only spanned 0.65 Z-scores; and the proportion stunted varied from 37 to 54%. WAZ varied somewhat less strongly with SES with a range from − 0.90 in SES1 to − 1.64 in SES5 ($P < 0.001$); the proportions of underweight children were 31 and 43% respectively. The range in WAZ between SES2 and SES5 was only 0.44, and the proportions of underweight children were 17 and 43%. WHZ did not vary at all across SES groupings.

Inspection of the data revealed a greater dispersion of HAZ and WAZ in SES1 (composed entirely of the more senior MRC staff) than the other groups suggesting that it remained a heterogeneous grouping that would merit further sub-division. We therefore performed a post hoc split of SES1 using the factor that seemed most likely to offer discriminatory power; namely whether or not the staff were resident within the MRC's fenced compound (and therefore living in better quality accommodation) (SES1A) or in the village (SES1B) (see Table 1 for descriptors). The analysis by the 6 groupings is listed in Table 3 and illustrated with interquartile ranges in Fig. 1. The children brought up in the MRC compound had HAZ = + 0.68, WAZ = + 0.36 and WHZ = − 0.03. None were stunted or underweight, and 1 was very marginally wasted. In SES1B, where the families lived in the village, mean HAZ was − 1.65, mean WAZ was − 1.64 and mean WHZ was − 1.07 despite their very high SES. Children in SES1A were significantly taller and heavier than children from each of the other groups even when parental heights were included in the model (Scheffé's post hoc tests, see Tables 2 and 3). WHZ did not differ between any of the groups.

Parental heights were correlated with offspring HAZ (mother's coefficient 0.66 (SE 0.13) Z-score per 10 cm ($P < 0.0001$); father's coefficient 0.52 (SE 0.15) Z-score per 10 cm ($P < 0.0001$). There was no difference in maternal heights across the 5 or 6 SES groups. Paternal heights in SES1 and 2 were greater than in SES4. When SES1 was subdivided, it was the father's in SES1B who were tallest and significantly taller than SES4. Father's heights in SES1A were not significantly different to any other group.

Discussion

The major WASH Benefits trials in Kenya and Bangladesh [11, 12] and the SHINE trial in Zimbabwe [13] have recently reported that promotion of improved water, supply, sanitation and handwashing had no effect on linear growth. These very disappointing results from large-scale, rigorously implemented trials in appropriate target populations require an explanation. Our current study suggests that the intent was correct but that the environmental hygiene threshold that permits normal child growth is far higher than achieved in WASH Benefits and SHINE. The original selection strategy of participants for the WHO MGRS [17] that forms the basis of the current WHO Growth Standards implicitly recognised this same point.

The key feature of this study is that the participant families had identical access to health care and, by virtue of living in the same small village, shared common exposures to many other health-determining factors. This allowed us to interrogate the influence of 5 socio-economic domains (occupation, income and possessions, education, access to water and sanitation, and housing) with far fewer confounders than would normally exist in such analyses. We were also able to examine a very steep gradient ranging from the poorest village families with very few resources to families in which one or both

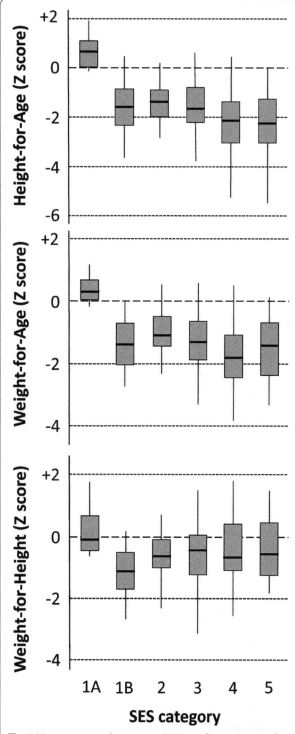

Fig. 1 Means, interquartile ranges and 95% confidence intervals for anthropometric scores at 24 m. Sample sizes, tests for trends and individual group comparisons by Scheffé's post hoc test are listed in Tables 2 and 3.

the villagers. Growth data was routinely measured and recorded for all children in the same anthropometric clinic, enabling an unbiased analysis of their attained size at 2 years of age; the growth nadir in this population.

The highly significant gradient in HAZ and WAZ across SES groups is unsurprising and validates the relevance of the SES metrics. The remarkable feature of the data is that the only children growing close to the WHO Growth Standard were those living in Western-type accommodation within the MRC campus (HAZ + 0.68, WAZ + 0.36, WHZ − 0.03). The children of staff of almost similar rank who, by virtue of a shortage of housing on the campus, lived in rented housing in the village fared substantially less well (HAZ − 1.65, WAZ − 1.64, WHZ − 1.07). The HAZ and WAZ advantage of children in SES1A was not explained by differences in parental heights suggesting that it is unlikely to reflect an intergenerational advantage.

Our analysis is unique to date and has the great strength of removing the influence of the healthcare and environmental variables listed in Box 1 that are concordant across all families and that otherwise would confound interpretation of the effects of the SES gradient studied. Its chief weakness is the limited sample size, and replication is needed if a similar natural experiment can be found elsewhere. The sample size limitation does not limit the key observation that child growth was far from desirable even in families with high levels of education, very good incomes and absolute food security. In a comparison of group SES1A and SES2 combined ($n = 57$) against the SES4 and SES5 groups combined ($n = 93$) HAZ varied by only 0.59 Z-scores from − 1.59 to − 2.18 and the prevalence of stunting from 39 to 54%. WAZ varied by only 0.38 Z-scores from − 1.28 to − 1.66. WHZ did not differ. An additional weakness is that the SES data were collected up to 15 year after the anthropometric data. This is of limited concern because we allocated occupation and salary ranking in MRC staff according to their grade when their child was 24 m and social mobility is very slow in villagers. Additionally, any misclassification would tend to nullify associations rather than introduce bias.

The modifiable components of children's growth (i.e. the non-genetic components) are influenced by a myriad of nutrition-specific factors (breast-feeding and complementary feeding practices, food availability and quality, and parental knowledge of the principles of child feeding) and nutrition-sensitive factors (sanitation and hygiene, access to health care, infections and stress). This likely explains why interventions aimed solely at improving complementary feeding, and diet have shown limited efficacy, even when conducted under the rigorously controlled conditions of research trials. Meta-analysis of trials involving feeding and/or educational interventions

parents had lived and trained in high-income countries and had advanced educational qualifications and incomes that were several orders of magnitude higher than

Table 3 Mean anthropometric scores at 24 m according to 6 post hoc SES categories

Variable	Mean per SES category						P value for Trend
	1A upper	1B upper	2 upper-middle	3 middle	4 lower-middle	5 lower	
N	8	11	46	72	65	28	
HAZ score	0.68 [1B,2,3,4,5]	− 1.65 [1A]	− 1.58 [1A]	− 1.69 [1A]	− 2.16 [1A]	− 2.23 [1A]	< 0.001
% stunted	0	45	37	44	54	54	
WAZ score	0.36 [1B,2,3,4,5]	− 1.64 [1A]	− 1.20 [1A]	− 1.35 [1A]	− 1.67 [1A]	− 1.64 [1A]	< 0.001
% underweight	0	55	17	19	34	43	
WHZ score	− 0.03	− 1.07	− 0.56	− 0.63	− 0.77	− 0.68	0.255
% wasted	12	9	4	4	9	4	
Mothers' heights	161.2	158.5	162.0	164.0	161.3	161.9	0.019
Fathers' heights	172.6	174.1 [4]	171.3	170.6	167.8 [1B]	170.4	< 0.001

Superscripts indicate the SES groups against which values are significantly different at $P < 0.01$ by Scheffé's post hoc test. For the children's anthropometry, their parents' heights were included in the model. Child sex was also included in the model

demonstrate average HAZ responses of less than 0.3 Z-scores; equivalent to about one sixth of the usual deficit by 2 years of age in LMICs [6]. Following these disappointments, it was argued that the quality of nutrition interventions had to be improved still further with the provision of a comprehensive range of micro- and macro-nutrients, and large trials of lipid-based nutritional supplements have recently been completed. Unfortunately, these have, by and large, also yielded disappointing outcomes ranging from no significant impact [18–21] to maximum benefits again not exceeding 0.3 Z-scores for height [22, 23]. Very recently, the WASH Benefits and SHINE trials have again confirmed this result. The groups receiving promotion of the WHO IYCF guidelines showed improvements of 0.13 (Kenya) and 0.25 (Bangladesh) Z-score in the nutrition group and of 0.16 (Kenya) and 0.13 (Bangladesh) Z-score in the nutrition plus WASH groups against the average HAZ in the control groups of − 1.54 in Kenya and − 1.79 in Bangladesh [11, 12]. The SHINE trial has recently reported very similar results with an improvement of 0.16 for HAZ in the IYCF group and 0.02 in the IYCF+WASH against a background level of − 1.59 Z-scores in the standard of care group [13].

A chief target of the WASH interventions has been to ameliorate the gut damage that is caused by poor living conditions [10]. Our previous work in The Gambia identified persistent and chronic damage to the gut (now commonly termed environmental enteric disease (EED)) as a likely mediating factor in growth failure [24, 25]. Enteropathy impairs nutrient absorption, increases energy and nutrient losses and causes chronic inflammation that suppresses the growth hormone/IGF1 somatotrophic axis [10, 26]. This chronic gut damage affects most children in poor settings and is believed to be initiated and sustained by repeated exposure to microorganisms (and possibly other aggravating factors) in a contaminated environment. A study in Bangladesh has found differences in biomarkers of EED between 'clean' and 'dirty' households and a 0.54 HAZ difference in growth in favour of the clean households, though it should be noted that average growth was still very poor at − 1.66 HAZ [27].

Overcoming such influences has formed the rationale for numerous WASH interventions. However, a Cochrane systematic review and meta-analysis of such trials published in 2013 concluded that efficacy was poor [28]. The analysis of randomised trials including over 4600 children studied over 9–12 m intervention periods revealed no evidence of any beneficial effect on weight-for-age or weight-for-height and only a marginally significant impact on height-for-age of less than one tenth of a standard deviation (+ 0.08 Z-score, 95%CI 0.00–0.16). An individual participant data analysis ($n = 5375$) was conducted for 5 RCTs. For HAZ, this identified a significant age interaction with children under 2 years gaining most benefit. Nonetheless, the benefit in this selected age band was still only 0.25 (95% CI 0.14–0.36) Z-scores [28]. The WASH Benefits and SHINE results are even more discouraging insofar as their null outcomes arose from very large, rigorously implemented trials in appropriate target populations [10–12].

One hypothesis about the lack of effects of the WASH interventions in WASH Benefits and SHINE is that they did not target the whole community; they only worked within individual households. Therefore, spillovers from the un-intervened households could still contribute to infection and inflammation in the study children. There is evidence that community-wide total sanitation interventions may have bigger effects [29–31], possibly related to herd protection. A similar effect may be at play within the MRC compound though it should be stressed that there is free movement into and out of the compound with multiple opportunities for cross-exposure between the SES1A children and villagers through social visits, markets, clinics and by sharing of transport.

The emergent consensus is that it has proven extremely difficult to shift child growth patterns by more than one sixth of the total deficit that accrues by age 2 years in LMICs. The Lancet Series on Maternal and Child Nutrition reinforces the conclusion that nutrition-related interventions will have limited impact [32]. The authors estimated that, even if scaled up to 90% coverage, the implementation of all of the currently identified evidence-based nutrition and nutrition-related interventions would eliminate around 20% of stunting globally.

The current study suggests a resolution to this paradox. Our data indicates that there is a very high threshold of living conditions that has to be surpassed for stunting to resolve. Our evidence suggests that despite adequate parental knowledge of the principles of hygiene and good nutrition within SES1B and SES2, and despite income levels allowing access to moderately good housing and virtually any foods, the children of such families still show profound growth faltering in early life. An explanation might lie in two domains. First, there are many fewer animals within the MRC compound and they are kept out of the houses, so it is much easier for parents to maintain their children in a setting with minimal faecal contamination; a factor considered a likely driver of infections and enteropathy [10, 33]. Second, studies have found that the volume of water usage is highly dependent upon time taken to access the water [33]. Even if water is available at an adjacent standpipe requiring just 2 min for collection, water usage has been found to average 20 l per person per day, whereas usage rises to 60 l per person per day when water is piped directly into the home [34]. We propose that the disappointing outcomes from the WASH trials [10–13] have arisen, not because the theoretical premise behind the trials is incorrect, but because the interventions have fallen short of the very high threshold indicated by our current data.

Conclusions

On the basis of these observations, we infer that improvements in housing conditions including, and perhaps especially, the provision of piped water into the home, may be a key factor in explaining why national stunting rates remain so persistent in low-income settings yet decline so markedly as countries pass through the economic transition. This could be tested using cluster-randomised or step-wedge intervention designs of what we term WASH+ + (and others are terming 'Transformative WASH') and, if true, would lead to a major shift in priorities for implementation of nutrition-specific and WASH-type interventions.

Abbreviations
HAZ: Height-for-age Z-score; LSHTM: London School of Hygiene & Tropical Medicine; MRC: Medical Research Council; SES: Socio-economic status; WASH: Water, sanitation and hygiene; WAZ: Weight-for-age Z-score; WHO: World Health Organisation; WHZ: Weight-for-height Z-score

Acknowledgements
We thank the participants for their willingness to join the study and share sensitive information, and two named reviewers (Drs Christine Stewart and Mahbubur Rahman) whose insightful comments have improved the analysis and discussion of the results.

Funding
The work was undertaken with support from the UK Medical Research Council (MRC) and Department for International Development (DFID) (grant ref. MCA760-5QX00) under the MRC/DFID Concordat.

Authors' contributions
MH, SEM and AMP conceived the study. MH conducted the fieldwork with the supervision and support of MD and HN. MH and AMP wrote the manuscript with input from all authors. All authors read and approved the final manuscript.

Competing interests
The authors declare that they have no competing interests.

Author details
[1]MRC Unit The Gambia at London School of Hygiene and Tropical Medicine, Atlantic Boulevard, Fajara, Banjul, The Gambia. [2]Regional Activity Centre for Sustainable Consumption and Production (SCP/RAC), Sant Pau Art Nouveau Site, Carrer Sant Antoni Maria Claret, 167, 08025 Barcelona, Spain. [3]Department of Women and Children's Health, King's College London, 10th Floor North Wing, St Thomas' Hospital, Westminster Bridge Road, London SE1 7EH, UK. [4]Centre for Maternal and Newborn Health, Liverpool School of Tropical Medicine, Pembroke Place, Liverpool L3 5QA, UK.

References
1. Victora CG, de Onis M, Hallal PC, Blössner M, Shrimpton R. Worldwide timing of growth faltering: revisiting implications for interventions. Pediatrics. 2010;125:e473–80.
2. Black RE, Victora CG, Walker SP, et al. Maternal and child undernutrition and overweight in low-income and middle-income countries. Lancet. 2013; 382:427–51.
3. Rayco-Solon P, Moore SE, Fulford AJ, Prentice AM. Fifty-year mortality trends in three rural African villages. Tropical Med Int Health. 2004;9:1151–60.
4. Poskitt EM, Cole TJ, Whitehead RG. Less diarrhoea but no change in growth: 15 years' data from three Gambian villages. Arch Dis Child. 1999;80:115–9.
5. Nabwera HM, Fulford AJ, Moore SE, Prentice AM. Growth faltering persists in rural Gambian children despite four decades of intervention. Lancet Global Health. 2017;5:e208–16.
6. Dewey KG, Adu-Afarwuah S. Systematic review of the efficacy and effectiveness of complementary feeding interventions in developing countries. Matern Child Nutr. 2008;4(Suppl 1):24–85.
7. Papageorghiou AT, Ohuma EO, Altman DG, et al. International standards for fetal growth based on serial ultrasound measurements: the Fetal Growth Longitudinal Study of the INTERGROWTH-21st project. Lancet. 2014;384:869–79.
8. World Health Organisation. WHO child growth standards based on length/height, weight and age. Acta Paediatr Suppl. 2006;450:76–85.
9. Stevens GA, Finucane MM, Paciorek CJ, Flaxman SR, White RA, Donner AJ, Ezzati M, and on behalf of Nutrition Impact Model Study Group (Child Growth). Trends in mild, moderate, and severe stunting and underweight, and progress towards MDG 1 in 141 developing countries: a systematic analysis of population representative data. Lancet. 2012;380:824–34.
10. Sanitation Hygiene Infant Nutrition Efficacy (SHINE) Trial Team, Humphrey JH, Jones AD, Manges A, Mangwadu G, Maluccio JA, Mbuya MN, Moulton LH, Ntozini R, Prendergast AJ, Stoltzfus RJ, Tielsch JM. The sanitation hygiene infant nutrition efficacy (SHINE) trial: rationale, design, and methods. Clin Infect Dis. 2015;61(Suppl 7):S685–702.
11. Null C, Stewart CP, Pickering AJ, et al. Effects or water quality, sanitation and handwashing, and nutritional interventions on diarrhoea and child growth in rural Kenya: a cluster-randomised trial. Lancet Global Helath. 2018;6:e316–29.

12. Luby SP, Rahman M, Arnold BF, et al. Effects or water quality, sanitation and handwashing, and nutritional interventions on diarrhoea and child growth in rural Bangladesh: a cluster-randomised trial. Lancet Global Helath. 2018;6:e302–15.
13. Humphrey JH, Mbuya MNN, Ntozini R, et al. Prendergast AJ for The Sanitation Hygiene Infant Nutrition Efficacy (SHINE) Trial Team. Independent and combined effects of improved water, sanitation and hygiene, and improved complementary feeding, on child stunting and anaemia in rural Zimbabwe: a cluster-randomised trial. Lancet Global Health. 2018. In press.
14. Hennig BJ, Unger SA, Dondeh BL, Hassan J, Hawkesworth S, Jarjou L, Jones KS, Moore SE, Nabwera HM, Ngum M, Prentice A, Sonko B, Prentice AM, Fulford AJ. Cohort profile: the Kiang West Longitudinal Population Study (KWLPS)—a platform for integrated research and health care provision in rural Gambia. Int J Epidemiol. 2015. https://doi.org/10.1093/ije/dyv206.
15. Ratcliffe AA, et al. Parent's socio-economic status and social support as risks for child mortality: consideration of health equity in The Gambia. In: de Savingy D, et al., editors. Measuring Health Equity in Small Areas: Findings from Demographic Surveillance Systems INDEPTH network. Hampshire: Ashgate; 2005. p. 109–26.
16. Prentice AM, Ward KA, Goldberg GR, Jarjou LM, Moore SE, Fulford AJ, Prentice A. Critical windows for nutritional interventions against stunting. Am J Clin Nutr. 2013;97:911–8.
17. de Onis M, Garza C, Victora CG, MK BB, Norum KR. The WHO multicentre growth reference study (MGRS): rationale, planning, and implementation. Food Nutr Bull. 2004;25(supplement 1):S3–S84.
18. Thakwalakwa CM, Ashorn P, Jawati M, Phuka JC, Cheung YB, Maleta KM. An effectiveness trial showed lipid-based nutrient supplementation but not corn-soya blend offered a modest benefit in weight gain among 6- to 18-month-old underweight children in rural Malawi. Public Health Nutr. 2012;15:1755–62.
19. Maleta KM, Phuka J, Alho L, et al. Provision of 10-40 g/d lipid-based nutrient supplements from 6 to 18 months of age does not prevent linear growth faltering in Malawi. J Nutr. 2015;145:1909–15.
20. Ashorn P, Alho L, Ashorn U, et al. Supplementation of maternal diets during pregnancy and for 6 months postpartum and infant diets thereafter with small-quantity lipid-based nutrient supplements does not promote child growth by 18 months of age in rural Malawi: a randomized controlled trial. J Nutr. 2015;145:1345–53.
21. Mangani C, Maleta K, Phuka J, Cheung YB, Thakwalakwa C, Dewey K, Manary M, Puumalainen T, Ashorn P. Effect of complementary feeding with lipid-based nutrient supplements and corn-soy blend on the incidence of stunting and linear growth among 6- to 18-month-old infants and children in rural Malawi. Matern Child Nutr. 2015;11(Suppl 4):132–43.
22. Iannotti LL, Dulience SJ, Green J, Joseph S, François J, Anténor ML, Lesorogol C, Mounce J, Nickerson NM. Linear growth increased in young children in an urban slum of Haiti: a randomized controlled trial of a lipid-based nutrient supplement. Am J Clin Nutr. 2014;99:198–208.
23. Hess SY, Abbeddou S, Jimenez EY, et al. Small-quantity lipid-based nutrient supplements, regardless of their zinc content, increase growth and reduce the prevalence of stunting and wasting in young Burkinabe children: a cluster-randomized trial. PLoS One. 2015;10:e0122242.
24. Lunn PG, Northrop-Clewes CA, Downes RM. Intestinal permeability, mucosal injury, and growth faltering in Gambian infants. Lancet. 1991;338:907–10.
25. Campbell DI, Elia M, Lunn PG. Growth faltering in rural Gambian infants is associated with impaired small intestinal barrier function, leading to endotoxemia and systemic inflammation. J Nutr. 2003;133:1332–8.
26. Humphrey JH. Child undernutrition, tropical enteropathy, toilets, and handwashing. Lancet. 2009;374:1032–5.
27. Lin A, Arnold BF, Afreen S, Goto R, Huda TM, Haque R, Raqib R, Unicomb L, Ahmed T, Colford JM Jr, Luby SP. Household environmental conditions are associated with enteropathy and impaired growth in rural Bangladesh. Am J Trop Med Hyg. 2013;89:130–7.
28. Dangour AD, Watson L, Cumming O, Boisson S, Che Y, Velleman Y, Cavill S, Allen E, Uauy R. Interventions to improve water quality and supply, sanitation and hygiene practices, and their effects on the nutritional status of children. Cochrane Database Syst Rev. 2013;8:CD009382.
29. Fuller JA, Villamor E, Cevallos W, Trostle J, Eisenberg JN. I get height with a little help from my friends: herd protection from sanitation on child growth in rural Ecuador. Int J Epidemiol. 2016;45:460–9.
30. Harris M, Alzua ML, Osbert N, Pickering A. Community-level sanitation coverage more strongly associated with child growth and household drinking water quality than access to a private toilet in rural Mali. Environ Sci Technol. 2017;51:7219–27.
31. Pickering AJ, Djebbari H, Lopez C, Coulibaly M, Alzua ML. Effect of a community-led sanitation intervention on child diarrhoea and child growth in rural Mali: a cluster-randomised controlled trial. Lancet Glob Health. 2015;3:e701–11.
32. Bhutta ZA, Das JK, Rizvi A, Gaffey MF, Walker N, Horton S, Webb P, Lartey A, Black RE, Lancet Nutrition Interventions Review Group; Maternal and Child Nutrition Study Group. Evidence-based interventions for improvement of maternal and child nutrition: what can be done and at what cost? Lancet. 2013;382:452–77.
33. Korpe PS, Petri WA Jr. Environmental enteropathy: critical implications of a poorly understood condition. Trends Mol Med. 2012;18:328–36.
34. Cairncross S, Feachem R. Environmental health engineering in the tropics: an introductory text. 2nd ed. Chichester: Wiley; 1993.

Determinants of the urinary and serum metabolome in children from six European populations

Chung-Ho E. Lau[1*], Alexandros P. Siskos[1,2], Léa Maitre[3,4,5], Oliver Robinson[6], Toby J. Athersuch[1,6], Elizabeth J. Want[1], Jose Urquiza[3,4,5], Maribel Casas[3,4,5], Marina Vafeiadi[7], Theano Roumeliotaki[7], Rosemary R. C. McEachan[9], Rafaq Azad[9], Line S. Haug[10], Helle M. Meltzer[10], Sandra Andrusaityte[11], Inga Petraviciene[11], Regina Grazuleviciene[11], Cathrine Thomsen[10], John Wright[9], Remy Slama[8], Leda Chatzi[12], Martine Vrijheid[3,4,5], Hector C. Keun[2] and Muireann Coen[1,13*]

Abstract

Background: Environment and diet in early life can affect development and health throughout the life course. Metabolic phenotyping of urine and serum represents a complementary systems-wide approach to elucidate environment–health interactions. However, large-scale metabolome studies in children combining analyses of these biological fluids are lacking. Here, we sought to characterise the major determinants of the child metabolome and to define metabolite associations with age, sex, BMI and dietary habits in European children, by exploiting a unique biobank established as part of the Human Early-Life Exposome project (http://www.projecthelix.eu).

Methods: Metabolic phenotypes of matched urine and serum samples from 1192 children (aged 6–11) recruited from birth cohorts in six European countries were measured using high-throughput ^{1}H nuclear magnetic resonance (NMR) spectroscopy and a targeted LC-MS/MS metabolomic assay (Biocrates Absolute*IDQ* p180 kit).

Results: We identified both urinary and serum creatinine to be positively associated with age. Metabolic associations to BMI z-score included a novel association with urinary 4-deoxyerythreonic acid in addition to valine, serum carnitine, short-chain acylcarnitines (C3, C5), glutamate, BCAAs, lysophosphatidylcholines (lysoPC a C14:0, lysoPC a C16:1, lysoPC a C18:1, lysoPC a C18:2) and sphingolipids (SM C16:0, SM C16:1, SM C18:1). Dietary-metabolite associations included urinary creatine and serum phosphatidylcholines (4) with meat intake, serum phosphatidylcholines (12) with fish, urinary hippurate with vegetables, and urinary proline betaine and hippurate with fruit intake. Population-specific variance (age, sex, BMI, ethnicity, dietary and country of origin) was better captured in the serum than in the urine profile; these factors explained a median of 9.0% variance amongst serum metabolites versus a median of 5.1% amongst urinary metabolites. Metabolic pathway correlations were identified, and concentrations of corresponding metabolites were significantly correlated ($r > 0.18$) between urine and serum.

(Continued on next page)

---

* Correspondence: esmond.lau06@imperial.ac.uk; m.coen@imperial.ac.uk
Chung-Ho E. Lau and Alexandros P. Siskos are joint first authors contributed equally to the work.
Hector C. Keun and Muireann Coen are joint senior authors.
[1]Division of Computational and Systems Medicine, Department of Surgery and Cancer, Faculty of Medicine, Imperial College London, London SW7 2AZ, UK
Full list of author information is available at the end of the article

(Continued from previous page)

Conclusions: We have established a pan-European reference metabolome for urine and serum of healthy children and gathered critical resources not previously available for future investigations into the influence of the metabolome on child health. The six European cohort populations studied share common metabolic associations with age, sex, BMI z-score and main dietary habits. Furthermore, we have identified a novel metabolic association between threonine catabolism and BMI of children.

Keywords: Exposome metabolomics, Metabonomics, Metabolic phenotyping, Epidemiology, Birth cohorts, Paediatrics, NMR spectroscopy, LC-MS, European children, Metabolic profile,

Background

Under-nutrition during gestation was first proposed in the early 1990s to explain the association observed between low birth weight in infancy and higher mortality rates from cardiovascular disease in male adults [1, 2]. Since then, it has been hypothesised that the origins of many diseases that manifest later in life may be traced back to fetal development—known as the DOHaD (Developmental Origins of Health and Disease) paradigm [3]. In addition, early-life environmental exposures may have wide-ranging consequences for health. Critical windows in development, such as the prenatal period and infancy, have been shown to be particularly susceptible to environmental risk factors that influence disease burden into adulthood [4–6]. For example, prenatal exposure to passive smoke and outdoor air pollutants are acknowledged risk factors for asthma and other allergies including eczema [7, 8], and exposure to endocrine-disrupting and household chemicals have been found to increase obesity risk in children [9, 10]. Moreover, childhood exposure to passive smoke has also been associated with lung cancer risk in adults [11], whilst prenatal infection and exposure to lead have been linked respectively to schizophrenia [12] and attention deficit hyperactivity disorder in children [13]. Growing evidence suggests environmental exposure in early life can also alter molecular phenotypes—such as the epigenome—which then persist throughout life [14, 15]. Consequently, the importance of measuring multiple environmental exposures simultaneously (the exposome) and the impact of this on health at different stages of life are increasingly being recognised [16–20]. Population cohort-based exposome research studies could help address the multi-dimensional interplay between various environmental factors and developmental health outcomes [21]. For example, a recent exposome study conducted in Greece has identified that proximity to landfill waste may impact neurodevelopment in children [22].

Metabolic profiling has been utilised to characterise markers of environmental exposures [23–27] and confer valuable information regarding early life health outcomes; from preterm birth [28] and fetal growth [29] to childhood disease [30–32]. Age, sex, body morphology, and dietary intakes all play important roles in determining the urine and serum metabolome, and whilst their contributions to metabolic phenotypes are relatively well characterised in the adult population [33–42], to date there are only a few studies, of relatively small sample size, in children [43–46]. In addition, epidemiological studies that permit evaluation of the complementarity of urine and serum metabolomics data are also lacking [47].

To address this knowledge gap, metabolomic analyses of serum and urine were performed as part of the Human Early-Life Exposome (HELIX) project, which seeks to define the environmental exposome from pregnancy to childhood, to associate these with child health outcomes and to define molecular 'omics' markers [48]. The project gathered samples and data from six longitudinal birth cohort studies across six European countries—France, Greece, Lithuania, Norway, Spain and the UK. Analyses were conducted on biofluid samples from the HELIX subcohort of children between 6 and 11 years of age to perform molecular phenotyping including metabolomics, proteomics, transcriptomics and genomics and also to measure chemical exposure levels in order to identify molecular markers of exposure [49]. Specifically in this current study, we aim to (a) characterise the major determinants of the child metabolome, (b) define metabolite associations to demographic factors, BMI and main dietary intake habits in European children, and (c) evaluate correlation patterns and complementarity between serum and urine metabolic profiles.

Methods

HELIX project multilevel study design

The HELIX study is a collaborative project across six established and longitudinal birth cohorts in Europe. A multilevel study design was employed. Level 1—the entire study population of HELIX consists of 31,472 mother-child pairs which were recruited between 1999 and 2010 during their pregnancies by the six cohorts. Level 2—the HELIX subcohort consists of 1301 mother-child pairs from which exposure data, 'omics' molecular profiles, and child health outcomes were measured at 6–11 years of age. Level 3—panel studies with repeated sampling periods from a cohort of 150 children and 150 pregnant women to understand temporal variability of the personal exposure data [49].

Current study sample population—the HELIX children subcohort

The children in the HELIX subcohort were followed up between December 2013 and February 2016; there were approximately 200 mother–child pairs from each of the six cohorts. Follow-up examinations for the subcohort took place either at local hospitals, primary care centres or the National Institute for Public Health (NIPH) in Oslo, during which mothers were interviewed and children checked and examined by trained nurses according to standardised operating procedures. Biological samples were also collected on the day of the examinations. Metabolic phenotypes of 1201 children's urine and sera samples from the HELIX subcohort were generated, of which complete matching metadata listed in Table 1 were available for 1192 children as follows: Born in Bradford, UK (BiB, $n = 199$) [50]; Study of determinants of pre- and postnatal developmental, France (EDEN, $n = 157$) [51]; Infancia y Medio Ambiente, Environment and Childhood, Spain (INMA, $n = 207$) [52]; Kaunas Cohort, Lithuania (KANC, $n = 201$) [53]; The Norwegian Mother and Child Cohort Study, Norway (MoBa, $n = 229$) [54]; Mother-Child Cohort in Crete, Greece (Rhea, $n = 199$) [55]. Hence, the number of samples carried forward for data analysis was 1192.

Body mass index and food dietary frequency data

zBMI

During the subcohort follow-up examinations, height and weight were respectively measured with a stadiometer and a digital weight scale both without shoes and with light clothing. Height and weight measurements were converted to body mass index (BMI in kg/m^2) for age and sex z-scores using the international World Health Organization (WHO) reference curves in order to allow for comparison with other studies [56].

Dietary frequency

Data on the food intake frequency of 44 food items from 11 main food groups were collected through a short food frequency questionnaire and the average number of times per week that each food item was consumed was recorded. The 11 main groups were sweets, which include chocolate (bars, bonbon, spreads, cacao), sugar, honey, jam or other sweets; meat, which includes processed meat, poultry and red meat; fish, which includes canned fish, oily fish, white fish and seafood; beverages, which include both high- and low-sugar soda, other soft and fizzy drinks; potatoes, which include also French fries; vegetables, which include both raw and cooked vegetables; dairy products, which include yogurt, cheese, milk and dairy desserts; cereal, which include bread, breakfast cereal, rice and pasta, rusks, crispy bread, rice and corn cakes; fruits, which include fruits, fresh juice, canned and dry fruits; bakery products which include biscuits, cookies and pastries; and total added lipids which include butter, margarine and vegetable oil.

Biofluid sample collection

Urine and sera samples were collected and processed according to identical pre-defined standardised protocols across all six cohorts. Urine samples were collected by family members at home, kept in a fridge overnight and transported in a temperature controlled environment. Samples were aliquoted and frozen within 3 h of arrival at the clinics. Two urine samples, representing last night-time and first morning voids, were collected on the evening and morning before the clinical examination and were subsequently pooled to generate a more representative sample of the last 24 h for metabolomic analysis ($n = 1107$) [57]. Either the night-time void ($n = 37$) or morning void ($n = 48$) sample was analysed in cases where a pooled sample was missing.

Serum sampling: Blood was collected during the follow-up visit at the end of the clinical examination. Blood samples were drawn using a 'butterfly' vacuum clip and local anaesthetic and were collected into 4 mL silica plastic tubes. Samples were inverted gently for 6–7 times and spun down at 2500 g for 15 min at 4 °C. The median serum sample processing time from sample collection to freezing was 1.8 h (IQR: 1.5–2.0), and the median postprandial interval (time between last

Table 1 Sample population characteristics in the HELIX subcohort study

	Overall	BiB	EDEN	INMA	KANC	MoBa	Rhea
Sample n	1192	199	157	207	201	229	199
Female (%)	45.4	46.2	42.0	44.9	45.8	48.0	44.2
Male (%)	54.6	53.8	58.0	55.1	54.2	52.0	55.8
White European (%)	89.6	42.7	100	100	100	95.6	100
BAME (%)	10.4	57.3	0	0	0	4.4	0
Age (years)	7.4 (6.5–8.9)	6.6 (6.4–6.8)	10.8 (10.3–11.2)	8.8 (8.4–9.3)	6.4 (6.1–6.8)	8.5 (8.2–8.8)	6.5 (6.4–6.6)
BMI (z-score)	0.3 (−0.4–1.2)	0.1 (−0.4–0.9)	0.2 (−0.5–1.2)	0.7 (−0.1–1.7)	0.4 (−0.3–1.2)	0.1 (−0.4–0.6)	0.6 (−0.3–1.6)

NB. BAME indicates Black and Asian Minority Ethnic group. For age and BMI, median values and interquartile range in parentheses are presented

meal and blood collection) was 3.3 h (IQR: 2.8–4.0, Additional file 1: Figure S1).

Urine metabolite NMR measurements

^{1}H NMR spectroscopy was chosen for urinary analysis for several reasons: it has inherently high reproducibility [58]; urinary metabolite concentrations are high, making the relatively low sensitivity of NMR spectroscopy less of a hindrance; the data processing workflow is well established [59]. One-dimensional 600 MHz ^{1}H NMR spectra of all 1192 urine samples were acquired on the same BrukerAvance III spectrometer operating at 14.1 Tesla within a period of 1 month. The spectrometer was equipped with a BrukerSampleJet system, and a 5-mm broad-band inverse configuration probe maintained at 300K. Prior to analysis, cohort samples were randomised to mitigate analytical bias, and individual samples were thawed and homogenised using a vortex mixer and centrifuged at 13,000 g for 10 min at 4 °C to remove insoluble material. Five hundred forty microliters of urine sample was mixed with 60 μL of a buffer solution (1.5 M KH$_2$PO$_4$, 2 mM NaN$_3$, 1% deuterated 3-(trimethylsilyl)-[2,2,3,3-d4]-propionic acid sodium salt (TSP) solution, pH 7.4) and was transferred into an NMR tube (5 mm Bruker SampleJet NMR tubes). Ninety-six-sample tube well plates were kept at 6 °C in the cooled Bruker SampleJet unit. Aliquots of the study quality control (QC) sample, made from pooled urine samples from 20 individuals included in this study, were used to monitor analytical performance throughout the run and were analysed at an interval of every 23 samples (i.e. 4 QC samples per well plate). The ^{1}H NMR spectra were acquired using a standard one-dimensional solvent suppression pulse sequence (relaxation delay - 90° pulse - 4 μs delay - 90° pulse - mixing time - 90° pulse - acquire FID). For each sample, 32 transients were collected into 64K data points using a spectral width of 12,000 Hz with a recycle delay of 4 s, a mixing time of 100 ms, and an acquisition time of 2.73 s. A line-broadening function of 0.3 Hz was applied prior to Fourier transformation. All ^{1}H NMR spectra were automatically phased and baseline-corrected using Topspin 3.2 software (Bruker-BioSpin, Rheinstetten, Germany). The ^{1}H NMR urine spectra were referenced to the TSP resonance at 0 ppm. NMR spectra were imported into the MATLAB 2014a (MathWorks, Massachusetts, USA) computing environment and aligned using the recursive segment-wise peak alignment method [60], an algorithm based on cross-correlation. The study QC sample spectrum was used as a reference for spectral alignment. A single representative resonance in the spectrum was selected for each assigned metabolite, based on its presence in a high proportion of the spectra, high signal-to-noise ratio, and limited overlap with other resonances. Metabolite resonance peak areas were estimated using trapezoidal numerical integration and were corrected for local spectral baseline, and 44 metabolites were obtained using this method. Quantification was achieved for 24 metabolites; 20 metabolites were semi-quantified using a method of signal integration and quantification as previously described in Maitre et.al [57]. Probabilistic quotient normalisation [61] was used to adjust for variable urine sample dilution.

Assignment of endogenous urinary metabolites was made by reference to online databases (HMDB) [62], statistical total correlation spectroscopy (STOCSY) [63] and using ChenomxNMRsuite 7.1 profiler (ChenomxInc, Edmonton, Canada) and/or confirmed by 2D NMR experiments on a selected sample including homonuclear ^{1}H-^{1}H correlation spectroscopy (COSY), and ^{1}H-^{1}H total correlation spectroscopy (TOCSY) and ^{1}H-^{13}C heteronuclear single quantum coherence spectroscopy (HSQC). Spike-in experiments using authentic chemical standards were also used to confirm novel metabolite annotations. A summary of signal annotation and assignment is shown in Additional file 1: Table S1.

Serum metabolite measurements

The Absolute*IDQ* p180 kit [64] was chosen for serum analysis as it is a widely used standardised, targeted LC-MS/MS assay, and its inter-laboratory reproducibility has been demonstrated by several independent laboratories [65]. It is increasingly employed for large-scale epidemiology studies [66] [67, 68], facilitating comparisons to thousands of metabolome profiles across other studies. Serum samples were quantified using the Absolute*IDQ* p180 kit following the manufacturer's protocol [64] using LC-MS/MS—and Agilent HPLC 1100 liquid chromatography coupled to a SCIEX QTRAP 6500 triple quadrupole mass spectrometer. Briefly, the kit allows for the targeted analysis of 188 metabolites in the classes of amino acids, biogenic amines, acylcarnitines, glycerophospholipids, sphingolipids and sum of hexoses, covering a wide range of analytes and metabolic pathways in one targeted assay. The kit consists of a single sample processing procedure, with two separate analytical runs, a combination of liquid chromatography (LC) and flow injection analysis (FIA) coupled to tandem mass spectrometry (MS/MS). Isotopically labelled and chemically homologous internal standards were used for quantification; in total, 56 analytes were fully quantified and validated. Of the total 188 metabolites measured, 42 metabolites were measured by LC-MS/MS and 146 metabolites by FIA-MS/MS. The amino acids and biogenic amines were analysed quantitatively by LC–ESI-MS/MS, with the use of an external seven-point calibration curve based on isotope-labelled internal standards. The quantification method for all amino acids and amines was fully validated. The acylcarnitines (40), glycerophospholipids

(90), sphingolipids (15), and sum of hexoses (1) were analysed by FIA-ESI-MS/MS, using a one-point internal standard calibration with representative internal standards. Metabolites were quantified (results shown in micromolar concentration units) according to the manufacturer's protocol using the MetIDQ™ Version 5.4.8 Boron software for targeted metabolomic data processing and management. Blank PBS (phosphate-buffered saline) samples (three technical replicates) were used for the calculation of the limits of detection (LOD). The median values of all PBS samples on the plate were calculated as approximation of the background noise per metabolite signal, and 3 times this value was calculated as the LOD.

LC-MS/MS data of serum samples were acquired in 18 batches. Every analytical batch, in a 96-well plate format, is included up to 76 randomised cohort samples. Also in every analytical batch, three sets of quality control samples were included, the NIST SRM 1950 plasma reference material (in 4 replicates), a commercial available serum QC material (CQC in 2 replicates, SeraLab, S-123-M-27485) and the QCs provided by the manufacturer in three concentration levels. The NIST SRM 1950 reference was used as the main quality control sample for the LC-MS/MS analysis.

Analytical performance of urinary and serum metabolites

Analytical performance in the urinary NMR and serum LC-MS/MS data was assessed by reference to the QC samples measured at regular intervals during the run, with 4 QC samples analysed in every 96-well plate batch. Coefficients of variation (CVs) for each metabolite were calculated based on the pooled QC for the NMR analysis and the NIST SRM 1950 for the LC-MS/MS. Moreover, for the LC-MS/MS serum analysis, the limits of detection (LODs) were also used to assess the analytical performance of individual metabolites. For the LC-MS/MS serum dataset, metabolite exclusion was based on a variable meeting two conditions: (1) CV of over 30% and (2) over 30% of the data are below LOD. Eleven out of the 188 serum metabolites detected were excluded as a result, leaving 177 serum metabolites to be used for further statistical analysis. Mean coefficients of variations across the 44 NMR detected urinary metabolites, and the 177 LC-MS/MS detected serum metabolites carried forward for data analysis were found to be 11 and 15%, respectively (Additional file 1: Tables S2 and S3).

Statistical analyses

Metabolite concentrations were $\log_{10}$ transformed to normalise data prior to statistical analyses, and the resultant distribution of the transformed data can be found in Additional files 2 and 3. To avoid log transform of zero values, the lowest non-zero value was added to the variable distribution as a constant before log transformation.

All statistical analyses were performed using R ('The R Project for Statistical Computing') software environment (v3.3.1) unless specified otherwise. Metabolome-wide association study (MWAS) analyses were performed using multiple linear regression models in the R package 'base'. Linear regression models were fitted for each metabolite with concentration as the outcome variable. Covariates included in the regression models were batch, run order, sex, age, zBMI and dietary intake habits of the 11 food groups; in addition, urine data models were adjusted for sampling type (night only, morning only or pooled sample) and the serum data models were adjusted for postprandial interval. Regression models were computed separately for each individual cohort and meta-analysis was used to combine the effect size estimates using a fixed-effect inverse variance weighting from the six cohorts with the R package 'meta', and I^2 statistics were used to assess the heterogeneity in the effect estimates between the cohorts. Bonferroni correction ($n = 177$ for serum data, $n = 44$ for urine data) was applied throughout to account for multiple test comparisons (p value threshold = 1.1×10^{-3} for urine and 2.8×10^{-4} for serum metabolites). For variance decomposition, analysis was performed using a partial R^2 approach, the variance in the urinary and serum data was partitioned according to the following 5 main categories: pre-analytical, analytical, demographic, dietary and cohort/country. The analysis was performed on each of the 44 urinary metabolites and 177 serum metabolites. In addition to the covariates used in the MWAS analyses—batch (analytical), run order (analytical), time of sampling (urine pre-analytical), postprandial interval (serum pre-analytical), sex (demographic), age (demographic), BMI z-score (demographic) and dietary intake frequencies; ethnicity (demographic), and serum and urine sample processing time variables (pre-analytical) were also included in the respective serum and urine variance decomposition analyses. For principal components analysis, metabolite data were also mean-centred and univariate scaled prior to PCA modelling. For serum and urine metabolic pairwise correlation analyses, data were pre-adjusted for analytical and pre-analytical variables and Pearson's correlation coefficients were calculated. Serum correlation networks were drawn using Cytoscape (version 3.5) software [69] and the MetScape plugin application (version 3) [70]. Additionally, we have examined the impact of applying alternative data transformation and imputation strategies on the MWAS analysis results. To this end, Box-Cox transformation [71] was used in conjunction with QRILC imputation (quantile regression approach for left-censored missing) [72] and the modelled results are shown in Additional file 1: Tables S12–S15. Box-Cox transformation and QRILC imputation were performed respectively using R packages 'MASS' and 'imputeLCMD'.

Results

Characteristics of the study population included in this analysis ($n = 1192$) are shown in Table 1. Around 200 children from each of the six cohorts participated in this study (54.6% male, 45.4% female), and the vast majority of the sample population were of White-European background with the notable exception of BiB (UK) where many were of Black and Asian Minority Ethnic group, mainly of South Asian origin. There were also significant age differences between the cohorts, with the children from the EDEN cohort being the oldest (median age in EDEN was 10.8 years whilst median ages in KANC, BiB, and Rhea were 6.4–6.6 years). In addition, there were substantial differences between the cohorts in BMI z-score and across dietary intake habits in the 11 food groups (Tables 1 and 2).

In our study, ^{1}H NMR spectroscopy and targeted LC-MS/MS were respectively used to perform metabolic profiling of the urine and serum samples. Estimates of the concentrations for urinary metabolites using NMR spectroscopy (μmol/mmol of creatinine) are provided in Additional file 1: Table S4 and for serum metabolite measurements using the LC-MS/MS Absolute*IDQ* p180 assay (μmol/L) in Additional file 1: Table S5.

Metabolic differences between cohorts

Differences in metabolite concentrations between cohorts were assessed by ANOVA after pre-adjusting for covariates through linear regression models. Metabolites with p values below the significance threshold after Bonferroni correction (p value threshold $= 1.1 \times 10^{-3}$ for urine and 2.8×10^{-4} for serum metabolites) are shown in Fig. 1. A large number of metabolites, 104 out of 177 serum metabolites and 10 of the 44 urine metabolites measured, were found to be significantly different between cohorts. In particular, serum amino acid levels were frequently found highest in the Rhea cohort, whilst a disproportionally high number of serum glycerophospholipid species were found to be most abundant in the MoBa cohort samples. Given the stark differences in the metabolic phenotypes between cohorts, we decided to perform stratified analyses followed by meta-analysis to combine the effect estimates from the six individual cohorts in many of the subsequent analyses.

Pre-analytical factors

None of the 177 serum metabolites were identified from meta-analysis to be significantly affected by serum sample processing time after adjusting for covariates and stratifying by country. Similarly, none of the 44 urinary metabolites were found to be associated with sample processing time. Thus, in subsequent analyses, urine and serum processing time were not included as covariates.

The majority of serum samples were collected 3 to 4 h postprandial (median was 3.3 h with IQR: 2.8–4.0), and there were no major differences in postprandial interval between the cohorts (Additional file 1: Figure S1). Postprandial effects could be observed in 21 out of 177 metabolites: 11 amino acids, one biogenic amine, two short-chain acylcarnitines, four long-chain acylcarnitines and three lysophosphatidylcholine species were found to be associated with postprandial interval (Fig. 2a). The 11 amino acids were negatively associated whilst the four long-chain acylcarnitines were positively associated with postprandial interval.

Comparing the urinary metabolite levels of night-time void ($n = 38$) and morning void ($n = 48$) samples, we found alanine and citrate concentrations to be elevated in the night-time void samples and N-methyl nicotinamide, N-acetyl-neuraminic acid and 4-deoxythreonic acid to be higher in the morning void samples (Fig. 2b).

Table 2 Dietary intake of 11 main food groups

	Overall	BiB	EDEN	INMA	KANC	MoBa	Rhea
Cereal	18.5 (12.5–26)	17 (13.1–23.5)	21.5 (13–27.5)	17 (11.4–24.1)	14 (9.3–22)	25 (19–29.6)	16 (12.1–23.5)
Meat	7.5 (5.1–10)	6 (4–9)	7.5 (5.5–10)	8 (7–12)	7.1 (5.1–10)	7.5 (5–10.5)	6.5 (5–7.6)
Fish	2 (1.1–3.5)	2 (1–3.3)	2.1 (1.5–3)	3.6 (2.4–5)	1.1 (0.4–1.6)	2.6 (1.6–5)	1.5 (1–2)
Dairy	19.8 (12.5–27.6)	24 (17.2–31.6)	24 (15–31)	18.1 (13.8–25.8)	11 (8–17)	20 (12.3–27)	22.5 (15.1–28.5)
Lipids	4.5 (1–8.5)	7 (4–10)	6 (3.1–9)	1 (0.3–3.1)	7 (4–11)	7.5 (4–15.5)	1 (0.1–3)
Potatoes	3.5 (2–4)	4 (3.1–6)	3.1 (1.5–4)	3.5 (2–4)	3.1 (3–5.6)	3.1 (1.1–3.1)	3.5 (2–4)
Vegetables	6.5 (4–10)	6 (4–10)	8 (4–11)	6 (3–8.5)	6 (3.5–8.5)	8.5 (6–14)	6.5 (4–10)
Fruits	8.8 (5.9–18)	15.5 (10–21)	6.6 (3.3–13.6)	7.5 (3.7–13.2)	7.4 (3.8–10)	14 (8.6–21)	8.5 (6.2–13.5)
Sweets	6.6 (3.5–10)	6.6 (3.6–10)	8.5 (5–14)	4.5 (2–8.1)	9.5 (7–15.5)	5 (3–7.5)	6 (3.3–7.5)
Bakery products	4 (1.5–6.5)	4 (2–7.5)	5.6 (2–8)	4 (3–6.5)	4 (2–6.5)	1.5 (1–2)	6 (4–8.5)
Beverages	0.5 (0–1)	0.5 (0–1.8)	1 (0.3–3)	0.5 (0–1.3)	0.5 (0.1–1)	0.6 (0.1–1.1)	0.1 (0–0.5)

Data represent portion consumed per week. Median values with interquartile range given in parentheses or percentages as indicated

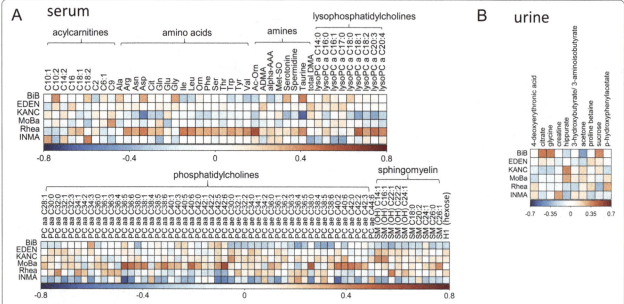

Fig. 1 Metabolic differences between the six cohorts. **a** Serum metabolites. **b** Urine metabolites. Colour represents standardised mean difference between cohorts; blue—metabolite levels lower than average, and red—metabolite levels higher than average. P values were assessed by ANOVA, and significant metabolites after multiple testing correction are shown. Using multiple linear regression models metabolic data were pre-adjusted for analytical batch and run order, age, sex, zBMI, frequency of weekly dietary intake of the 11 food groups, and a sampling type in the case of urine and postprandial interval in the case of serum, prior to ANOVA analysis. BiB (UK), EDEN (France), KANC (Lithuania), MoBa (Norway), Rhea (Greece), INMA (Spain)

Demographic factors and BMI for the HELIX children

Both urinary and serum creatinine levels (Additional file 1: Figures S3, S4 and Table S6) were found to be significantly associated with age after adjusting for multiple testing using Bonferroni correction. An increase of 1 year in the child's age was associated with increases of 0.39 standard deviation (SD) in urinary creatinine level (95% CI 0.26 to 0.53) and 0.30 SD in serum creatinine level (95% CI 0.17 to 0.43). A positive association between creatinine concentration and age was identified as a common phenotype amongst our six different study cohorts (Additional file 1: Figures S3 and S4); effect sizes between urine creatinine level and age were 0.40 SD/year for BiB, 0.27 SD/year for EDEN, 0.35 SD/year for KANC, 0.33 SD/year for MoBa, 0.84 SD/year for Rhea and 0.45 SD/year for INMA. No other urine or serum metabolites measured were associated with age.

Metabolic associations with sex, adjusted for covariates and multiple testing, are shown in Fig. 3. Variation in effect size between cohorts was assessed using I^2 statistic, which measures the percentage of variation across cohorts that is due to heterogeneity rather than chance. Fifteen out of 18 urine or serum metabolites identified as associated with sex have $I^2 < 50\%$ (Additional file 1: Table S7). Urinary isoleucine was found at lower concentrations (− 0.24 SD lower; 95% CI − 0.37 to − 0.12) while 5-oxoproline (0.23 SD higher; CI 0.11 to 0.36) and tyrosine (0.43 SD higher; CI 0.31 to 0.55) were higher in males. Amongst the serum metabolites, the neurotransmitter serotonin (0.32 SD higher; CI 0.20 to 0.44) was found to be higher in males while serine (− 0.26; CI − 0.39 to − 0.14), lysine (− 0.24; CI − 0.35 to − 0.12), ornithine (− 0.35; CI − 0.47 to − 0.23), putrescine (− 0.21; CI − 0.33 to − 0.10), six median-to-long chain acylcarnitines (C10, C12, C14:1, C14:1–OH, C14:2 and C16:1) and three sphingolipids (SM C16:1, SM C18:0, SM C18:1) were found higher in females.

Based on regression models adjusted for covariates, we found 45 urine or serum metabolites to be associated with BMI z-score and 44 of the 45 associations have $I^2 < 50\%$ (Fig. 4 and Additional file 1: Table S8). Urinary 4-deoxyerythronic acid (metabolite SD per unit zBMI: 0.21; 95% CI 0.16 to 0.26) and valine (BCAA, metabolite SD/zBMI: 0.09; CI 0.04 to 0.15) were positively associated with BMI z-score, and urinary p-cresol sulphate (a microbial metabolite and uremic toxicant [73], metabolite SD/zBMI: − 0.10; CI − 0.16 to − 0.05) and pantothenate (vitamin B_5—required for synthesis of coenzyme A, metabolite SD/zBMI: − 0.12; CI − 0.17 to − 0.07) were negatively associated with BMI z-score. Positive associations between urine 4-deoxyerythronic acid and valine levels and zBMI could be observed consistently in five of the six different study cohorts with the exception of MoBa (Additional file 1: Figures S5 and S6); effect sizes between urine 4-deoxyerythronic acid level and zBMI were 0.25 SD/unit score for BiB, 0.25 SD/unit score for

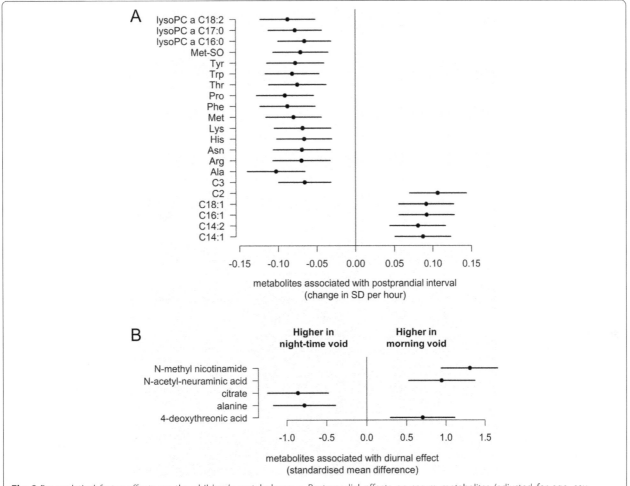

Fig. 2 Pre-analytical factor effects on the children's metabolome. **a** Postprandial effects on serum metabolites (adjusted for age, sex, zBMI)—meta-analysis after stratifying by cohorts with estimates representing the change in metabolite SD per hour postprandial and error bar indicating 95% confidence interval. **b** Diurnal effects on urine metabolites. Only t test adjusted $p < 0.05$ are shown ($n = 48$ for morning and $n = 37$ for night samples). The estimates indicate the standardised mean differences between the morning and night samples, with the error bars indicating the 95% confidence intervals. Metabolites found higher in the morning void samples are shown as positive and metabolites found higher in night-time void samples are shown as negative

EDEN, 0.25 SD/unit score for KANC, 0.00 SD/unit score for MoBa (not significant), 0.22 SD/unit score for Rhea and 0.19 SD/unit score for INMA. Interestingly, children from MoBa have the lowest BMI z-score amongst the six cohorts (Table 1).

Amongst serum metabolites, significant positive associations with BMI z-score included free carnitine, (metabolite SD/zBMI: 0.18; CI 0.13 to 0.24), short-chain acylcarnitines (C3, C5), seven amino acids including glutamate, BCAAs valine and leucine and sphingolipids (SM C16:0, SM C16:1, SM C18:1). A large number of phosphatidylcholine species (20) and four lysophosphatidylcholines (lysoPC a C14:0, lysoPC a C16:1, lysoPC a C18:1, lysoPC a C18:2) were also found to be strongly associated with BMI z-score in the study (Fig. 4 and Additional file 1: Table S8). Again, associations between serum metabolites and zBMI could be observed consistently in our study cohorts, for example both serum glutamate (Additional file 1: Figure S7) and carnitine (Additional file 1: Figure S8) levels were positively associated with zBMI in all six cohorts.

Dietary intake

Figure 5 and Additional file 1: Table S9 summarise the significant urine and serum metabolite associations with the 11 dietary food group intake after adjusting for multiple testing (p value threshold = 1.1×10^{-3} for urine and 2.8×10^{-4} for serum metabolites) and covariates including analytical batch and run order, age, sex, BMI z-score and postprandial interval for serum and urine sampling type for urine models. We identified 57 diet-metabolite associations and 40 of the 57 associations have $I^2 < 50\%$.

For urinary metabolites, we identified creatine to be positively associated with meat intake (SD per portion

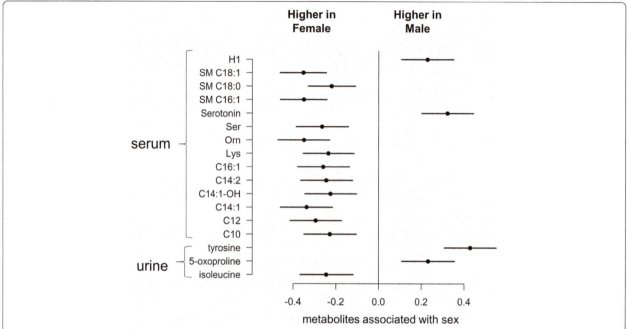

Fig. 3 Sex associations with ¹H NMR urine and serum metabolites in children—meta-analysis after stratifying by cohorts. Regression models were adjusted for covariates, and Bonferroni correction was used to adjust for multiple testing. The estimates represent the metabolite standardised mean difference between males and females with the error bars indicating the 95% confidence intervals. Metabolites found higher in male children are shown as positive, and metabolites found higher in female children are shown as negative

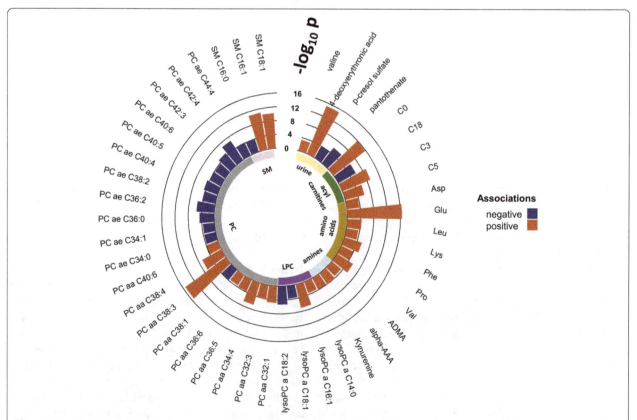

Fig. 4 Urine and serum metabolites associated with BMI z-score—meta-analysis after stratifying by cohorts. Regression models were adjusted for analytical batching, postprandial effect (for serum), sampling (urine), age, sex and dietary intakes of the 11 main food groups

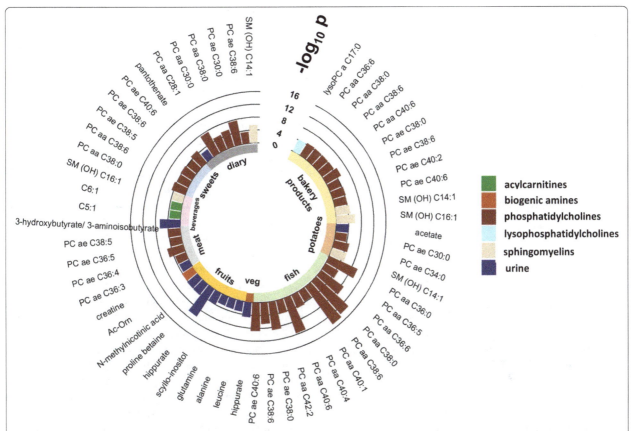

Fig. 5 Metabolites associated with dietary intake frequencies (weekly). Weekly dietary frequency intake data of the 11 main food groups (cereal, meat, fish, dairy, lipids, potatoes, vegetables, fruits, sweets, bakery products, beverages) were collected via food frequency questionnaire, and multiple linear regression analysis followed by meta-analysis were performed on each metabolite—dietary factor pair. Regression models were adjusted for analytical batching, postprandial effect (for serum), sampling (urine), age, sex and zBMI score

per week: 0.025; 95% CI 0.012 to 0.039). Hippurate was positively associated with both fruit (SD per portion per week: 0.026; 95% CI 0.018 to 0.034) and vegetable consumption (SD per portion per week: 0.021; 95% CI 0.011 to 0.031). Proline betaine, N-methylnicotinic acid and *scyllo*-inositol were positively associated with fruit intake, whilst glutamine, alanine and leucine were negatively associated with fruit intake. In addition, pantothenate and acetate were respectively found positively associated with dairy and potato intake.

For serum metabolites, we found 12 glycerophosphatidylcholine species to be associated with fish consumption (Fig. 5), 4 glycerophosphatidylcholine species (PC ae 36:3, PC ae 36:4, PC ae 36:5 and PC ae 38:5) to be positively associated with meat consumption and 5 glycerophosphatidylcholine species (PC aa C38:0, PC aa C38:6, PC ae C38:5, PC ae C38:6, PC ae C40:6) to be negatively associated with sweet consumption. In addition, we found acetylornithine to be positively associated with fruit intake, and two acylcarnitines (C5:1, C6:1) and one sphingolipid (SM (OH) C16:1) to be negatively associated with beverages (soft and fizzy drinks).

Variance decomposition analysis of LC-MS/MS serum and NMR urine metabolic profiles

Using principal components analysis, we found that metabolites in LC-MS/MS serum metabolic profiles were inherently more collinear when compared to NMR urine profiles; only 6 principal components were required to describe half of the variance in the 177 serum metabolites as opposed to 12 principal components required to describe the same proportion of the variance in the 44 urinary metabolites (Additional file 1: Figure S9). Secondly, as metabolic profiles often capture information derivable from various sources that may be analysis-specific or individual-specific, we performed variance decomposition analysis to discover and compare the volume of information contained in the two metabolic datasets that were attributable to the various factors. Using a partial R^2 approach, we partitioned the variance in the urinary and serum data according to the following 5 main categories: pre-analytical, analytical, demographic, dietary and cohort/country. The analysis was performed on each of the 44 urinary metabolites and on each of the 177 serum metabolites, and Fig. 6 illustrates the distributions of the

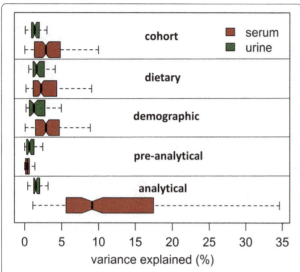

Fig. 6 Variance decompositions of LC-MS/MS serum and NMR urine metabolic profiles. Using a partial R^2 approach, regression models were performed on each of the 44 urinary metabolites and on each of the 177 serum metabolites. Variables included in the model: batch (analytical), run order (analytical), time of sampling (urine pre-analytical), postprandial interval (serum pre-analytical), sample processing time (pre-analytical), sex (demographic), age (demographic), BMI z-score (demographic), ethnicity (demographic), 11 dietary intake frequencies (dietary) and cohort

percentages of variance explained by the 5 categories. Our data indicate that whilst analytical biases accounted for only a small fraction (median of 1.5%) of the explained variance in the NMR urinary profile, they accounted for a much larger portion of the explained variance (median of 9.1%) in the LC-MS/MS serum profile. Dietary information accounted for the largest proportion of the explained variance in the urinary metabolic profile (median of 1.6%), and overall, we found that demographic, dietary and information about country of origin are better reflected in the serum dataset, as these factors together explain a median of 9.0% amongst serum metabolites versus a median of 5.1% amongst urine metabolites (breakdown by individual metabolite can be found in Additional file 1: Tables S10 and S11).

Serum and urine metabolic pairwise correlations

Metabolite inter-correlations often convey biological pathway information; thus, metabolite pairwise correlation analyses were performed separately for serum and urine datasets. Significant correlations were observed between serum metabolites which belong to the same compound classes (Fig. 7), and in particular, strong correlation clusters are found for glycerophospholipids species (maximum Pearson's correlation coefficient $r = 0.94$), amino acids (maximum $r = 0.97$) and acylcarnitines (maximum $r = 0.88$). Other notable correlations included positive correlations between valine, leucine and isoleucine (all BCAA, $r > 0.92$), alpha-AAA (α-aminoadipic acid) with BCAA and lysine, positive correlations between valine and short chain acylcarnitines (C5, C3, C4, $r = 0.65$ between valine and C5) and negative correlations between alanine and acetylcarnitine (C2, $r = -0.54$). Significant positive correlations between urine metabolites are shown as a heatmap in Fig. 8 (p value threshold of 5.3×10^{-5}). Positive correlations included leucine with valine ($r = 0.56$), acetate with succinate ($r = 0.32$), formate with acetate ($r = 0.17$), trimethylamine oxide and dimethylamine ($r = 0.44$), 3-indoxylsulfate and p-cresol sulphate ($r = 0.43$), alanine and glycine and threonine/lactate ($r = 0.52–0.65$), 4-deoxyerythronic acid with alanine ($r = 0.17$) and threonine/lactate ($r = 0.21$), and creatine with carnitine/choline ($r = 0.30$). Significant negative correlations included 4-deoxythreonic acid with the following amino acids: threonine/lactate, alanine, tyrosine, glutamine and glycine ($r = -0.17$ to -0.42). Pairwise correlation between metabolite concentrations across the two biological fluid types were also examined (Additional file 1: Figure S10, p value threshold of 6.4×10^{-6}). Significant correlations were found in 391/7788 serum-urine metabolite pairs. Significant positive correlations were found in the cases when a metabolite has been measured in both urine and serum. Specifically creatinine ($r = 0.39$), glycine ($r = 0.35$), alanine ($r = 0.29$), valine ($r = 0.18$), serum carnitine and urine carnitine/choline ($r = 0.23$), and serum threonine and urinary threonine/lactate ($r = 0.26$) are all individually strongly correlated across the two biological fluid matrices. Other notable correlations include serum threonine with urine 4-deoxyerythronic acid ($r = 0.31$), which is consistent with the proposition that threonine is the main source of 4-deoxyerythronic acid [74]. Urine N-methylnicotinic acid was correlated ($r = 0.23$) with serum Ac-Orn (acetylornithine), and additionally, we also found urine acetone and 4-deoxythreonic acid to be positively associated with multiple serum acylcarnitines, while urine alanine was negatively associated with multiple serum acylcarnitines (Additional file 1: Figure S10). Amongst the 391 significant serum-urine metabolite pairs, the median correlation r^2 was 2.7% whilst across all 7788 serum-urine metabolite pairs the median correlation r^2 was only 0.15% indicating that, even if a subset of serum-urine metabolic correlations are significant, information contained in our urine and serum profiles was largely orthogonal to one another.

Discussion

Utilising two reproducible and well-characterised metabolic profiling platforms, ^{1}H NMR spectroscopy and LC-MS/MS, we have characterised the urine and serum metabolic phenotypes in European children from six cohort populations representing different demographic and sample characteristics. Little is known regarding the normal concentration ranges of urinary and serum metabolites in healthy European children at present, and in this study, we have used a sample size of approximately 1200

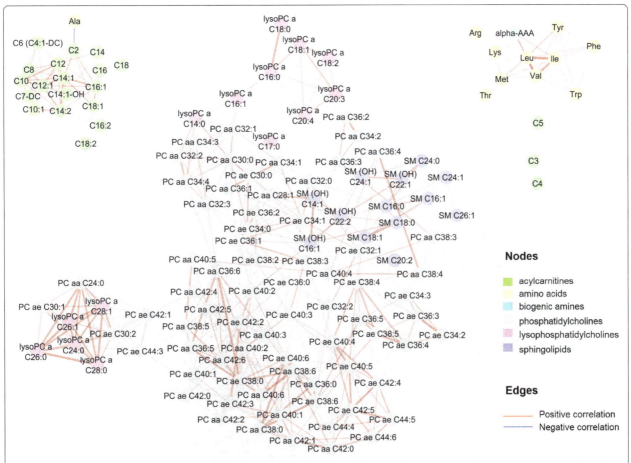

Fig. 7 Serum metabolic correlation network diagram generated using MetScape (Cytoscape) based on metabolite pairwise correlations ("edge") either < − 0.5 or > 0.65

individuals spread across six European countries and embedded the work in a population with rich metadata on diet, anthropometry and environmental exposure. ^{1}H NMR spectroscopy and targeted LC-MS/MS (the Absolute*IDQ* p180 kit) were chosen for the analysis of urine, and serum samples correspondingly in this study, as they offer good sensitivity, broad dynamic range and metabolite coverage, are widely applied and have been used previously for epidemiological studies in the respective bio fluids [75].

Sample handling and pre-analytical effects

Sample handling in such a large population and across six different centres would be expected to impact on metabolite levels. Stability of serum metabolites are considered lower when compared to those found in urine, and it has been reported that concentrations of many blood metabolites are altered by 12 h pre-storage delay at room temperature [76]. Thus, great care was taken when the study sample collection protocol was developed to help ensure that the sample processing time was kept short (< 2 h). Two separate studies have previously found that urine or serum samples stored at 4 °C for up to 24 h before being frozen were comparable to those frozen immediately [77, 78], and in our study, we have confirmed that neither urine nor serum sample processing time appear to bias our subsequent data analysis. Also, the design of the urine sample collection benefited from our previous pilot work [57] and we took advantage of a pooled sample design, combining the last sample before bedtime with the first morning void sample in the following day, to reduce diurnal variations. Morning or night void samples were only included in analyses as replacements for the pooled samples when pooled samples were missing (7% of the total). Levels of several metabolites, including citrate and *N*-methyl nicotinamide, were found to be significantly different between morning or night-time void samples; these are consistent with findings from our earlier pilot panel study which examined the diurnal and day-to-day variability of urine sampling [57]. Whilst fasting-state samples reduce temporal within-day sampling variability compared to non-fasted samples [75], such sample collections are not always feasible, as was the case for

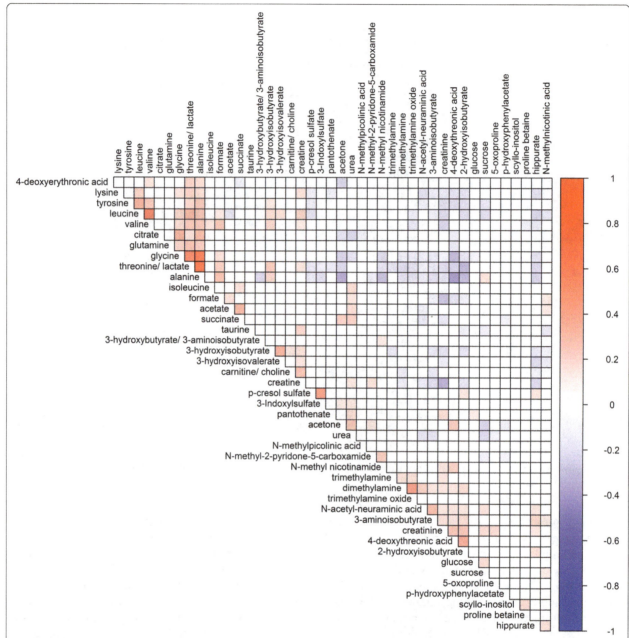

Fig. 8 Urinary metabolic correlation heatmap diagram. Colour represents Pearson correlation coefficients and only significant correlations after Bonferroni correlations (p value threshold = 5.3×10^{-5}) are shown

the HELIX project. Thus, most of the serum samples analysed were from non-fasting states with a median postprandial period of 3.3 h, and we have found large number of amino acids and acylcarnitines to be associated with postprandial intervals. Similarly, in a previous study of healthy female volunteers [79], using the Absolute*IDQ* p180 kit, significantly altered postprandial concentrations of amino acids and acylcarnitines were reported, likely as a result of changes in fatty acid oxidation and ketogenesis.

Demographic factors, BMI and the child metabolome

Overall, we found the serum metabolite concentrations from the HELIX children population to be remarkably similar to reference values obtained in a study of healthy French adults [66]. However, there are some notable differences; for example, the serum creatinine level is lower in the HELIX children compared with adult populations, probably reflecting differences in lean muscle mass between adults and children [80]—a well-studied phenomenon [81] that was replicated in our study.

Likewise, the urinary creatinine level was lower in the HELIX children population compared to reference values for adult populations [82, 83], and our cohort-stratified regression models also identified both urinary and serum creatinine to be positively associated with a child's age, reaffirming creatinine as a valid indicator of muscle development in children [81, 82, 84].

Body anthropometry is an important predictor of molecular profiles and is of intense interest for disease risk stratification in epidemiological studies. The standardised BMI z-score calculated for a given age and sex has been established as a reliable measure in accessing obesity burden in child populations [85]. We observed positive associations between urinary and serum BCAAs and standardised BMI z-score, which have previously been reported in other children or young adult populations [43, 86, 87]. BCAAs are important nutrient signals [88], and increased circulating BCAAs levels have been suggested to predict future insulin resistance [43] as well as increased cardio-metabolic risk independent to adiposity in young adults [86]. Also, we identified two sphingolipids (SM C16:1 and SM C18:1) to be both higher in females and positively associated with BMI z-score, possibly reflecting differences in body fat composition and physical development between boys and girls. Also, two of the lysophosphatidylcholines (lysoPC a C16:1, lysoPC a C18:1) associated with BMI z-score in this study have recently been shown to be correlated to infant birth weight [89]. Moreover, out of the 41 serum metabolites found to be associated with BMI z-score in our HELIX children cohort, 14 metabolites (including kynurenine, glutamate, lysoPC a C18:1, lysoPC a C18:2) have also previously been reported in the EPIC study in an adult population, where the Absolute*IDQ* p180 kit was also used [90], demonstrating that many serum metabolic associations with BMI observed in adulthood can also be found in childhood.

A key finding of our study was novel evidence for a positive association between urinary 4-deoxyerythronic acid and child BMI z-score, a threonine catabolite [91, 92] found elevated during pregnancy [93]. Whilst very little is currently known about the biology of 4-deoxyerythronic acid, it is present and has been found to be inversely associated with age in adults [27, 74, 94], and higher levels of this and related metabolites have been observed in children with early onset type I diabetes [95]. Threonine is an essential amino acid, and threonine dehydrogenase has been reported as a relatively minor (~ 10%) contributor to threonine oxidation in humans when compared to other species (up to 80%) [77]—indicating that exogenous sources or symbiotic microbial metabolism may be playing an important role in 4-deoxyerythronic acid exposure. Interestingly, it has been reported that formula-fed infants have a lower capacity to oxidise threonine than do infants fed breast milk [96] and that catabolism of threonine can lead to methylglyoxal production which contributes to the pathophysiology of obesity and diabetes [97] and can reduce health span in model systems [98]. Urinary 4-deoxyerythronic acid was found positively associated with child BMI in five of the six participating cohorts, with the exception of MoBa which has the lowest BMI z-score distribution amongst the six cohorts. It is possible that 4-deoxyerythronic acid association to BMI is more discernable in overweight populations. We report herein a correlation between serum threonine and urinary 4-deoxyerythronic acid which supports the hypothesis that endogenous catabolism of threonine is a source of this metabolite. However, further work is required to understand the relationship between 4-deoxyerythronic acid and metabolic health.

Habitual dietary intake and the child metabolome

We have confirmed in children a number of known diet-metabolite associations in adults, including meat (which has high creatine content) with urine creatine [99], vegetables and fruits with urine hippurate [100, 101], fruits with proline betaine and *scyllo*-inositol [47, 102]. It is also of note that all 12 metabolites associated with fish intake in the study were serum glycerophosphatidylcholine metabolites; oily fish in the diet alters glycerophospholipid composition and is an important nutrient source for polyunsaturated fatty acids [103, 104]. The extent to which metabolic phenotypes mediate the impact of dietary behaviour on childhood adiposity and cardiovascular indicators will be a focus of our future work. We anticipate that the metabolic phenotyping dataset acquired on the HELIX study population will provide a useful molecular resource to help elucidate the complex interactions between childhood environmental and dietary exposures and adverse health outcomes.

Complementarity between the serum and urine metabolome

In the HELIX study, matched urine and serum samples across six European cohorts were collected according to well-defined protocols, providing a valuable resource for uncovering metabolic relationships across the two most accessible biological fluid types. Whilst NMR spectroscopy and LC-MS/MS-based metabolic profiling have been widely applied in epidemiological studies [34, 68, 83, 105, 106], our study is one of very few that allows comparison of the effects of pre-analytical, analytical, demographic, dietary and geographic variation between the two biofluid types from the same sample population. It has previously been reported that biological variations are more robustly captured in a blood metabolic profile compared to urine [107]. In our study, we confirm that the combined information from demographics, diet and cohort accounts for greater variance in the LC-MS/MS serum profile compared to NMR urine profile, even if the LC-MS/MS serum profile is more susceptible to analytical batch effects. However, with respect to dietary habits specifically, these are better reflected in the urinary metabolome presumably due to high metabolite turnover, and it has previously been reported in a colon adenoma case-control study ($n = 253$) that more metabolites in urine were uniquely associated with diet than in serum [47]. Our pairwise metabolite correlation analyses also potentially confer information about metabolic pathway activities: urinary acetate with formate and succinate (TCA cycle activity and gut bacterial metabolism); urinary creatine with choline/carnitine (meat diet); 3-indoxylsulfate and p-cresol sulphate (both sulphated uremic solutes produced by gut bacteria); urinary dimethylamine with trimethylamine, and trimethylamine oxide (amine derivatives), and urinary and serum valine with leucine (branched-chain amino acid metabolism). Our correlation analysis between metabolite concentrations across the two biological fluid types confirmed that for many compounds, metabolite concentrations between urine and serum are positively correlated and also confirmed metabolic pathway associations with serum threonine and urinary 4-deoxyerythronic acid (threonine catabolism) [74].

Limitations
Our study had a number of important limitations. Firstly, the sample size from each of the six individual cohorts was relatively small ($n\sim200$) for observational studies, limiting the statistical power available to uncover novel metabolic associations, particularly when effect sizes were generally small. There were also notable differences in sample characteristics between the cohorts, particularly in age, with the median cohort child age varying from 6 to 11 years old, making it difficult to disentangle cohort level differences from other covariates in our variance decomposition analyses, as those confounders were heavily correlated. Our study also lacks 24-h dietary recall data, and serum samples were collected from non-fasting states. In addition, we acknowledge the inherent limitations in the use of food frequency questionnaire which include the potential for dietary intake misclassifications and that categorising distinct food sources into groups may be imperfect. For example, cocoa could be considered as a vegetable but was classified as sweets in this study. We intend to follow up the metabolite—diet associations identified in this study with detailed food subgroup analyses as part of a future publication.

To make certain the timely completion of an annotated metabolome resource, we have decided to acquire and to process the serum and urine metabolic data using analytical methods which quantify omnipresent metabolites that were typically detected well in this study. Whilst this approach had the advantage of improving the sensitivity and specificity of the quantitation and provide explicit metabolite identification, it limited the number of metabolites that were measured and resulted in only partial coverage of the serum and urine metabolome. Also, the serum metabolic assay only provided partial specificity in the assignment of lipid species as the locations of double bonds or the length of the fatty acid chains remain ambiguous. Supplementing the current study with other complementary metabolomic approaches such as untargeted LC-MS and GC-MS analyses in future would help enhance metabolite coverage and greatly augment the metabolome resource of healthy children available at present.

Conclusions
We have characterised the major components of the urine and serum metabolome in the HELIX subcohort. Typically but not universally, metabolic associations with age, sex, BMI z-score and dietary habits were common to the six populations studied. Also, a novel metabolic association between threonine catabolism and BMI of children was identified. Inter-metabolite correlation analyses for both urine and serum metabolic phenotypes revealed potential pathway associations, and population-specific variance (demographic, dietary and country of origin) was better captured in the serum than in the urine metabolic profile. This study establishes a reference metabolome resource in multiple European populations for urine and serum from healthy children. This provides a critical foundation for future work to define the utility of metabolic profiles to monitor or predict the impact of environmental and other exposures on human biology and child health.

Abbreviations
BCAA: Branched-chain amino acids; BiB: Born in Bradford, UK; BLD: Below the limit of detection; BMI: Body mass index; CI: Confidence interval; EDEN: Study of determinants of pre- and postnatal developmental, France; HELIX: The Human Early-Life Exposome project; HPLC: High-performance liquid chromatography; INMA: Infancia y Medio Ambiente, Environment and Childhood, Spain; IQR: Interquartile range; KANC: Kaunas Cohort, Lithuania; LC-MS/MS: Liquid chromatography tandem mass spectrometry; LOD: Limit of detection; LPC: Lysophosphatidylcholine; MoBa: The Norwegian Mother and Child Cohort Study, Norway; NMR: Nuclear magnetic resonance; PC: Phosphatidylcholine; PCA: Principal component analysis; QRILC: Quantile

regression approach for left-censored missing; Rhea: Mother-Child Cohort in Crete, Greece; SM: Sphingomyelin

Acknowledgements
This research received funding from the EU European Commission's Seventh Framework Programme (FP7/2007-2013) under grant agreement no. 308333—the HELIX project. We would like to thank all the study participants and the full list of the HELIX Project Investigators that can be found at http://www.projecthelix.eu. The Norwegian Mother and Child Cohort Study is supported by the Norwegian Ministry of Health and Care Services and the Ministry of Education and Research, NIH/NIEHS (contract no. N01-ES-75558), NIH/NINDS (grant no. 1 UO1 NS 047537-01 and grant no. 2 UO1 NS 047537-06A1). Dr. Maribel Casas received funding from Instituto de Salud Carlos III (Ministry of Economy and Competitiveness) (MS16/00128).
We are grateful to all the participating families in Norway who take part in this on-going cohort study, but especially those families who came in for a clinical examination of their child, who in addition donated blood and urine to this specific study.
Born in Bradford is only possible because of the enthusiasm and commitment of the children and parents in BiB. We are grateful to all the participants, health professionals and researchers who have made Born in Bradford happen.

Funding
The research leading to these results has received funding from the European Community's Seventh Framework Programme (FP7/2007-2013) under grant agreement no. 308333—the HELIX project.

Authors' contributions
CEL and APS performed the metabolomics experiments, conducted the data analyses and drafted the manuscript. MC, HCK, TJA and EW conceived this study, participated in the metabolomics experimental design and coordination and drafted the manuscript. MVrijheid coordinated the HELIX project and supervised the project data collection. LC prepared the clinical examination protocols and contributed to the interpretation of the dietary intake habits data. LM coordinated the data collection and harmonisation for the HELIX project, and participated in the urine metabolomics NMR data acquisition. OR coordinated the biofluid sample and data collection for the HELIX project and prepared questionnaires and protocols. JU managed the HELIX project database. HMM was involved in designing the MoBa cohort and oversaw all aspects of the subcohort data collection for MoBa. OR, MCasas, MVafeiadi, TR, RM, RA, LSH, HMM, SA, IP, RG, CT, JW, RS, LC, and MVrijheid were involved in development of the protocols and contributed to the biobank sample or data collection, or the management at the six participating cohorts. All authors read and approved the final manuscript.

Competing interests
The authors declare that they have no competing interests.

Author details
[1]Division of Computational and Systems Medicine, Department of Surgery and Cancer, Faculty of Medicine, Imperial College London, London SW7 2AZ, UK. [2]Division of Cancer, Department of Surgery and Cancer, Faculty of Medicine, Imperial College London, London W12 0NN, UK. [3]ISGlobal, Barcelona, Spain. [4]Universitat Pompeu Fabra (UPF), Barcelona, Spain. [5]CIBER Epidemiologa y Salud Pública (CIBERESP), Madrid, Spain. [6]MRC-PHE Centre for Environment and Health, School of Public Health, Faculty of Medicine, Imperial College London, London W2 1PG, UK. [7]Department of Social Medicine, Faculty of Medicine, University of Crete, Heraklion, Crete, Greece. [8]Inserm, Univ. Grenoble Alpes, CNRS, IAB (Institute of Advanced Biosciences), Grenoble, France. [9]Bradford Institute for Health Research, Bradford Teaching Hospitals NHS Foundation Trust, Bradford, UK. [10]Norwegian Institute of Public Health, Oslo, Norway. [11]Department of Environmental Sciences, Vytautas Magnus University, Kaunas, Lithuania. [12]Department of Preventive Medicine, Keck School of Medicine, University of Southern California, Los Angeles, USA. [13]Oncology Safety, Drug Safety and Metabolism, IMED Biotech Unit, AstraZeneca, 1 Francis Crick Avenue, Cambridge CB2 0RE, UK.

References
1. Leon DA, Lithell HO, Vagero D, Koupilova I, Mohsen R, Berglund L, Lithell UB, McKeigue PM. Reduced fetal growth rate and increased risk of death from ischaemic heart disease: cohort study of 15 000 Swedish men and women born 1915-29. Br Med J. 1998;317(7153):241–5.
2. Barker DJP, Gluckman PD, Godfrey KM, Harding JE, Owens JA, Robinson JS. Fetal nutrition and cardiovascular-disease in adult life. Lancet. 1993; 341(8850):938–41.
3. Wadhwa PD, Buss C, Entringer S, Swanson JM. Developmental origins of health and disease: brief history of the approach and current focus on epigenetic mechanisms. Semin Reprod Med. 2009;27(5):358–68.
4. Thacher JD, Gruzieva O, Pershagen G, Neuman A, Wickman M, Kull I, Melen E, Bergstrom A. Pre- and postnatal exposure to parental smoking and allergic disease through adolescence. Pediatrics. 2014;134(3):428–34.
5. Berends LM, Ozanne SE. Early determinants of type-2 diabetes. Best Pract Res Clin Endocrinol Metab. 2012;26(5):569–80.
6. Burbank AJ, Sood AK, Kesic MJ, Peden DB, Hernandez ML. Environmental determinants of allergy and asthma in early life. J Allergy Clin Immunol. 2017;140(1):1–12.
7. Burke H, Leonardi-Bee J, Hashim A, Pine-Abata H, Chen YL, Cook DG, Britton JR, McKeever TM. Prenatal and passive smoke exposure and incidence of asthma and wheeze: systematic review and meta-analysis. Pediatrics. 2012; 129(4):735–44.
8. Deng QH, Lu C, Li YG, Sundell J, Norback D. Exposure to outdoor air pollution during trimesters of pregnancy and childhood asthma, allergic rhinitis, and eczema. Environ Res. 2016;150:119–27.
9. Vafeiadi M, Roumeliotaki T, Myridakis A, Chalkiadaki G, Fthenou E, Dermitzaki E, Karachaliou M, Sarri K, Vassilaki M, Stephanou EG, et al. Association of early life exposure to bisphenol A with obesity and cardiometabolic traits in childhood. Environ Res. 2016;146:379–87.
10. Agay-Shay K, Martinez D, Valvi D, Garcia-Esteban R, Basagana X, Robinson O, Casas M, Sunyer J, Vrijheid M. Exposure to endocrine-disrupting chemicals during pregnancy and weight at 7 years of age: a multi-pollutant approach. Environ Health Perspect. 2015;123(10):1030–7.
11. Boffetta P, Tredaniel J, Greco A. Risk of childhood cancer and adult lung cancer after childhood exposure to passive smoke: a meta-analysis. Environ Health Perspect. 2000;108(1):73–82.
12. Gilmore JH, Jarskog LF, Vadlamudi S, Lauder J. Prenatal infection and risk for schizophrenia: IL-I beta, IL-6, and TNF alpha inhibit cortical neuron dendrite development. Neuropsychopharmacology. 2004;29(7):1221–9.
13. Braun JM, Kahn RS, Froehlich T, Auinger P, Lanphear BP. Exposures to environmental toxicants and attention deficit hyperactivity disorder in US children. Environ Health Perspect. 2006;114(12):1904–9.
14. Heijmans BT, Tobi EW, Stein AD, Putter H, Blauw GJ, Susser ES, Slagboom PE, Lumey LH. Persistent epigenetic differences associated with prenatal exposure to famine in humans. Proc Natl Acad Sci U S A. 2008;105(44):17046–9.
15. Ghantous A, Hernandez-Vargas H, Byrnes G, Dwyer T, Herceg Z. Characterising the epigenome as a key component of the fetal exposome in evaluating in utero exposures and childhood cancer risk. Mutagenesis. 2015;30(6):733–42.
16. Lioy PJ, Rappaport SM. Exposure science and the exposome: an opportunity for coherence in the environmental health sciences. Environ Health Perspect. 2011;119(11):A466–7.
17. Wild CP. The exposome: from concept to utility. Int J Epidemiol. 2012; 41(1):24–32.
18. Vineis P, van Veldhoven K, Chadeau-Hyam M, Athersuch TJ. Advancing the application of omics-based biomarkers in environmental epidemiology. Environ Mol Mutagen. 2013;54(7):461–7.
19. Robinson O, Martinez D, Aurrekoetxea JJ, Estarlich M, Somoano AF, Iniguez C, Santa-Marina L, Tardon A, Torrent M, Sunyer J, et al. The association between passive and active tobacco smoke exposure and child weight status among Spanish children. Obesity. 2016;24(8):1767–77.
20. Robinson O, Basagana X, Agier L, de Castro M, Hernandez-Ferrer C, Gonzalez JR, Grimalt JO, Nieuwenhuijsen M, Sunyer J, Slama R, et al. The pregnancy exposome: multiple environmental exposures in the INMA-Sabadell birth cohort. Environ Sci Technol. 2015;49(17):10632–41.
21. Bisgaard H, Vissing NH, Carson CG, Bischoff AL, Folsgaard NV, Kreiner-Moller E, Chawes BLK, Stokholm J, Pedersen L, Bjarnadottir E, et al. Deep phenotyping of the unselected COPSAC2010 birth cohort study. Clin Exp Allergy. 2013;43(12):1384–94.

22. Sarigiannis DA. Assessing the impact of hazardous waste on children's health: the exposome paradigm. Environ Res. 2017;158:531–41.
23. Athersuch TJ, Keun HC. Metabolic profiling in human exposome studies. Mutagenesis. 2015;30(6):755–62.
24. Athersuch TJ. The role of metabolomics in characterizing the human exposome. Bioanalysis. 2012;4(18):2207–12.
25. Baker MG, Simpson CD, Lin YS, Shireman LM, Seixas N. The use of metabolomics to identify biological signatures of manganese exposure. Ann Work Expo Health. 2017;61(4):406–15.
26. Ladva CN, Golan R, Greenwald R, Yu TW, Sarnat SE, Flanders WD, Uppal K, Walker DI, Tran V, Liang DH, et al. Metabolomic profiles of plasma, exhaled breath condensate, and saliva are correlated with potential for air toxics detection. J Breath Res. 2018;12(1):016008.
27. Ellis JK, Athersuch TJ, Thomas LDK, Teichert F, Perez-Trujillo M, Svendsen C, Spurgeon DJ, Singh R, Jarup L, Bundy JG, et al. Metabolic profiling detects early effects of environmental and lifestyle exposure to cadmium in a human population. BMC Med. 2012;10:61.
28. Wilson K, Hawken S, Ducharme R, Potter BK, Little J, Thebaud B, Chakraborty P. Metabolomics of prematurity: analysis of patterns of amino acids, enzymes, and endocrine markers by categories of gestational age. Pediatr Res. 2014;75(2):367–73.
29. Maitre L, Villanueva CM, Lewis MR, Ibarluzea J, Santa-Marina L, Vrijheid M, Sunyer J, Coen M, Toledano MB. Maternal urinary metabolic signatures of fetal growth and associated clinical and environmental factors in the INMA study. BMC Med. 2016;14:177.
30. Overgaard AJ, Kaur S, Pociot F. Metabolomic biomarkers in the progression to type 1 diabetes. Curr Diab Rep. 2016;16(12):127.
31. Smolinska A, Klaassen EMM, Dallinga JW, van de Kant KDG, Jobsis Q, Moonen EJC, van Schayck OCP, Dompeling E, van Schooten FJ. Profiling of volatile organic compounds in exhaled breath as a strategy to find early predictive signatures of asthma in children. PLoS One. 2014;9(4):e95668.
32. James SJ, Cutler P, Melnyk S, Jernigan S, Janak L, Gaylor DW, Neubrander JA. Metabolic biomarkers of increased oxidative stress and impaired methylation capacity in children with autism. Am J Clin Nutr. 2004;80(6):1611–7.
33. Yu ZH, Zhai GJ, Singmann P, He Y, Xu T, Prehn C, Roemisch-Margl W, Lattka E, Gieger C, Soranzo N, et al. Human serum metabolic profiles are age dependent. Aging Cell. 2012;11(6):960–7.
34. Elliott P, Posma JM, Chan Q, Garcia-Perez I, Wijeyesekera A, Bictash M, Ebbels TMD, Ueshima H, Zhao LC, van Horn L, et al. Urinary metabolic signatures of human adiposity. Sci Transl Med. 2015;7(285):285ra62.
35. Guertin KA, Moore SC, Sampson JN, Huang WY, Xiao Q, Stolzenberg-Solomon RZ, Sinha R, Cross AJ. Metabolomics in nutritional epidemiology: identifying metabolites associated with diet and quantifying their potential to uncover diet-disease relations in populations. Am J Clin Nutr. 2014;100(1):208–17.
36. Jourdan C, Petersen AK, Gieger C, Doring A, Illig T, Wang-Sattler R, Meisinger C, Peters A, Adamski J, Prehn C, et al. Body fat free mass is associated with the serum metabolite profile in a population-based study. PLoS One. 2012;7(6):e40009.
37. Kochhar S, Jacobs DM, Ramadan Z, Berruex F, Fuerhoz A, Fay LB. Probing gender-specific metabolism differences in humans by nuclear magnetic resonance-based metabonomics. Anal Biochem. 2006;352(2):274–81.
38. Moore SC, Matthews CE, Sampson JN, Stolzenberg-Solomon RZ, Zheng W, Cai QY, Tan YT, Chow WH, Ji BT, Liu DK, et al. Human metabolic correlates of body mass index. Metabolomics. 2014;10(2):259–69.
39. Stella C, Beckwith-Hall B, Cloarec O, Holmes E, Lindon JC, Powell J, van der Ouderaa F, Bingham S, Cross AJ, Nicholson JK. Susceptibility of human metabolic phenotypes to dietary modulation. J Proteome Res. 2006;5(10):2780–8.
40. Holmes E, Loo RL, Stamler J, Bictash M, Yap IKS, Chan Q, Ebbels T, De Iorio M, Brown IJ, Veselkov KA, et al. Human metabolic phenotype diversity and its association with diet and blood pressure. Nature. 2008;453(7193):396–U350.
41. Wurtz P, Wang Q, Kangas AJ, Richmond RC, Skarp J, Tiainen M, Tynkkynen T, Soininen P, Havulinna AS, Kaakinen M, et al. Metabolic signatures of adiposity in young adults: Mendelian randomization analysis and effects of weight change. PLoS Med. 2014;11(12):e1001765.
42. Dunn WB, Lin WC, Broadhurst D, Begley P, Brown M, Zelena E, Vaughan AA, Halsall A, Harding N, Knowles JD, et al. Molecular phenotyping of a UK population: defining the human serum metabolome. Metabolomics. 2015;11(1):9–26.
43. McCormack SE, Shaham O, McCarthy MA, Deik AA, Wang TJ, Gerszten RE, Clish CB, Mootha VK, Grinspoon SK, Fleischman A. Circulating branched-chain amino acid concentrations are associated with obesity and future insulin resistance in children and adolescents. Pediatric Obesity. 2013;8(1):52–61.
44. Knip M, Virtanen SM, Akerblom HK. Infant feeding and the risk of type 1 diabetes. Am J Clin Nutr. 2010;91(5):1506S–13S.
45. Freemark M. Metabolomics in nutrition research: biomarkers predicting mortality in children with severe acute malnutrition. Food Nutr Bull. 2015;36:S88–92.
46. Chiu CY, Yeh KW, Lin G, Chiang MH, Yang SC, Chao WJ, Yao TC, Tsai MH, Hua MC, Liao SL, et al. Metabolomics reveals dynamic metabolic changes associated with age in early childhood. PLoS One. 2016;11(2):e0149823.
47. Playdon MC, Sampson JN, Cross AJ, Sinha R, Guertin KA, Moy KA, Rothman N, Irwin ML, Mayne ST, Stolzenberg-Solomon R, et al. Comparing metabolite profiles of habitual diet in serum and urine. Am J Clin Nutr. 2016;104(3):776–89.
48. Vrijheid M, Slama R, Robinson O, Chatzi L, Coen M, van den Hazel P, Thomsen C, Wright J, Athersuch TJ, Avellana N, et al. The human early-life exposome (HELIX): project rationale and design. Environ Health Perspect. 2014;122(6):535–44.
49. Maitre L, de Bont J, Casas M, Robinson O, Aasvang GM, Agier L, Andrušaitytė S, Ballester F, Basagaña X, Borràs E, et al. Human Early Life Exposome (HELIX) study: a European population-based exposome cohort. BMJ Open. 2018;8(9):e021311.
50. Wright J, Small N, Raynor P, Tuffnell D, Bhopal R, Cameron N, Fairley L, Lawlor DA, Parslow R, Petherick ES, et al. Cohort profile: the Born in Bradford multi-ethnic family cohort study. Int J Epidemiol. 2013;42(4):978–91.
51. Heude B, Forhan A, Slama R, Douhaud L, Bedel S, Saurel-Cubizolles MJ, Hankard R, Thiebaugeorges O, De Agostini M, Annesi-Maesano I, et al. Cohort profile: the EDEN mother-child cohort on the prenatal and early postnatal determinants of child health and development. Int J Epidemiol. 2016;45(2):353–63.
52. Guxens M, Ballester F, Espada M, Fernandez MF, Grimalt JO, Ibarluzea J, Olea N, Rebagliato M, Tardon A, Torrent M, et al. Cohort profile: the INMA-INfancia y Medio Ambiente-(environment and childhood) project. Int J Epidemiol. 2012;41(4):930–40.
53. Grazuleviciene R, Nieuwenhuijsen MJ, Vencloviene J, Kostopoulou-Karadanelli M, Krasner SW, Danileviciute A, Balcius G, Kapustinskiene V. Individual exposures to drinking water trihalomethanes, low birth weight and small for gestational age risk: a prospective Kaunas cohort study. Environ Health. 2011;10:32.
54. Magnus P, Birke C, Vejrup K, Haugan A, Alsaker E, Daltveit AK, Handal M, Haugen M, Hoiseth G, Knudsen GP, et al. Cohort profile update: the Norwegian mother and child cohort study (MoBa). Int J Epidemiol. 2016;45(2):382–8.
55. Chatzi L, Leventakou V, Vafeiadi M, Koutra K, Roumeliotaki T, Chalkiadaki G, Karachaliou M, Daraki V, Kyriklaki A, Kampouri M, et al. Cohort profile: the mother-child cohort in Crete, Greece (Rhea study). Int J Epidemiol. 2017;46(5):1392–1393k.
56. de Onis M, Onyango AW, Borghi E, Siyam A, Nishida C, Siekmann J. Development of a WHO growth reference for school-aged children and adolescents. Bull World Health Organ. 2007;85(9):660–7.
57. Maitre L, Lau CE, Vizcaino E, Robinson O, Casas M, Siskos AP, Want EJ, Athersuch T, Slama R, Vrijheid M, et al. Assessment of metabolic phenotypic variability in children's urine using 1H NMR spectroscopy. Sci Rep. 2017;7:46082.
58. Dona AC, Jimenez B, Schafer H, Humpfer E, Spraul M, Lewis MR, Pearce JTM, Holmes E, Lindon JC, Nicholson JK. Precision high-throughput proton NMR spectroscopy of human urine, serum, and plasma for large-scale metabolic phenotyping. Anal Chem. 2014;86(19):9887–94.
59. Karaman I, Ferreira DLS, Boulange CL, Kaluarachchi MR, Herrington D, Dona AC, Castagne R, Moayyeri A, Lehne B, Loh M, et al. Workflow for integrated processing of multicohort untargeted H-1 NMR metabolomics data in large-scale metabolic epidemiology. J Proteome Res. 2016;15(12):4188–94.
60. Veselkov KA, Lindon JC, Ebbels TMD, Crockford D, Volynkin VV, Holmes E, Davies DB, Nicholson JK. Recursive segment-wise peak alignment of biological H-1 NMR spectra for improved metabolic biomarker recovery. Anal Chem. 2009;81(1):56–66.
61. Dieterle F, Ross A, Schlotterbeck G, Senn H. Probabilistic quotient normalization as robust method to account for dilution of complex biological mixtures. Application in H-1 NMR metabonomics. Anal Chem. 2006;78(13):4281–90.

62. Wishart DS, Tzur D, Knox C, Eisner R, Guo AC, Young N, Cheng D, Jewell K, Arndt D, Sawhney S. HMDB: the human metabolome database. Nucleic Acids Res. 2007;35(Database):D521–6.
63. Cloarec O, Dumas ME, Craig A, Barton RH, Trygg J, Hudson J, Blancher C, Gauguier D, Lindon JC, Holmes E, et al. Statistical total correlation spectroscopy: an exploratory approach for latent biomarker identification from metabolic H-1 NMR data sets. Anal Chem. 2005;77(5):1282–9.
64. User Manual UM_p180_AB SCIEX_9. Biocrates Life Sciences AG. Innsbruck; 2014.
65. Siskos AP, Jain P, Romisch-Margl W, Bennet M, Achaintre D, Asad Y, Marney L, Richardson L, Koulman A, Griffin JL, et al. Interlaboratory reproducibility of a targeted metabolomics platform for analysis of human serum and plasma. Anal Chem. 2017;89(1):656–65.
66. Trabado S, Al-Salameh A, Croixmarie V, Masson P, Corruble E, Feve B, Colle R, Ripoll L, Walther B, Boursier-Neyret C, et al. The human plasma-metabolome: reference values in 800 French healthy volunteers; impact of cholesterol, gender and age. PLoS One. 2017;12(3):e0173615.
67. Merz B, Nothlings U, Wahl S, Haftenberger M, Schienkiewitz A, Adamski J, Suhre K, Wang-Sattler R, Grallert H, Thorand B, et al. Specific metabolic markers are associated with future waist-gaining phenotype in women. PLoS One. 2016;11(6):e0157733.
68. Yet I, Menni C, Shin SY, Mangino M, Soranzo N, Adamski J, Suhre K, Spector TD, Kastenmuller G, Bell JT. Genetic influences on metabolite levels: a comparison across metabolomic platforms. PLoS One. 2016;11(4):e0153672.
69. Smoot ME, Ono K, Ruscheinski J, Wang PL, Ideker T. Cytoscape 2.8: new features for data integration and network visualization. Bioinformatics. 2011;27(3):431–2.
70. Basu S, Duren W, Evans CR, Burant CF, Michailidis G, Karnovsky A. Sparse network modeling and MetScape-based visualization methods for the analysis of large-scale metabolomics data. Bioinformatics. 2017;33(10):1545–53.
71. Sakia RM. The Box-Cox transformation technique - a review. J R Stat Soc Ser D. 1992;41(2):169–78.
72. Wei RM, Wang JY, Su MM, Jia E, Chen SQ, Chen TL, Ni Y. Missing value imputation approach for mass spectrometry-based metabolomics data. Sci Rep. 2018;8:663.
73. Vanholder R, Schepers E, Pletinck A, Nagler EV, Glorieux G. The uremic toxicity of Indoxyl sulfate and p-Cresyl sulfate: a systematic review. J Am Soc Nephrol. 2014;25(9):1897–907.
74. Darling PB, Grunow J, Rafii M, Brookes S, Ball RO, Pencharz PB. Threonine dehydrogenase is a minor degradative pathway of threonine catabolism in adult humans. Am J Physiol Endocrinol Metab. 2000;278(5):E877–84.
75. Carayol M, Licaj I, Achaintre D, Sacerdote C, Vineis P, Key TJ, Moret NCO, Scalbert A, Rinaldi S, Ferrari P. Reliability of serum metabolites over a two-year period: a targeted metabolomic approach in fasting and non-fasting samples from EPIC. PLoS One. 2015;10(8):e0135437.
76. Anton G, Wilson R, Yu ZH, Prehn C, Zukunft S, Adamski J, Heier M, Meisinger C, Romisch-Margl W, Wang-Sattler R, et al. Pre-analytical sample quality: metabolite ratios as an intrinsic marker for prolonged room temperature exposure of serum samples. PLoS One. 2015;10(3):e0121495.
77. Dunn WB, Broadhurst D, Ellis DI, Brown M, Halsall A, O'Hagan S, Spasic I, Tseng A, Kell DB. A GC-TOF-MS study of the stability of serum and urine metabolomes during the UK Biobank sample collection and preparation protocols. Int J Epidemiol. 2008;37:23–30.
78. Barton RH, Nicholson JK, Elliott P, Holmes E. High-throughput H-1 NMR-based metabolic analysis of human serum and urine for large-scale epidemiological studies: validation study. Int J Epidemiol. 2008;37:31–40.
79. Shrestha A, Mullner E, Poutanen K, Mykkanen H, Moazzami AA. Metabolic changes in serum metabolome in response to a meal. Eur J Nutr. 2017;56(2):671–81.
80. Baxmann AC, Ahmed MS, Marques NC, Menon VB, Pereira AB, Kirsztajn GM, Heilberg IP. Influence of muscle mass and physical activity on serum and urinary creatinine and serum cystatin C. Clin J Am Soc Nephrol. 2008;3(2):348–54.
81. Savory DJ. Reference ranges for serum creatinine in infants, children and adolescents. Ann Clin Biochem. 1990;27:99–101.
82. Sugita O, Uchiyama K, Yamada T, Sato T, Okada M, Takeuchi K. Reference values of serum and urine creatinine, and of creatinine clearance by a new enzymatic method. Ann Clin Biochem. 1992;29:523–8.
83. Bouatra S, Aziat F, Mandal R, Guo AC, Wilson MR, Knox C, Bjorndahl TC, Krishnamurthy R, Saleem F, Liu P, et al. The human urine metabolome. PLoS One. 2013;8(9):e73076.
84. Richmond W, Colgan G, Simon S, Stuart-Hilgenfeld M, Wilson N, Alon US. Random urine calcium/osmolality in the assessment of calciuria in children with decreased muscle mass. Clin Nephrol. 2005;64(4):264–70.
85. Must A, Anderson SE. Body mass index in children and adolescents: considerations for population-based applications. Int J Obes. 2006;30(4):590–4.
86. Mangge H, Zelzer S, Pruller F, Schnedl WJ, Weghuber D, Enko D, Bergsten P, Haybaeck J, Meinitzer A. Branched-chain amino acids are associated with cardiometabolic risk profiles found already in lean, overweight and obese young. J Nutr Biochem. 2016;32:123–7.
87. Perng W, Gillman MW, Fleisch AF, Michalek RD, Watkins SM, Isganaitis E, Patti ME, Oken E. Metabolomic profiles and childhood obesity. Obesity. 2014;22(12):2570–8.
88. Lynch CJ, Adams SH. Branched-chain amino acids in metabolic signalling and insulin resistance. Nat Rev Endocrinol. 2014;10(12):723–36.
89. Robinson O, Keski-Rahkonen P, Chatzi L, Kogevinas M, Nawrot T, Pizzi C, Plusquin M, Richiardi L, Robinot N, Sunyer J, et al. Cord blood metabolic signatures of birth weight: a population-based study. J Proteome Res. 2018;17(3):1235–47.
90. Carayol M, Leitzmann MF, Ferrari P, Zamora-Ros R, Achaintre D, Stepien M, Schmidt JA, Travis RC, Overvad K, Tjonneland A, et al. Blood metabolic signatures of body mass index: a targeted metabolomics study in the EPIC cohort. J Proteome Res. 2017;16(9):3137–46.
91. Edgar AJ. The human L-threonine 3-dehydrogenase gene is an expressed pseudogene. BMC Genet. 2002;3:18.
92. Van Winkle LJ, Galat V, Iannaccone PM. Threonine appears to be essential for proliferation of human as well as mouse embryonic stem cells. Front Cell Dev Biol. 2014;2:18.
93. Diaz SO, Barros AS, Goodfellow BJ, Duarte IF, Carreira IM, Galhano E, Pita C, Almeida MD, Gil AM. Following healthy pregnancy by nuclear magnetic resonance (NMR) metabolic profiling of human urine. J Proteome Res. 2013;12(2):969–79.
94. Thompson JA, Markey SP, Fennessey PV. Gas-chromatographic-mass-spectrometric identification and quantitation of tetronic and deoxytetronic acids in urine from normal adults and neonates. Clin Chem. 1975;21(13):1892–8.
95. Kassel DB, Martin M, Schall W, Sweeley CC. Urinary metabolites of L-threonine in type-1 diabetes determined by combined gas-chromatography chemical ionization mass-spectrometry. Biomed Environ Mass Spectrom. 1986;13(10):535–40.
96. Darling PB, Dunn M, Sarwar G, Brookes S, Ball RO, Pencharz PB. Threonine kinetics in preterm infants fed their mothers' milk or formula with various ratios of whey to casein. Am J Clin Nutr. 1999;69(1):105–14.
97. Matafome P, Sena C, Seica R. Methylglyoxal, obesity, and diabetes. Endocrine. 2013;43(3):472–84.
98. Ravichandran M, Priebe S, Grigolon G, Rozanov L, Groth M, Laube B, Guthke R, Platzer M, Zarse K, Ristow M. Impairing L-threonine catabolism promotes healthspan through methylglyoxal-mediated proteohormesis. Cell Metab. 2018;27(4):914–25 e915.
99. Nair S, O'Brien SV, Hayden K, Pandya B, Lisboa PJG, Hardy KJ, Wilding JPH. Effect of a cooked meat meal on serum creatinine and estimated glomerular filtration rate in diabetes-related kidney disease. Diabetes Care. 2014;37(2):483–7.
100. Krupp D, Doberstein N, Shi LJ, Remer T. Hippuric acid in 24-hour urine collections is a potential biomarker for fruit and vegetable consumption in healthy children and adolescents. J Nutr. 2012;142(7):1314–20.
101. Edmands WMB, Beckonert OP, Stella C, Campbell A, Lake BG, Lindon JC, Holmes E, Gooderham NJ. Identification of human urinary biomarkers of cruciferous vegetable consumption by metabonomic profiling. J Proteome Res. 2011;10(10):4513–21.
102. Heinzmann SS, Brown IJ, Chan Q, Bictash M, Dumas ME, Kochhar S, Stamler J, Holmes E, Elliott P, Nicholson JK. Metabolic profiling strategy for discovery of nutritional biomarkers: proline betaine as a marker of citrus consumption. Am J Clin Nutr. 2010;92(2):436–43.
103. Glaser C, Demmelmair H, Koletzko B. High-throughput analysis of fatty acid composition of plasma glycerophospholipids. J Lipid Res. 2010;51(1):216–21.
104. Careaghouck M, Sprecher H. Effect of a fish oil diet on the composition of rat neutrophil lipids and the molecular-species of choline and ethanolamine glycerophospholipids. J Lipid Res. 1989;30(1):77–87.
105. Psychogios N, Hau DD, Peng J, Guo AC, Mandal R, Bouatra S, Sinelnikov I, Krishnamurthy R, Eisner R, Gautam B, et al. The human serum metabolome. PLoS One. 2011;6(2):e16957.

Quantifying the risk of local Zika virus transmission in the contiguous US during the 2015–2016 ZIKV epidemic

Kaiyuan Sun[1], Qian Zhang[1], Ana Pastore-Piontti[1], Matteo Chinazzi[1], Dina Mistry[1], Natalie E Dean[2], Diana Patricia Rojas[2], Stefano Merler[3], Piero Poletti[3], Luca Rossi[4], M Elizabeth Halloran[5,6], Ira M Longini Jr[2] and Alessandro Vespignani[1,4]*

Abstract

Background: Local mosquito-borne Zika virus (ZIKV) transmission has been reported in two counties in the contiguous United States (US), prompting the issuance of travel, prevention, and testing guidance across the contiguous US. Large uncertainty, however, surrounds the quantification of the actual risk of ZIKV introduction and autochthonous transmission across different areas of the US.

Methods: We present a framework for the projection of ZIKV autochthonous transmission in the contiguous US during the 2015–2016 epidemic using a data-driven stochastic and spatial epidemic model accounting for seasonal, environmental, and detailed population data. The model generates an ensemble of travel-related case counts and simulates their potential to have triggered local transmission at the individual level in the 2015–2016 ZIKV epidemic.

Results: We estimate the risk of ZIKV introduction and local transmission at the county level and at the 0.025° × 0.025° cell level across the contiguous US. We provide a risk measure based on the probability of observing local transmission in a specific location during a ZIKV epidemic modeled after the epidemic observed during the years 2015–2016. The high spatial and temporal resolution of the model allows us to generate statistical estimates of the number of ZIKV introductions leading to local transmission in each location. We find that the risk was spatially heterogeneously distributed and concentrated in a few specific areas that account for less than 1% of the contiguous US population. Locations in Texas and Florida that have actually experienced local ZIKV transmission were among the places at highest risk according to our results. We also provide an analysis of the key determinants for local transmission and identify the key introduction routes and their contributions to ZIKV transmission in the contiguous US.

Conclusions: This framework provides quantitative risk estimates, fully captures the stochasticity of ZIKV introduction events, and is not biased by the under-ascertainment of cases due to asymptomatic cases. It provides general information on key risk determinants and data with potential uses in defining public health recommendations and guidance about ZIKV risk in the US.

Keywords: Zika virus, Risk assessment, Computational modeling

---

* Correspondence: a.vespignani@neu.edu
[1]Laboratory for the Modeling of Biological and Socio-technical Systems, Northeastern University, Boston 02115, USA
[4]Institute for Scientific Interchange Foundation, 10126 Turin, Italy
Full list of author information is available at the end of the article

Background

From 2015 to 2016, the Zika virus (ZIKV) epidemic spread across most countries in the Americas, including the United States (US) [1–3]. As of July 3, 2018, three US territories, including Puerto Rico, have reported 37,255 ZIKV cases mostly due to widespread local transmission [3, 4]. Laboratory evidence of possible ZIKV infections has been found in 4900 pregnant women from US territories, 167 of whom have had pregnancy outcomes with ZIKV-related birth defects [3, 5, 6]. The US states and District of Columbia have reported 5710 travel-associated ZIKV cases, including 2474 pregnant women with evidence of ZIKV infection and 116 ZIKV-related birth defects [3]. Two geographical locations have experienced local transmission of ZIKV in the contiguous US: Miami-Dade County, in Florida, and Cameron County, in Texas [7, 8]. While the outbreaks in Florida and Texas were limited, the indirect impact on the local economy has been remarkable [9].

Concerns have been raised that several other locations in the contiguous US were at risk of ZIKV transmission, thus triggering a number of studies aimed at identifying populations at highest risk of local transmission [10–20]. In particular, detailed studies based on environmental suitability, epidemiological factors, and travel-related case importations have been used to estimate the risk for specific counties in the US [21, 22]. In this study, we quantify the risk of local ZIKV transmission by using a data-driven stochastic and spatial epidemic model accounting for seasonal, environmental, and detailed population data. The model also accounts for the association between socioeconomic status and the risk of exposure to mosquitoes, and it has been previously used to estimate the introduction of Zika in the Americas and the spatial and temporal dynamics of the epidemic [23]. By using an extensive likelihood analysis with data from places with a reliable epidemiological surveillance system, the model generates a stochastic ensemble of simulations estimating the place and time of introduction of ZIKV in Brazil and the unfolding of the epidemic in the Americas. For each simulation, the individual-level scale of the model allows for the construction of daily travel-related case counts (TCCs) tracking the number of infected individuals in the contiguous US at the county level and at the finer spatial resolution of 0.025° × 0.025° corresponding approximately to 2.5 km × 2.5 km cells, comparable in size to the ZIKV active transmission areas identified in Florida by the Centers for Disease Control and Prevention (CDC) [24]. Using the time series of county-specific TCCs and the mechanistic transmission model, it is possible to estimate the probability that a specific location would experience local ZIKV transmission during the 2015–2016 time window. The methodology proposed here provides a statistical estimate of ZIKV transmission risk that is not biased by the under-ascertainment of infections and the single historical occurrence of the case importation timeline that fail to account for the full stochasticity of transmission. The TCC database also allows us to identify key sources and routes of ZIKV introductions. Results from our study can provide guidance to public health agencies in their efforts to identify populations and seasons at high risk of ZIKV transmission, so that resources towards outbreak prevention and response can be allocated more efficiently.

Methods

We consider three major factors associated with local ZIKV transmission in the contiguous US: the intensity of travel-related infection importations, the environmental suitability for ZIKV transmission, and the socioeconomic risk of exposure to mosquitoes. In this study, we develop a data-driven computational framework (Fig. 1) to quantitatively account for these three factors and to evaluate their impact on ZIKV transmission. Based on this framework, we assess the risk of local ZIKV transmission across the contiguous US through the full course of the 2015–2016 ZIKV epidemic.

The starting point of our methodology is the construction of a synthetic database of TCC entering the US through airport transportation hubs. The database is generated from simulations based on a large-scale spatial model simulating the 2015–2016 ZIKV epidemics, where both symptomatic and asymptomatic ZIKV infections are considered [23]. The synthetic database of TCC contains for each infected individual the time of arrival, stage of ZIKV infection, airports of origin and arrival, and location of residence in the contiguous US[1] [25]. A schematic sample of the database is shown in Table 1.

Each infected individual's likelihood of exposure to mosquito bites and his/her capability of triggering local ZIKV transmission is affected by the ecological presence of mosquitoes in his/her location of residence. Indeed, our model integrates mosquito abundance data (*Ae. aegypti* and *Ae. albopictus*) [26, 27] that takes into account for temperature suitability, precipitation, vegetation, and urbanization and considers seasonal variations in the mosquito density determined by daily temperature. The individual's socioeconomic status, which is strongly associated with factors such as sanitation conditions, accessibility to air conditioning, and level of disease awareness, also affects the likelihood of exposure to mosquitoes [14, 28, 29]. Our computational framework considers a data layer based on global socioeconomic indicators [30], which is calibrated with historical mosquito-borne disease outbreaks in naive populations to provide a likelihood map of the individual's exposure to mosquitoes [23]. This map serves as a spatial filter (Fig. 1c-II) that probabilistically selects individuals exposed to mosquito bites down to the resolution of a 0.25° × 0.25° cell containing his/her location

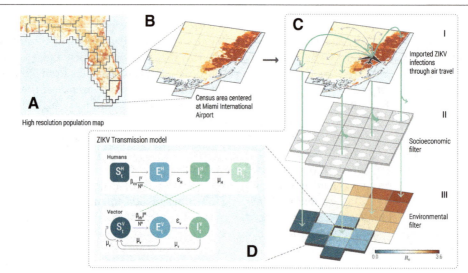

Fig. 1 A schematic illustration of the computational framework to assess the risk of ZIKV introductions into the contiguous US. **a** High-resolution (0.025° × 0.025°~2.5 km × 2.5 km) population density map [59] and Voronoi tessellation of the contiguous US into census areas with a major airport transportation hub at each of their centers [60]. **b** An example of the census area centered at Miami International Airport. **c** I: Travel-associated ZIKV infections entering the Miami International Airport. Location of residence of each ZIKV infection is randomly assigned with likelihood proportional to the population density within each census area. II: The probabilistic filter of the risk of exposure to mosquitoes due to socioeconomic factors such as housing conditions, sanitation, and disease awareness. III: Spatiotemporal specific ZIKV transmission dynamics are influenced by environmental factors that are temperature sensitive, including the spatial distribution of Aedes mosquitoes, seasonal mosquito abundance, and ZIKV transmissibility. **d** Compartmental stochastic ZIKV transmission model used to evaluate the environmental suitability of ZIKV transmission. Humans are divided into susceptible S^H, exposed E^H, infectious I^H, and recovered R^H compartments, and mosquitoes are divided into susceptible S^V, exposed E^V, and infectious I^V compartments

of residence. Each of the exposed individuals can potentially trigger detectable local ZIKV transmissions (Fig. 1c-III, d), according to the stochastic mechanistic ZIKV transmission model that takes into account mosquito abundance, the current temperature in the area, and the transmission dynamics of ZIKV (see Additional file 1: Supplementary Information). We define a detectable local transmission as the generation of 20 or more autochthonous transmission infections triggered by a single ZIKV infection introduction. Smaller outbreaks would likely go unnoticed assuming a 5% to 10% detection rate of infections due to the large proportion of asymptomatic cases [31–33]. Due to fine spatial and temporal resolution, the transmission model is able to account for the significant variability in the ZIKV basic reproduction number (R_0) across locations, as well as the variability within the same location at different times. These differences in R_0 are driven by temperature and the mosquito abundance, among other variables. The details of the mechanistic model and the calculation of the socioeconomic risk of exposure to mosquitoes are reported in Additional file 1. More technically, we can define the following procedure:

(1) We randomly sample one out of the simulated TCC from the statistical ensemble output of the ZIKV model [23].
(2) For each infected individual in the TCC, we stochastically determine whether he/she is potentially exposed to mosquito bites based on the probability of exposure p_e at the location of residence x. p_e is calibrated based on socioeconomic indicators and x identifies a specific county or spatial cell. In each location x, these individuals could potentially trigger local transmission.
(3) Based on the individual's stage of infection (exposed or infectious), time of introduction, and location of residence (at 0.025° × 0.025° resolution), we simulate local ZIKV transmission with the same stochastic

Table 1 A sample of the database containing simulated travel-related ZIKV-infected individuals entering the US

Case ID	Time of arrival	Airport of arrival	Stage of infection	Airport of origin	Location of residence (latitude, longitude)
0001	2015-12-01	MIA	Exposed	BOG	(25.864, −80.257)
0101	2016-07-15	JFK	Infectious	SJU	(40.729, −73.991)
0212	2016-11-23	MIA	Infectious	SJU	(25.808, −80.130)

transmission model used in the global model (described in Additional file 1: Supplementary Information) with the specific parameters calibrated to each 0.25° × 0.25° cell in the US.

(4) For each simulated TCC, the above procedure identifies all the infections triggering detectable local transmission. For every time interval Δt and geographical area x of interest, we can associate variable $n(x, \Delta t) = 1$ if there is at least one imported infection from the TCC that triggers detectable local transmission, and $n(x, \Delta t) = 0$ otherwise.

In order to provide a probabilistic risk measurement, we execute $N = 10^6$ resamplings from the ensemble of simulated TCC generated by the model and repeat the above procedure. The resampling procedure accounts for the many possible TCCs compatible with the observed ZIKV epidemic and stochastic effects in the local transmission. This is because not all case importations will result in local outbreaks, even in areas where transmission is favored. The risk of local ZIKV transmission for area x during time window Δt can be thus defined as

$$r_{tr}(x, \Delta t) = \frac{1}{N} \sum_{i=1}^{N} n_i(x, \Delta t) \qquad (1)$$

where i indexes the 10^6 outcomes from the resampled TCCs. This definition of the risk can be aggregated at various spatial (0.025° × 0.025°) and temporal resolutions (≥ 1 day), and it can be used to generate risk maps of ZIKV introduction across the contiguous US. Unless otherwise specified, we consider in this study the local transmission risk $r_{tr}(x)$ that is defined on the Δt referring to the time window spanning from January 1, 2015 to December 31, 2016. This definition of risk can be interpreted as the probability of observing a detectable local transmission in a specific area per ZIKV epidemic.

Results

By using the methodology outlined in the previous section, we provide quantitative estimates of $r_{tr}(x)$ both at the county level and at 0.025° × 0.025° cell resolution. Figure 2a shows the risk of ZIKV introduction at county level in the contiguous US through the full course of the simulated 2015–2016 ZIKV epidemics. We consider four main brackets for the risk and the associated population sizes. At the county level, the highest risk bracket $r_{tr}(x) > 0.5$ includes only 0.71% of the total population in the contiguous US. In these areas, one would expect to observe detectable local transmission events with a probability above 50% during the simulated 2015–2016 ZIKV epidemic. Even when we extend the high-risk bracket to include counties with $r_{tr}(x) > 1/8$, this includes only 2.56% of the total population in the contiguous US. Thus, the risk of local transmission is extremely concentrated to specific geographical locations. Figure 2d shows the population living in counties with different risk brackets of ZIKV introduction and their percentage with respect to the total population in the contiguous US.

The counties of Miami-Dade, Florida, and Cameron, Texas, where local transmission was observed in the year 2016, were both estimated to be high-risk locations (risk bracket, greater than 1/4). Densely populated areas along the Gulf Coast also show up as high-risk locations, in agreement with estimates from other models [12]. The risk of ZIKV introduction and local transmission $r_{tr}(x)$ is highly spatially heterogeneous (Fig. 2a, b). This heterogeneity persists even within the state of Florida, where most areas are estimated to be environmentally suitable for ZIKV transmission all year long [12, 34]. This is mostly because of socioeconomic and local climate heterogeneities. At a spatial granularity of 0.025° × 0.025°, it is possible to perform a statistical analysis of the risk distribution. In Fig. 2c, we report the distribution of cell-specific risks $r_{tr}(x)$. The distribution has a very right-skewed heavy tail extending over more than four orders of magnitude, a clear signature of the large heterogeneity of the risk in the contiguous US.

It is worth stressing that the source of ZIKV introductions in each location is time-dependent, since the TCC is determined by both the magnitude of the epidemic in the regions of the Americas affected by ZIKV and travel patterns from these areas. Our model explicitly simulates individual ZIKV-infected travelers, with detailed information about the traveler's origin and destination at the daily scale. This allows us to decompose the relative contribution of potential ZIKV introductions from different epidemic regions and to identify routes of high risk with high spatio-temporal resolution. In Table 2, we report the likelihood of local ZIKV transmission in Miami-Dade, Florida, for the year 2015 and 2016 triggered by infection importations from the Caribbean, Central America and Mexico, and South America. The likelihood accounts for intensity of ZIKV transmission in epidemic regions, the travel volume between the source regions and Miami-Dade, and the time-dependent environmental suitability of local transmission in Miami-Dade. In Fig. 3, we report the daily risk of ZIKV infections in Miami-Dade from different geographical regions as well as the time-dependent relative contributions of different regions to the risk throughout the years 2015 and 2016.

As shown in both Table 2 and Fig. 3, in 2015, countries in the Caribbean and South America were major contributors to ZIKV introduction risk in Miami-Dade. On the other hand, countries in Central America and Mexico became major contributors in 2016. This reflects the fact that the ZIKV epidemic started earlier in South

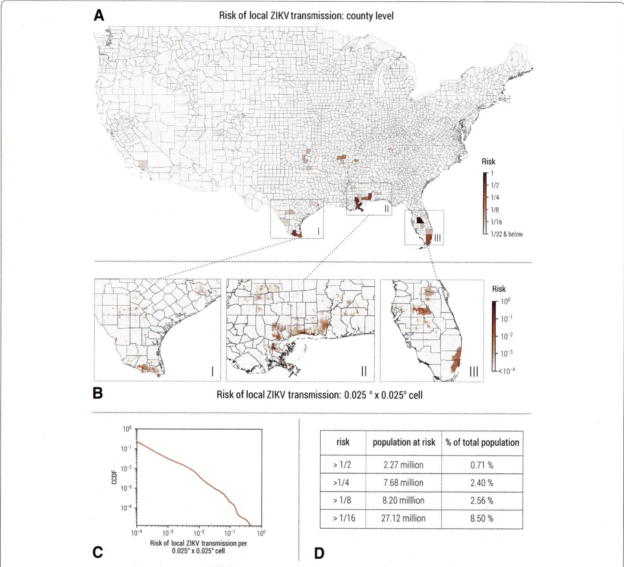

Fig. 2 The cumulative risk of local ZIKV transmission in the contiguous US. The cumulative risk of local ZIKV transmission at different spatial resolutions is evaluated through the full course of the simulated 2015–2016 ZIKV epidemic. **a** The cumulative risk map of local ZIKV transmission for each county in the contiguous US. The color scale indicates for any given county the probability of experiencing at least one ZIKV outbreak with more than 20 infections (details in Additional file 1). **b** High spatial resolution estimates (0.025° × 0.025°) of the cumulative risk of local ZIKV transmission through the full course of the simulated 2015–2016 ZIKV epidemic. **c** The complementary cumulative distribution function of the local ZIKV transmission risk for all 0.025° × 0.025°cells (on a log-log scale). The heavy tail feature of the distribution reflects strong spatial heterogeneity in terms of local ZIKV transmission risk. **d** The total population in the counties of the US with different risk levels of local ZIKV transmission and their percentage with respect to the total population in the contiguous US

Table 2 The likelihood of a given local ZIKV transmission event in Miami-Dade, Florida, from different geographical regions (Caribbean, South America, Central America and Mexico) for the years 2015 and 2016

Region	Year 2015		Year 2016	
	Likelihood (%)	95% CI (%)	Likelihood (%)	95% CI (%)
Caribbean	43.81	(10.47–61.98)	40.15	(14.09–59.79)
South America	27.67	(27.87–78.42)	27.67	(16.10–47.31)
Central America and Mexico	10.50	(3.61–20.39)	30.02	(17.54–48.52)

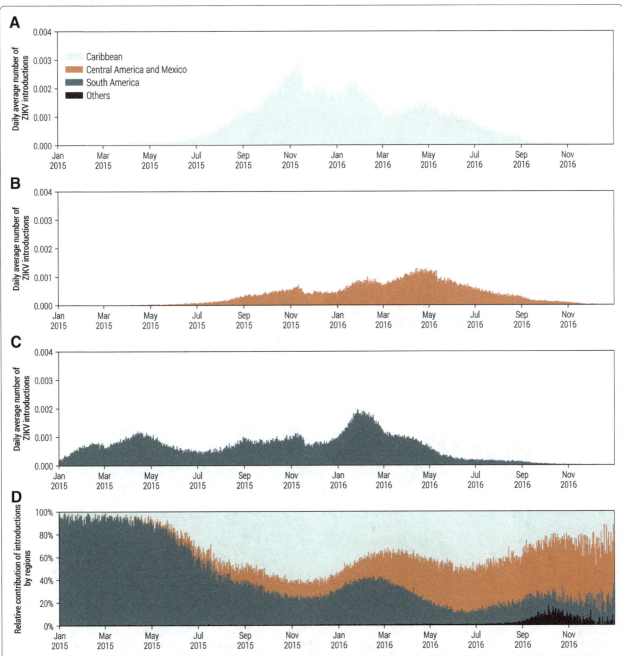

Fig. 3 A breakdown of local ZIKV transmission events by the geographical origins of travel-associated ZIKV infections in Miami-Dade, Florida. **a–c** The daily average number of ZIKV imported infections per day that trigger outbreaks with more than 20 infections, originating from the Caribbean, Central America and Mexico, and South America. **d** The relative contributions to the expected number of local ZIKV transmission events by different geographical regions

American countries, including Brazil and Colombia, and later on spread to countries in Central America and Mexico. Caribbean countries, however, remained a major source of infection importation in both 2015 and 2016. This is possibly due to the high travel volumes between Florida and the Caribbean, as well as high incidence rate and weak seasonality of ZIKV transmission in that region. This is in line with epidemiological data from Florida's Department of Health, as well as phylogenetic analysis based on sequenced ZIKV genomes from both infected humans and mosquitoes in Florida [35].

In Fig. 4, we zoom in on three representative areas to disentangle the key determinants shaping the spatiotemporal risk of local ZIKV transmission. Panels a, b, and c in Fig. 4 represent geographical areas covering Miami-Dade, Florida; Cameron, Texas; and New York City, New York.

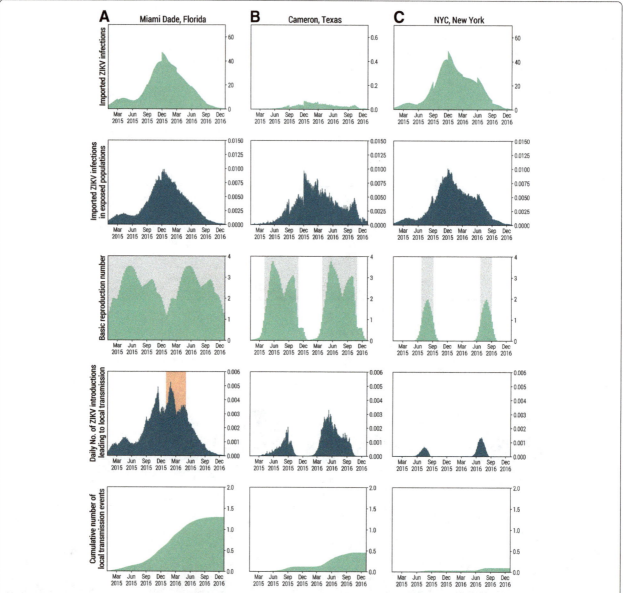

Fig. 4 Factors which co-shape the spatiotemporal risk of local ZIKV transmission in three different regions in the contiguous US. Columns from left to right represent **a** Miami-Dade, Florida; **b** Cameron, Texas; and **c** New York City, New York. Row 1 shows the average daily number of imported ZIKV infections. Note that for Cameron, Texas, the scale on the y-axis is different than that of Miami-Dade, Florida, and NYC, New York. Row 2 shows the average number of imported ZIKV infections that pass through the socioeconomic filter p_e and reside in areas potentially exposed to mosquitoes. Row 3 shows the basic reproduction number (weekly average) calculated based on the ZIKV transmission model. Gray-shaded time windows indicate when the basic reproduction number $R_0 > 1$ and sustainable ZIKV transmission is possible. Row 4 shows the expected daily number of ZIKV introductions with the red-shaded time window indicating the estimated time of local ZIKV transmission based on phylogenetic analysis [35]. Row 5 shows the average cumulative number of local ZIKV transmission events since January 1, 2015

Both Miami-Dade and New York City experienced a high volume of ZIKV infection importations due to high population density and close proximity to major international transportation hubs. Cameron, Texas, on the other hand, had far fewer ZIKV infection importations. However, due to socioeconomic factor (among other factors), the population in Cameron, Texas, is more likely to be exposed to mosquitoes than the populations of Miami-Dade and New York City. Consequently, the volume of Cameron's imported infections that were exposed to mosquito bites is comparable to those of Miami-Dade and New York City.

The environmental suitability of ZIKV transmission in the three areas is remarkably different. The basic reproduction number R_0 is above the epidemic threshold ($R_0 > 1$) in Miami-Dade throughout the year, indicating ZIKV transmission is environmentally suitable all year long. Cameron, Texas, has moderate environmental suitability, where R_0 drops below the threshold in winter seasons. New York City is far less environmentally suitable for ZIKV transmission, with a narrow time window of approximately 2 months during summer when R_0 is larger than 1.

Given the individual-level resolution of the model, we can focus on the daily average number of travel-associated ZIKV infections leading to local transmission. This is a different indicator than risk. The latter is defined as the probability of observing at least one event of detectable local transmission in the area, thus overlooking the number of different introduction events that trigger local transmission. The profile of daily ZIKV introductions that would lead to local transmission (Fig. 4, row 4) is jointly shaped by ZIKV infection importations, socioeconomic risk of exposure to mosquitoes, and the environmental suitability of ZIKV transmission. The cumulative number of ZIKV introductions leading to local transmission was high in both Miami-Dade, Florida, and Cameron, Texas, where local transmission occurred in the year 2016. The time of ZIKV introduction in Miami-Dade, Florida, is estimated to have occurred between January and May 2016 based on phylogenetic analysis of sequenced ZIKV genomes from infected patients and *Ae. aegypti* mosquitoes [35]. Our model suggests (Fig. 4, row 4) high risk of ZIKV introduction during the same time window, despite relatively low environmental suitability. The high risk of introduction in Miami-Dade between January and May 2016 was mainly driven by a high influx of imported ZIKV infections. Based on our simulations, Miami-Dade county has on average 1.29 cumulative introductions leading to local transmission events (95%CI (0–9)) throughout 2015 and 2016 (Fig. 4, row 5, insert). However, the distribution of the number of introductions is positively skewed (skewness $\gamma_1 = 4.40$), with a maximum of 55 introductions. This indicates the possibility of multiple introductions during the ZIKV outbreak in Miami-Dade, Florida, in line with estimates from phylogenetic analysis [35].

To investigate to what extent the spatial variation of local ZIKV transmission is driven by key socioeconomic and environmental determinants, we first consider a regression model exploring the relation between the average number of local ZIKV transmissions ($\log(n_{tr})$ is the dependent variable) and three key determinants: the number of ZIKV importations, average temperature, and the GDP per capita. Specifically, the explanatory variables include:

- $\log(N_{im})$, the logarithm of the cumulative average number of TCC for each 0.25° × 0.25° cell from January 1, 2015, to December 31, 2016.
- $\log(f_{20°})$, the logarithm of the fraction of days over the year with an average temperature larger than 20 °C for each 0.25° × 0.25° cell.
- $\log(GDP)$, the gross domestic product per capita in terms of purchasing power parity for each 0.25° × 0.25° cell.

In Table 3, we show that if all three explanatory variables are included in the regression (model 1), the model can explain 73.9% of the variance in the number of average introductions leading to local transmission in each cell x. While only considering $\log(N_{im})$ and $\log(f_{20°})$ (model 2), we can explain 56.2% of the variance, and using $\log(N_{im})$ (model 3) alone can explain 47.5% of the variance. It is worth remarking that such a simple statistical analysis cannot fully explain the variance of $\log(n_{tr})$ due to the nonlinear dependency between ZIKV transmission, vector population dynamics, and temperature. It is also due to the highly nonlinear nature of the disease transmission dynamics captured by the epidemic threshold (where the basic reproduction number (R_0) needs to be larger than one to be able to spread in a population). In addition, more than 90% of the geographical areas in the contiguous US are not included in the regression because the simulations project no local transmission events in those areas. However, 77% (in terms of areas) of these "risk-free" areas are not environmentally suitable for ZIKV transmission according to our model.

To better illustrate the role of the three main drivers of Zika transmission, we conduct a sensitivity analysis considering three counterfactual scenarios. In each counterfactual scenario, we modify one of the three drivers across the contiguous US to uniformly mimic the conditions in Miami-Dade, Florida, while keeping the other two drivers intact. Specifically:

- In counterfactual scenario 1, the environmental suitability (the temperature and thus all temperature-modulated disease parameters) and socioeconomic risk of exposure remain the same, while for all airports in the US, the ZIKV infection importations are set to be the same as those of the airport in Miami-Dade, Florida.
- In counterfactual scenario 2, the ZIKV infection importations and the socioeconomic risk of exposure to mosquitoes remain the same. However, in this scenario, the temperature and consequently all temperature-modulated parameters of ZIKV transmission model across the contiguous US are set to be the same as those in Miami-Dade, Florida.
- In counterfactual scenario 3, the ZIKV infection importations and the environmental suitability are kept intact, while the socioeconomic risks of exposure to mosquitoes across the contiguous US are set to be the same as that in Miami-Dade, Florida.

Table 3 Regression analysis between log(n_{tr}) and explanatory variables including log(N_{im}), log($f_{20}°$), and log(GDP)

	Model 1	Model 2	Model 3
log(N_{im})	0.72*** (0.69, 0.74)	0.48*** (0.45, 0.51)	0.49*** (0.46, 0.52)
log($f_{20}°$)	2.18*** (1.89, 2.48)	3.40*** (3.01, 3.78)	
log(GDP)	−13.29*** (−14.20, −12.38)		
R squared	74.9%	57.9%	47.5%

In model 1, all three explanatory variables log(N_{im}), log($f_{20}°$), and log(GDP) are included. Model 2 includes log(N_{im}) and log($f_{20}°$). Model 3 only includes log(N_{im}). For each model, we report the regression coefficient (95% CI) for each of the explanatory variables along with R squared, based on n = 1220 cells

n_{tr} average number of local ZIKV transmissions within each 0.25° × 0.25° cell from January 1, 2015, to December 31, 2016, N_{im} number of ZIKV importations, $f_{20}°$ fraction of days with temperature higher than 20 °C, GDP gross domestic product per capita in purchasing power parity

***$p < 0.001$

For each of the three counterfactual scenarios, we repeat the analysis performed with the real data and generate the cumulative county-level risk map of local ZIKV transmission during the years 2015–2016 (see Additional file 1: Supplementary Information, Section 4). All three risk maps of the counterfactual scenarios are distinctly different from the risk map of Fig. 2a. Particularly, in counterfactual scenario 1, under unrealistic high intensity of ZIKV infection importations, all areas with overlapping favorable environmental and socioeconomic determinants are at high risk of local ZIKV transmission. In counterfactual scenario 2, with unrealistic favorable environmental suitabilities of ZIKV across the US, the areas at high risk are no longer restricted to the proximity of the US southern border. Many counties with low average yearly temperature and absence of Aedes mosquitos in the real world present significant risks of local ZIKV transmission. In counterfactual scenario 3, with high socioeconomic status equivalent to Miami-Dade, Florida, both southern Texas and populated areas along the Gulf Coast were relieved from high probability of encountering Zika, leaving southern Florida as the only focus of high risk. Thus, all three drivers are necessarily required to evaluate the risk of local ZIKV transmission in the contiguous US.

Discussion

A prominent feature of our findings is the spatiotemporal heterogeneity of ZIKV transmission risk across the contiguous US. Spatially, our model estimates that approximately 68.9% of the people in the contiguous US live in areas that are environmentally suitable for ZIKV transmission, in line with other models' estimates [36]. However, taking all ZIKV introduction and transmission determinants into consideration, areas with non-negligible risk (greater than 1/8) are concentrated in densely populated areas along the Gulf Coast, capturing 2.56% of the US population. From a temporal perspective, certain areas experience strong seasonality of ZIKV environmental suitability, with a narrow time window when ZIKV transmission is possible. Given limited resources, identifying seasons and regions of high risk may help guide resource allocation for high-risk population screening, intervention, and vector control. Our model is also able to identify the high-risk routes of ZIKV importations through air travel. Imported infections originating from Caribbean countries served as a major contributor to trigger local ZIKV transmission in Florida. Although it has the highest number of estimated ZIKV infections among all countries, Brazil is not a major contributor overall (5.75% of potential introductions leading to local transmission across the contiguous US). This is due to Rio de Janeiro and Sao Paulo, two of the largest transportation hubs in Brazil which make up 65% of the international travel to US from Brazil, being located in the Southern region where ZIKV transmission activity is relatively low. In addition, Rio de Janeiro and Sao Paulo have the opposite seasonality compared to the contiguous US. When it is environmentally suitable for ZIKV transmission in Rio de Janerio and Sao Paulo, it is not suitable for ZIKV transmission in most of the US. Thus, imported ZIKV infections from Brazil were less likely to fuel potential transmissions in the US.

Our model also suggests that in Miami-Dade, Florida, the overall risk of ZIKV introduction in 2015 is comparable to that in 2016, while local transmission is only observed in 2016. This could be explained by the stochasticity of transmission events. Another possibility is that because of the high asymptomatic rate of ZIKV infections, limited local transmission events occurred in 2015 without being picked up by the surveillance system. Awareness of ZIKV was low in 2015 as the World Health Organization declared ZIKV as a Public Health Emergency of International Concerns only in early 2016. Around the same time, the CDC announced a Health Alert Network advisory for Zika virus [3], marking the start of active monitoring of ZIKV activities in the US.

The proposed model has several limitations. The high volume of cruise ship stops along coastal areas of Florida to the Caribbean may elevate the risk of ZIKV transmissions beyond what is estimated in our model. Sexual transmission and transmission through other routes, not considered by our model, may facilitate the risk of local transmission even further. From January 1, 2015, to August 9, 2017, there were 49 reported ZIKV cases in the contiguous US acquired through other routes, including sexual transmission [3, 37–39]. This indicates that a larger population may be affected by ZIKV [40–42]. In addition, ZIKV RNA was detected in semen as long as 92 days after symptom onset and is able to be sexually transmitted 31–42 days after symptom onset [43]. ZIKV's ability to persist in infected males and the potential to infect through sexual transmission long after symptom onset are troublesome. However, the specific risk through sexual transmission or other transmission routes are not well understood, and the overall impact of ZIKV infections acquired through other routes remains unclear. As such, we do not include them in our study [44]. Risk of exposure to mosquitoes associated with socioeconomic factors is widely recognized but poorly quantified. In our model, we utilize seroprevalence studies from nine chikungunya outbreaks on confined, naive populations to estimate this association, in line with other approaches used to estimate the ZIKV attack rate [14]. Further studies however are needed to advance our understanding of the association between risk of exposure to mosquitoes and socioeconomic status.

Our model assumes the mosquito abundance is explicitly modulated by temperature, since many studies suggest that temperature is the main driver of the seasonal variation of mosquito abundance [45–48]. The effect of rainfall as an environmental driver is indirectly included into our model through incorporating the mosquito presence data created by Kraemer et al. [27]. The study suggests that for both *Ae. aegypti* and *Ae. albopictus*, maximum and minimum precipitation make significant contributions to explain the spatial distribution of *Aedes* mosquitoes, consequently affecting the environmental suitability of local ZIKV transmission. However, a full mechanistic modeling of the influence of rainfall (i.e., daily timescale) on the mosquito lifecycle, while interesting, is still out of reach on a global scale. Along with rainfall, human water supplies may also affect the availability of stagnant water, especially in urban settings [45, 49]. Without controlling for the effect of human water supplies, the effect of precipitation could be positive [50–52], negative [53], or no effect at all [54, 55]. In Additional file 1: Supplementary Information, we provide a figure illustrating the seasonal abundance provided by our model.

In our model, we consider both *Ae. aegpyti* and *Ae. albopictus* as competent vectors to transmit the ZIKV. However, the competence of *Ae. albopictus* to transmit ZIKV is debated, and the notable differences in the spatial distributions of *Ae. aegpyti* and *Ae. albopictus* make it crucial for evaluating the global risk of ZIKV [27, 56]. However, these differences are less relevant when limiting the risk assessment within the spatial range of the contiguous US. This is because the geographical distribution of the environmental suitability of *Ae. aegpyti* and *Ae. albopictus* is largely overlapping within the contiguous US, based on the studies by Johnson et al. [57]. The environmental suitability distribution of *Ae. albopictus* extends a bit further north when compared to that of *Ae. aegypti*. In the areas where only *Ae. albopictus* are present, the overall environmental suitability of ZIKV transmission is very low due to the presence of strong seasonality, and our model estimates that those areas would have minimal risk of experiencing local ZIKV transmission in the years 2015–2016 (Fig. 2).

In 2017–2018, ZIKV transmission activities in most countries throughout the Americas has plummeted [2], in agreement with model estimates [23, 58]. The risk of ZIKV introduction in the contiguous US would be expected to be negligible as imported infections triggering the local transmission would be drastically reduced. However, one should exercise caution as vector-transmitted diseases are known to show strong spatial heterogeneity and seasonality and are affected by socioeconomic factors. The stochastic nature of ZIKV transmission could leave a considerable amount of naive populations living in regions at risk of ZIKV transmission. Furthermore, expansion of the *Aedes* mosquito distribution, human migration, and shifts in socioeconomic status could lead to more populations being at risk for local ZIKV transmission. It is more likely that ZIKV transmission activities in the future may resemble the current situation of chikungunya, where transmission activities could flare up sporadically. The possible sporadic outbreaks of ZIKV would continue to pose a risk to the contiguous US, where most of the population is naive to the virus and a large fraction live in areas environmentally suitable for ZIKV transmission.

Conclusion

In this study, we show that the overall risk of ZIKV introduction and local transmission during the 2015–2016 outbreak is jointly determined by the intensity of ZIKV importations, environmental suitability for ZIKV transmissions, and the socioeconomic risk of exposure to mosquitoes. Our estimates suggest that the risk of ZIKV introductions has a very strong spatial and temporal heterogeneity. The areas in the contiguous US at non-negligible risk (that is, greater than 1/8) only account for 2.6% of the total population in the contiguous US. The model is able to identify the hotspots for ZIKV introductions, and it reveals the relative contributions of ZIKV introductions from different geographical regions over time. The results of our study have the potential to guide the development of ZIKV prevention and response strategies in the contiguous US.

Endnotes

[1]Although there has been reporting in the media about the traffic to and from Latin and Caribbean countries, airline traffic in 2016 has been stable with a mere 4.4% increase.

Abbreviations
CDC: Centers for Disease Control and Prevention; GDP: Gross domestic product; PPP: Purchasing power parity; TCCs: Travel-related case counts; US: United States; ZIKV: Zika virus

Acknowledgements
Not applicable

Funding
This work was supported by the Models of Infectious Disease Agent Study, National Institute of General Medical Sciences Grant U54GM111274 and the NIH supplement Grant R01 AI102939-05.

Authors' contributions
KS, MEH, IML, and AV designed the research. KS, QZ, MC, APyP, SM, DM, PP, LR, and AV performed the research. KS, QZ, MC, APyP, DM, NED, DPR, and AV analyzed the data. KS, QZ, MC, APyP, NED, DPR, SM, DM, PP, LR, MEH, IML, and AV wrote the paper. All authors read and approved the final manuscript.

Competing interests
AV has received research support unrelated to this paper (through his employer Northeastern University) from Metabiota Inc. The other authors declare that they have no competing interests.

Author details
[1]Laboratory for the Modeling of Biological and Socio-technical Systems, Northeastern University, Boston 02115, USA. [2]Department of Biostatistics, College of Public Health and Health Professions, University of Florida, Gainesville 32611, USA. [3]Bruno Kessler Foundation, 38123 Trento, Italy. [4]Institute for Scientific Interchange Foundation, 10126 Turin, Italy. [5]Vaccine and Infectious Disease Division, Fred Hutchinson Cancer Research Center, Seattle 98109, USA. [6]Department of Biostatistics, University of Washington, Seattle 98195, USA.

References
1. World Health Organization. Zika virus and complications: 2016 Public Health Emergency of International Concern: World Health Organization; 2017. http://www.who.int/emergencies/zika-virus/en/ Accessed 17 Sept 2017
2. Pan American Health Organization. Zika virus infection: Pan American Health Organization; 2017. https://goo.gl/oABMtf Accessed 17 Sept 2017
3. Centers for Disease Control and Prevention. Zika virus: Centers for Disease Control and Prevention; 2017. https://www.cdc.gov/zika/index.html Accessed 17 Sept 2017
4. Walker WL. Zika virus disease cases—50 states and the District of Columbia, January 1–July 31, 2016. Morb Mortal Wkly Rep. 2016;65(36):983.
5. Reynolds MR, Jones AM, Petersen EE, Lee EH, Rice ME, Bingham A, Ellington SR, Evert N, Reagan-Steiner S, Oduyebo T, et al. Vital signs: update on Zika virus-associated birth defects and evaluation of all US infants with congenital Zika virus exposure-US Zika Pregnancy Registry, 2016. Morb Mortal Wkly Rep. 2017;66(13):366–73.
6. Honein MA, Dawson AL, Petersen EE, Jones AM, Lee EH, Yazdy MM, Ahmad N, Macdonald J, Evert N, Bingham A, et al. Birth defects among fetuses and infants of US women with evidence of possible Zika virus infection during pregnancy. JAMA. 2017;317(1):59–68.
7. Centers for Disease Control and Prevention. Advice for people living in or traveling to Brownsville, Texas: Centers for Disease Control and Prevention; 2017. https://www.cdc.gov/zika/intheus/texas-update.html Accessed 17 Sept 2017
8. Centers for Disease Control and Prevention. Advice for people living in or traveling to South Florida: Centers for Disease Control and Prevention; 2017. https://www.cdc.gov/zika/intheus/florida-update.html Accessed 17 Sept 2017
9. Lee BY, Alfaro-Murillo JA, Parpia AS, Asti L, Wedlock PT, Hotez PJ, Galvani AP. The potential economic burden of Zika in the continental United States. PLoS Negl Trop Dis. 2017;11(4):0005531.
10. Keegan LT, Lessler J, Johansson MA. Quantifying Zika: advancing the epidemiology of Zika with quantitative models. J Infect Dis. 2017;216(suppl 10):884–90.
11. Monaghan AJ, Morin CW, Steinhoff DF, Wilhelmi O, Hayden M, Quattrochi DA, Reiskind M, Lloyd AL, Smith K, Schmidt CA, et al. On the seasonal occurrence and abundance of the Zika virus vector mosquito Aedes aegypti in the contiguous United States. PLoS Curr. 2016;8. https://doi.org/10.1371/currents.outbreaks.50dfc7f46798675fc63e7d7da563da76.
12. Messina JP, Kraemer MU, Brady OJ, Pigott DM, Shearer FM, Weiss DJ, Golding N, Ruktanonchai CW, Gething PW, Cohn E, et al. Mapping global environmental suitability for Zika virus. Elife. 2016;5:15272.
13. Bogoch II, Brady OJ, Kraemer MU, German M, Creatore MI, Brent S, Watts AG, Hay SI, Kulkarni MA, Brownstein JS, et al. Potential for Zika virus introduction and transmission in resource-limited countries in Africa and the Asia-Pacific region: a modelling study. Lancet Infect Dis. 2016;16(11):1237–45.
14. Perkins TA, Siraj AS, Ruktanonchai CW, Kraemer MU, Tatem AJ. Model-based projections of Zika virus infections in childbearing women in the Americas. Nat Microbiol. 2016;1:16126.
15. Alfaro-Murillo JA, Parpia AS, Fitzpatrick MC, Tamagnan JA, Medlock J, Ndeffo-Mbah ML, Fish D, Ávila-Agüero ML, Marín R, Ko AI, et al. A cost-effectiveness tool for informing policies on Zika virus control. PLoS Negl Trop Dis. 2016;10(5):0004743.
16. Dinh L, Chowell G, Mizumoto K, Nishiura H. Estimating the subcritical transmissibility of the Zika outbreak in the State of Florida, USA, 2016. Theor Biol Med Model. 2016;13(1):20.
17. Rocklöv J, Quam MB, Sudre B, German M, Kraemer MU, Brady O, Bogoch II, Liu-Helmersson J, Wilder-Smith A, Semenza JC, et al. Assessing seasonal risks for the introduction and mosquito-borne spread of Zika virus in Europe. EBioMedicine. 2016;9:250–6.
18. Lourenço J, de Lima MM, Faria NR, Walker A, Kraemer MU, Villabona-Arenas CJ, Lambert B, de Cerqueira EM, Pybus OG, Alcantara LC, et al. Epidemiological and ecological determinants of Zika virus transmission in an urban setting. eLife. 2017;6:e29820.
19. Ajelli M. Modeling mosquito-borne diseases in complex urban environments. Acta Trop. 2017;176:332–4.
20. Ajelli M, Moise IK, Hutchings TCS, Brown SC, Kumar N, Johnson NF, Beier JC. Host outdoor exposure variability affects the transmission and spread of Zika virus: insights for epidemic control. PLoS Negl Trop Dis. 2017;11(9):0005851.
21. Castro LA, Fox SJ, Chen X, Liu K, Bellan SE, Dimitrov NB, Galvani AP, Meyers LA. Assessing real-time Zika risk in the United States. BMC Infect Dis. 2017;17(1):284.
22. Fox SJ, Bellan SE, Perkins TA, Johansson MA, Meyers LA. Downgrading disease transmission risk estimates using terminal importations. bioRxiv. 2018:265942. https://doi.org/10.1101/265942.
23. Zhang Q, Sun K, Chinazzi M, y Piontti AP, Dean NE, Rojas DP, Merler S, Mistry D, Poletti P, Rossi L, et al. Spread of Zika virus in the Americas. Proc Natl Acad Sci. 2017;114(22):4334–43.
24. Centers for Disease Control and Prevention. Guidance for areas with local Zika virus transmission in the continental United States and Hawaii: Centers for Disease Control and Prevention; 2017. https://www.cdc.gov/zika/geo/domestic-guidance.html Accessed 17 Sept 2017
25. The International Civil Aviation Organization (ICAO): The world of air transport in 2016 (2016). https://www.icao.int/annual-report-2016/Pages/the-world-of-air-transport-in-2016.aspx Accessed 17 Sept 2017.
26. Centers for Disease Control and Prevention. Estimated range of *Aedes aegypti* and *Aedes albopictus* in the United States, 2017: Centers for Disease Control and Prevention; 2017. https://www.cdc.gov/zika/vector/range.html Accessed 17 Sept 2017
27. Kraemer MU, Sinka ME, Duda KA, Mylne AQ, Shearer FM, Barker CM, Moore CG, Carvalho RG, Coelho GE, Van Bortel W, et al. The global distribution of the arbovirus vectors Aedes aegypti and Ae. albopictus. Elife. 2015;4:08347.
28. Sissoko D, Moendandze A, Malvy D, Giry C, Ezzedine K, Solet JL, Pierre V. Seroprevalence and risk factors of chikungunya virus infection in Mayotte Indian Ocean, 2005-2006: a population-based survey. PLoS One. 2008;3(8):3066. https://doi.org/10.1371/journal.pone.0003066.
29. Reiter P, Lathrop S, Bunning M, Biggerstaff B, Singer D, Tiwari T, Baber L, Amador M, Thirion J, Hayes J, et al. Texas lifestyle limits transmission of dengue virus. Emerg Infect Dis. 2003;9(1):86.
30. Nordhaus, W.D., Chen, X.: Global gridded geographically based economic data (G-econ), version 4 (2016).

31. Duffy MR, Chen T-H, Hancock WT, Powers AM, Kool JL, Lanciotti RS, Pretrick M, Marfel M, Holzbauer S, Dubray C, et al. Zika virus outbreak on Yap Island, federated states of Micronesia. N Engl J Med. 2009;360(24):2536–43.
32. Russell SP, Ryff KR, Gould CV, Martin SW, Johansson MA. Detecting local Zika virus transmission in the continental United States: a comparison of surveillance strategies. PLOS Currents Outbreaks. 2017:145102. Edition 1. https://doi.org/10.1371/currents.outbreaks.cd76717676629d47704170ecbdb5f820.
33. Moghadas SM, Shoukat A, Espindola AL, Pereira RS, Abdirizak F, Laskowski M, Viboud C, Chowell G. Asymptomatic transmission and the dynamics of Zika infection. Sci Rep. 2017;7(1):5829.
34. Marini G, Guzzetta G, Rosà R, Merler S. First outbreak of Zika virus in the continental United States: a modelling analysis. Euro Surveill. 2017;22(37).
35. Grubaugh ND, Ladner JT, Kraemer MU, Dudas G, Tan AL, Gangavarapu K, Wiley MR, White S, Thézé J, Magnani DM, et al. Genomic epidemiology reveals multiple introductions of Zika virus into the United States. Nature. 2017;546(7658):401–5.
36. Bogoch II, Brady OJ, Kraemer M, German M, Creatore MI, Kulkarni MA, Brownstein JS, Mekaru SR, Hay SI, Groot E, et al. Anticipating the international spread of Zika virus from Brazil. Lancet. 2016;387(10016):335–6.
37. Foy BD, Kobylinski KC, Foy JLC, Blitvich BJ, da Rosa AT, Haddow AD, Lanciotti RS, Tesh RB. Probable non–vector-borne transmission of Zika virus, Colorado, USA. Emerg Infect Dis. 2011;17(5):880.
38. Russell K, Hills SL, Oster AM, Porse CC, Danyluk G, Cone M, Brooks R, Scotland S, Schiffman E, Fredette C, et al. Male-to-female sexual transmission of Zika virus—United States, January-April 2016. Clin Infect Dis. 2016;64(2):211–3.
39. McCarthy M. Zika virus was transmitted by sexual contact in Texas, health officials report. BMJ. 2016;352:i720.
40. Gao D, Lou Y, He D, Porco TC, Kuang Y, Chowell G, Ruan S. Prevention and control of Zika as a mosquito-borne and sexually transmitted disease: a mathematical modeling analysis. Sci Rep. 2016;6:28070.
41. Allard A, Althouse BM, Hébert-Dufresne L, Scarpino SV. The risk of sustained sexual transmission of Zika is underestimated. PLoS Pathog. 13(9):1006633–2017.
42. Yakob L, Kucharski A, Hue S, Edmunds WJ. Low risk of a sexually-transmitted Zika virus outbreak. Lancet Infect Dis. 2016;16(10):1100–2.
43. Gaskell KM, Houlihan C, Nastouli E, Checkley AM. Persistent Zika virus detection in semen in a traveler returning to the United Kingdom from Brazil, 2016. Emerg Infect Dis. 2017;23(1):137.
44. Kim CR, Counotte M, Bernstein K, Deal C, Mayaud P, Low N, Broutet N, et al. Investigating the sexual transmission of Zika virus. Lancet Glob Health. 2018;6(1):24–5.
45. Tran A, L'Ambert G, Lacour G, Benoît R, Demarchi M, Cros M, Cailly P, Aubry-Kientz M, Balenghien T, Ezanno P. A rainfall- and temperature-driven abundance model for Aedes albopictus populations. Int J Environ Res Public Health. 2013;10(5):1698–719. https://doi.org/10.3390/ijerph10051698.
46. Alto BW, Juliano SA. Precipitation and temperature effects on populations of Aedes albopictus (Diptera: Culicidae): implications for range expansion. J Med Entomol. 2001;38(5):646–56.
47. Gomes AF, Nobre AA, Cruz OG. Temporal analysis of the relationship between dengue and meteorological variables in the city of Rio de Janeiro, Brazil, 2001-2009. Cad Saude Publica. 2012;28(11):2189–97.
48. Xu L, Stige LC, Chan K-S, Zhou J, Yang J, Sang S, Wang M, Yang Z, Yan Z, Jiang T, et al. Climate variation drives dengue dynamics. Proc Natl Acad Sci. 2017;114(1):113–8.
49. Barrera R, Amador M, Mackay AJ. Population dynamics of Aedes aegypti and dengue as influenced by weather and human behavior. PLoS Negl Trop Dis. 2011;5(12):1378. https://doi.org/10.1371/journal.pntd.0001378.
50. Lourenço-de-Oliveira R, Castro MG, Braks MAH, Lounibos LP. The invasion of urban forest by dengue vectors in Rio de Janeiro. J Vector Ecol. 2004;29:94–100.
51. Reiskind M, Lounibos L. Spatial and temporal patterns of abundance of Aedes aegypti L.(Stegomyia aegypti) and Aedes albopictus (Skuse)[Stegomyia albopictus (Skuse)] in southern Florida. Med Vet Entomol. 2013;27(4):421–9.
52. Li M-T, Sun G-Q, Yakob L, Zhu H-P, Jin Z, Zhang W-Y. The driving force for 2014 dengue outbreak in Guangdong, China. PLoS One. 2016;11(11): 0166211.
53. Roiz D, Rosà R, Arnoldi D, Rizzoli A. Effects of temperature and rainfall on the activity and dynamics of host-seeking Aedes albopictus females in northern Italy. Vector Borne Zoonotic Dis. 2010. https://doi.org/10.1089/vbz.2009.0098.
54. Luciano T, Severini IF, Di Luca IM, Bella IA, ryP Roberto R. Seasonal patterns of oviposition and egg hatching rate of Aedes albopictus in Rome. J Am Mosq Control Assoc. 2003;19(1):100.
55. Azil AH, Long SA, Ritchie SA, Williams CR. The development of predictive tools for pre-emptive dengue vector control: a study of Aedes aegypti abundance and meteorological variables in North Queensland, Australia. Tropical Med Int Health. 2010;15(10):1190–7.
56. Gardner LM, Chen N, Sarkar S. Global risk of Zika virus depends critically on vector status of Aedes albopictus. Lancet Infect Dis. 2016;16(5):522–3.
57. Johnson TL, Haque U, Monaghan AJ, Eisen L, Hahn MB, Hayden MH, Savage HM, McAllister J, Mutebi J-P, Eisen RJ. Modeling the environmental suitability for Aedes (Stegomyia) aegypti and Aedes (Stegomyia) albopictus (Diptera: Culicidae) in the contiguous United States. J Med Entomol. 2017; 54(6):1605–14.
58. Ferguson NM, Cucunubá ZM, Dorigatti I, Nedjati-Gilani GL, Donnelly CA, Basáñez M-G, Nouvellet P, Lessler J. Countering the Zika epidemic in Latin America. Science. 2016;353(6297):353–4.
59. CIESIN-Columbia University: Global population count grid time series estimates (2017). https://doi.org/10.7927/H4CC0XNV Accessed 31 Dec 2017.
60. Balcan D, Gonçalves B, Hu H, Ramasco JJ, Colizza V, Vespignani A. Modeling the spatial spread of infectious diseases: the GLobal Epidemic and Mobility computational model. J Comput Sci. 2010;1(3):132–45.

Permissions

All chapters in this book were first published in MEDICINE, by BioMed Central; hereby published with permission under the Creative Commons Attribution License or equivalent. Every chapter published in this book has been scrutinized by our experts. Their significance has been extensively debated. The topics covered herein carry significant findings which will fuel the growth of the discipline. They may even be implemented as practical applications or may be referred to as a beginning point for another development.

The contributors of this book come from diverse backgrounds, making this book a truly international effort. This book will bring forth new frontiers with its revolutionizing research information and detailed analysis of the nascent developments around the world.

We would like to thank all the contributing authors for lending their expertise to make the book truly unique. They have played a crucial role in the development of this book. Without their invaluable contributions this book wouldn't have been possible. They have made vital efforts to compile up to date information on the varied aspects of this subject to make this book a valuable addition to the collection of many professionals and students.

This book was conceptualized with the vision of imparting up-to-date information and advanced data in this field. To ensure the same, a matchless editorial board was set up. Every individual on the board went through rigorous rounds of assessment to prove their worth. After which they invested a large part of their time researching and compiling the most relevant data for our readers.

The editorial board has been involved in producing this book since its inception. They have spent rigorous hours researching and exploring the diverse topics which have resulted in the successful publishing of this book. They have passed on their knowledge of decades through this book. To expedite this challenging task, the publisher supported the team at every step. A small team of assistant editors was also appointed to further simplify the editing procedure and attain best results for the readers.

Apart from the editorial board, the designing team has also invested a significant amount of their time in understanding the subject and creating the most relevant covers. They scrutinized every image to scout for the most suitable representation of the subject and create an appropriate cover for the book.

The publishing team has been an ardent support to the editorial, designing and production team. Their endless efforts to recruit the best for this project, has resulted in the accomplishment of this book. They are a veteran in the field of academics and their pool of knowledge is as vast as their experience in printing. Their expertise and guidance has proved useful at every step. Their uncompromising quality standards have made this book an exceptional effort. Their encouragement from time to time has been an inspiration for everyone.

The publisher and the editorial board hope that this book will prove to be a valuable piece of knowledge for researchers, students, practitioners and scholars across the globe.

List of Contributors

Clara H. Mulder
Population Research Centre, Faculty of Spatial Sciences, University of Groningen, Groningen, The Netherlands

Matias Reus-Pons
Population Research Centre, Faculty of Spatial Sciences, University of Groningen, Groningen, The Netherlands
Interface Demography, Department of Sociology, Vrije Universiteit Brussel, Brussels, Belgium

Eva U. B. Kibele
Statistical Office Bremen, Bremen, Germany

Fanny Janssen
Population Research Centre, Faculty of Spatial Sciences, University of Groningen, Groningen, The Netherlands
Netherlands Interdisciplinary Demographic Institute, The Hague, The Netherlands

Mary O'Reilly
Eastern Health, Level 2/5 Arnold Street, VIC 3128, Australia

Katherine E. Harding, Annie K. Lewis, David A. Snowdon and Nicholas F. Taylor
Eastern Health, Level 2/5 Arnold Street, VIC 3128, Australia
La Trobe University, Kingsbury Drive, Bundoora, VIC 3086, Australia

Sandra G. Leggat, Luke Prendergast and Leila Karimi
La Trobe University, Kingsbury Drive, Bundoora, VIC 3086, Australia

Jennifer J. Watts
Deakin University, 221 Burwood Highway, Burwood, VIC 3125, Australia

Bridie Kent
University of Plymouth, Drake Circus, Plymouth, Devon PL4 8AA, UK

Michelle Kotis
Victorian Department of Health and Human Services, 50 Lonsdale Street, Melbourne, VIC 3000, Australia

Benjamin Fletcher, Joseph Lee, Oliver Van Hecke, Brian D. Nicholson and Sarah Stevens
Nuffield Department of Primary Care Health Sciences, University of Oxford, Radcliffe Observatory Quarter, Woodstock Road, Oxford OX2 6GG, United Kingdom

Niklas Bobrovitz, Carl Heneghan, Igho Onakpoya, David Nunan, Jack O'Sullivan and Kamal R. Mahtani
Nuffield Department of Primary Care Health Sciences, University of Oxford, Radcliffe Observatory Quarter, Woodstock Road, Oxford OX2 6GG, United Kingdom
Centre for Evidence-Based Medicine, University of Oxford, Oxford, United Kingdom

Dylan Collins
Nuffield Department of Primary Care Health Sciences, University of Oxford, Radcliffe Observatory Quarter, Woodstock Road, Oxford OX2 6GG, United Kingdom
Faculty of Medicine, University of British Columbia, Vancouver, Canada

Alice Tompson
Nuffield Department of Primary Care Health Sciences, University of Oxford, Radcliffe Observatory Quarter, Woodstock Road, Oxford OX2 6GG, United Kingdom
Faculty of Public Health and Policy, London School of Hygiene and Tropical Medicine, London, United Kingdom

Rebecca Fisher
Nuffield Department of Primary Care Health Sciences, University of Oxford, Radcliffe Observatory Quarter, Woodstock Road, Oxford OX2 6GG, United Kingdom
The Health Foundation, London, United Kingdom

Brittney Scott
Department of Critical Care Medicine, University of Calgary, Calgary, Canada
Snyder Institute for Chronic Diseases, University of Calgary, Calgary, Canada

Nia Roberts
Bodelian Libraries, University of Oxford, Oxford, UK

Alexander Doroshenko
Division of Preventive Medicine, Department of Medicine, Faculty of Medicine and Dentistry and School of Public Health, University of Alberta, Edmonton, Canada

Caitlin S. Pepperell, Tatum D. Mortimer, Tracy M. Smith and Hailey E. Bussan
Departments of Medicine (Infectious Diseases) and Medical Microbiology and Immunology, School of Medicine and Public Health, University of Wisconsin–Madison, Madison, USA

Courtney Heffernan, Mary Lou Egedahl and Richard Long
Department of Medicine, Faculty of Medicine and Dentistry and TB Program Evaluation and Research Unit, University of Alberta, Edmonton, Canada

Gregory J. Tyrrell
Department of Laboratory Medicine and Pathology, University of Alberta, Provincial Laboratory for Public Health, Alberta Health Services, Edmonton, Canada

Ines Stevic, Klaus Pantel and Heidi Schwarzenbach
Department of Tumor Biology, University Medical Center Hamburg-Eppendorf, Martinistraße 52, 20246 Hamburg, Germany

Volkmar Müller
Department of Gynecology, University Medical Center Hamburg-Eppendorf, Hamburg, Germany

Karsten Weber and Sibylle Loibl
GBG Forschungs GmbH, Neu-Isenburg, Germany

Peter A. Fasching
Department of Gynecology and Obstetrics, University Hospital Erlangen, Comprehensive Cancer Center Erlangen-EMN, Friedrich-Alexander University Erlangen-Nuremberg, Erlangen, Germany

Thomas Karn
University Women's Hospital, Frankfurt, Germany

Frederic Marmé
Center for Gynecological Oncology at University Women's Hospital, Heidelberg, Germany

Christian Schem
Mammazentrum Hamburg, Hamburg, Germany

Elmar Stickeler
Universitätsklinikum Aachen, Aachen, Germany

Carsten Denkert
Charite Berlin, Institute of Pathology and German Cancer Consortium (DKTK), Partner Site, Berlin, Germany

Marion van Mackelenbergh
Universitätsklinikums Schleswig-Holstein Kiel, Kiel, Germany

Christoph Salat
Hämatoonkologische Schwerpunktpraxis, Munich, Germany

Andreas Schneeweiss
Universitätsklinikum Heidelberg, Heidelberg, Germany

Michael Untch
Helios Kliniken Berlin-Buch, Berlin, Germany

Hsien-Yen Chang
Department of Health Policy and Management, Johns Hopkins Bloomberg School of Public Health, Baltimore, MD, USA
Center for Drug Safety and Effectiveness, Johns Hopkins University, Baltimore, MD, USA
Center for Population Health Information Technology, Johns Hopkins University, Baltimore, MD, USA

Hadi Kharrazi, Dave Bodycombe and Jonathan P. Weiner
Department of Health Policy and Management, Johns Hopkins Bloomberg School of Public Health, Baltimore, MD, USA
Center for Population Health Information Technology, Johns Hopkins University, Baltimore, MD, USA

G. Caleb Alexander
Center for Drug Safety and Effectiveness, Johns Hopkins University, Baltimore, MD, USA
Department of Epidemiology, Johns Hopkins Bloomberg School of Public Health, 615 N. Wolfe Street W6035, Baltimore, MD 21205, USA
Division of General Internal Medicine, Department of Medicine, Johns Hopkins Medicine, Baltimore, MD, USA

Hla Phyo Wai, Aung Myat Thu, Zay Soe Khant and Chanida Indrasuta
Medical Action Myanmar, Yangon, Myanmar

Elizabeth A. Ashley
Myanmar Oxford Clinical Research Unit (MOCRU), Yangon, Myanmar

Alistair R. D. McLean
Medical Action Myanmar, Yangon, Myanmar
Myanmar Oxford Clinical Research Unit (MOCRU), Yangon, Myanmar

Thar Tun Kyaw
Department of Public Health, Ministry of Health and Sports, Nay Pyi Taw, Myanmar

Nicholas P. J. Day, Arjen Dondorp and Nicholas J. White
Mahidol-Oxford Tropical Medicine Research Unit (MORU), Faculty of Tropical Medicine, Mahidol University, Bangkok, Thailand
Centre for Tropical Medicine and Global Health, Nuffield Department of Clinical Medicine, University of Oxford, Oxford, UK

List of Contributors

Frank M. Smithuis
Medical Action Myanmar, Yangon, Myanmar
Myanmar Oxford Clinical Research Unit (MOCRU), Yangon, Myanmar
Centre for Tropical Medicine and Global Health, Nuffield Department of Clinical Medicine, University of Oxford, Oxford, UK

James D. Munday and W. John Edmunds
Centre for Mathematical Modelling of Infectious Diseases, London School of Hygiene and Tropical Medicine, London, UK
Department of Infectious Disease Epidemiology, Faculty of Epidemiology and Population Health, London School of Hygiene and Tropical Medicine, London, UK

Albert Jan van Hoek
Centre for Mathematical Modelling of Infectious Diseases, London School of Hygiene and Tropical Medicine, London, UK
Department of Infectious Disease Epidemiology, Faculty of Epidemiology and Population Health, London School of Hygiene and Tropical Medicine, London, UK
National Institute for Public Health and the Environment (RIVM), Bilthoven, The Netherlands

Katherine E. Atkins
Centre for Mathematical Modelling of Infectious Diseases, London School of Hygiene and Tropical Medicine, London, UK
Department of Infectious Disease Epidemiology, Faculty of Epidemiology and Population Health, London School of Hygiene and Tropical Medicine, London, UK
Centre for Global Health, Usher Institute of Population Health Sciences and Informatics, Edinburgh Medical School, The University of Edinburgh, Edinburgh, UK

Danielle I. Stanisic, Xue Q. Liu, Ibrahim El-Deeb, Ingrid B. Rodriguez, Jessica Powell, Nicole M. Willemsen, Sai Lata De, Mei-Fong Ho and Michael F. Good
Institute for Glycomics, Griffith University, Parklands Drive, Southport, Queensland, Australia

James Fink, Johanna Mayer, Sarah Coghill, Letitia Gore and John Gerrard
Gold Coast University Hospital, 1 Hospital Blvd, Southport, Queensland, Australia

Stephen L. Hoffman
Sanaria Inc., Gaithersburg, MD, USA

Joel Glynn
Health Economics at Bristol, Population Health Sciences, Bristol Medical School, University of Bristol, Bristol, UK

Myles-Jay Linton, Joanna Coast and William Hollingworth
Health Economics at Bristol, Population Health Sciences, Bristol Medical School, University of Bristol, Bristol, UK
The National Institute for Health Research Collaboration for Leadership in Applied Health Research and Care West (NIHR CLAHRC West), University Hospitals Bristol NHS Foundation Trust, Bristol, UK

Tim Jones
The National Institute for Health Research Collaboration for Leadership in Applied Health Research and Care West (NIHR CLAHRC West), University Hospitals Bristol NHS Foundation Trust, Bristol, UK

Amanda Owen-Smith
Health Economics at Bristol, Population Health Sciences, Bristol Medical School, University of Bristol, Bristol, UK
Centre for Academic Primary Care, Population Health Sciences, Bristol Medical School, University of Bristol, Bristol, UK

Rupert A. Payne
Centre for Academic Primary Care, Population Health Sciences, Bristol Medical School, University of Bristol, Bristol, UK

S. E. Murthy, M. E. Murphy, Kasha P. Singh and T. D. McHugh
UCL Centre for Clinical Microbiology, Department of Infection, University College London, Royal Free Campus, Rowland Hill Street, London NW3 2PF, UK

F. Chatterjee
Department of Radiology, Barts Health NHS Trust, The Royal London Hospital, Whitechapel Road, London E1 1BB, UK

A. Crook, A. J. Nunn and P. P. J. Phillips
Medical Research Council UK Clinical Trials Unit at University College London, Aviation House, 125 Kingsway, London WC2B 6NH, UK

R. Dawson
University of Cape Town Lung Institute, George Street, Mowbray, Cape Town, South Africa

C. Mendel and S. R. Murray
Global Alliance for Tuberculosis Drug Development, New York, NY 10005, USA

S. H. Gillespie
Medical and Biological Sciences, School of Medicine, University of St Andrews, North Haugh, St Andrews KY16 9TF, UK

D Das, K Stepniewska, R Mansoor and P J Guerin
World Wide Antimalarial Resistance Network (WWARN), Oxford, UK
Centre for Tropical Medicine and Global Health, Nuffield Department of Clinical Medicine, University of Oxford, Oxford, UK

J Tarning
WorldWide Antimalarial Resistance Network (WWARN), Oxford, UK
Centre for Tropical Medicine and Global Health, Nuffield Department of Clinical Medicine, University of Oxford, Oxford, UK
Mahidol Oxford Tropical Medicine Research Unit, Faculty of Tropical Medicine, Mahidol University, Bangkok, Thailand

R F Grais
Epicentre, Paris, France

S van der Kam
Médecins Sans Frontières, Amsterdam, Netherlands

E A Okiro
Kemri Wellcome Trust Research Programme, Kilifi, Kenya

K I Barnes
Division of Clinical Pharmacology, Department of Medicine, University of Cape Town, Cape Town, South Africa
WorldWide Antimalarial Resistance Network (WWARN) Pharmacology, University of Cape Town, Cape Town, South Africa

D J Terlouw
Liverpool School of Tropical Medicine, Liverpool, UK
Malawi-Liverpool Wellcome Trust Clinical Research Programme, Blantyre, Malawi
College of Medicine, University of Malawi, Blantyre, Malawi

Eleanor Barry, Trisha Greenhalgh and Nicholas Fahy
Nuffield Department of Primary Care Health Sciences, University of Oxford, Radcliffe Primary Care Building, Radcliffe Observatory Quarter Woodstock Road, Oxford OX2 6GG, UK

Joanne R. Winter, Helen R. Stagg, Colette J. Smith and Ibrahim Abubakar
Institute for Global Health, University College London, 30 Guildford Street, London WC1N 1EH, UK

Jennifer A. Davidson, Alison E. Brown and Valerie Delpech
National Infections Service, Public Health England, 61 Colindale Avenue, London NW9 5EQ, UK

Maeve K. Lalor and Dominik Zenner
Institute for Global Health, University College London, 30 Guildford Street, London WC1N 1EH, UK
National Infections Service, Public Health England, 61 Colindale Avenue, London NW9 5EQ, UK

James Brown
Royal Free London National Health Service Foundation Trust, Royal Free Hospital, Pond Street, London NW3 2QG, UK

Marc Lipman
Royal Free London National Health Service Foundation Trust, Royal Free Hospital, Pond Street, London NW3 2QG, UK
UCL Respiratory, Division of Medicine, University College London, Royal Free Campus, Pond Street, London NW3 2PF, UK

Anton Pozniak
Chelsea and Westminster Hospital, 369 Fulham Road, London SW10 9NH, UK

Duncan McNab
NHS Education for Scotland, 2 Central Quay, Glasgow, Scotland G3 8BW, UK
NHS Ayrshire and Arran, Ayr, UK
Institute of Health and Wellbeing, University of Glasgow, Glasgow, UK

John Freestone
NHS Ayrshire and Arran, Ayr, UK

Chris Black
NHS Education for Scotland, 2 Central Quay, Glasgow, Scotland G3 8BW, UK
NHS Ayrshire and Arran, Ayr, UK

Paul Bowie
NHS Education for Scotland, 2 Central Quay, Glasgow, Scotland G3 8BW, UK
Institute of Health and Wellbeing, University of Glasgow, Glasgow, UK

Andrew Carson-Stevens
Division of Population Medicine, School of Medicine, Cardiff University, Cardiff, UK

Department of Family Practice, University of British Columbia, Vancouver, Canada
Australian Institute of Health Innovation, Macquarie University, Sydney, Australia

Youri Yordanov
INSERM, U1153, Hôpital Hôtel-Dieus, 1, place du parvis Notre Dame, 75004 Paris, France
Sorbonne Universités, UPMC Paris Univ-06, Paris, France
Service des Urgences - Hôpital Saint Antoine, Assistance Publique–Hôpitaux de Paris (APHP), Paris, France
Centre d'Épidémiologie Clinique, Hôpital Hôtel Dieu, Assistance Publique–Hôpitaux de Paris (APHP), Paris, France

Agnes Dechartres and Isabelle Boutron
INSERM, U1153, Hôpital Hôtel-Dieus, 1, place du parvis Notre Dame, 75004 Paris, France
Centre d'Épidémiologie Clinique, Hôpital Hôtel Dieu, Assistance Publique–Hôpitaux de Paris (APHP), Paris, France
Faculté de Médecine, Université Paris Descartes, Sorbonne Paris Cité, Paris, France
Cochrane France, Paris, France

Ignacio Atal, Viet-Thi Tran and Perrine Crequit
INSERM, U1153, Hôpital Hôtel-Dieus, 1, place du parvis Notre Dame, 75004 Paris, France
Centre d'Épidémiologie Clinique, Hôpital Hôtel Dieu, Assistance Publique–Hôpitaux de Paris (APHP), Paris, France

Philippe Ravaud
INSERM, U1153, Hôpital Hôtel-Dieus, 1, place du parvis Notre Dame, 75004 Paris, France
Centre d'Épidémiologie Clinique, Hôpital Hôtel Dieu, Assistance Publique–Hôpitaux de Paris (APHP), Paris, France
Faculté de Médecine, Université Paris Descartes, Sorbonne Paris Cité, Paris, France
Cochrane France, Paris, France
Department of Epidemiology, Columbia University, Mailman School of Public Health, New York, USA

Momodou K Darboe and Andrew M Prentice
MRC Unit The Gambia at London School of Hygiene and Tropical Medicine, Atlantic Boulevard, Fajara, Banjul, The Gambia

Mayya Husseini
MRC Unit The Gambia at London School of Hygiene and Tropical Medicine, Atlantic Boulevard, Fajara, Banjul, The Gambia

Regional Activity Centre for Sustainable Consumption and Production (SCP/RAC), Sant Pau Art Nouveau Site, Carrer Sant Antoni Maria Claret, 167, 08025 Barcelona, Spain

Sophie E Moore
MRC Unit The Gambia at London School of Hygiene and Tropical Medicine, Atlantic Boulevard, Fajara, Banjul, The Gambia
Department of Women and Children's Health, King's College London, 10th Floor North Wing, St Thomas' Hospital, Westminster Bridge Road, London SE1 7EH, UK

Helen M Nabwera
Centre for Maternal and Newborn Health, Liverpool School of Tropical Medicine, Pembroke Place, Liverpool L3 5QA, UK

Chung-Ho E. Lau and Elizabeth J. Want
Division of Computational and Systems Medicine, Department of Surgery and Cancer, Faculty of Medicine, Imperial College London, London SW7 2AZ, UK

Hector C. Keun
Division of Cancer, Department of Surgery and Cancer, Faculty of Medicine, Imperial College London, London W12 0NN, UK

Alexandros P. Siskos
Division of Computational and Systems Medicine, Department of Surgery and Cancer, Faculty of Medicine, Imperial College London, London SW7 2AZ, UK
Division of Cancer, Department of Surgery and Cancer, Faculty of Medicine, Imperial College London, London W12 0NN, UK

Léa Maitre, Jose Urquiza, Maribel Casas and Martine Vrijheid
ISGlobal, Barcelona, Spain
Universitat Pompeu Fabra (UPF), Barcelona, Spain
CIBER Epidemiologa y Salud Pública (CIBERESP), Madrid, Spain

Oliver Robinson
MRC-PHE Centre for Environment and Health, School of Public Health, Faculty of Medicine, Imperial College London, London W2 1PG, UK

Toby J. Athersuch
Division of Computational and Systems Medicine, Department of Surgery and Cancer, Faculty of Medicine, Imperial College London, London SW7 2AZ, UK

MRC-PHE Centre for Environment and Health, School of Public Health, Faculty of Medicine, Imperial College London, London W2 1PG, UK

Marina Vafeiadi and Theano Roumeliotaki
Department of Social Medicine, Faculty of Medicine, University of Crete, Heraklion, Crete, Greece

Remy Slama
Inserm, Univ. Grenoble Alpes, CNRS, IAB (Institute of Advanced Biosciences), Grenoble, France

Rosemary R. C. McEachan, Rafaq Azad and John Wright
Bradford Institute for Health Research, Bradford Teaching Hospitals NHS Foundation Trust, Bradford, UK

Line S. Haug, Helle M. Meltzer and Cathrine Thomsen
Norwegian Institute of Public Health, Oslo, Norway

Sandra Andrusaityte, Inga Petraviciene and Regina Grazuleviciene
Department of Environmental Sciences, Vytautas Magnus University, Kaunas, Lithuania

Leda Chatzi
Department of Preventive Medicine, Keck School of Medicine, University of Southern California, Los Angeles, USA

Muireann Coen
Division of Computational and Systems Medicine, Department of Surgery and Cancer, Faculty of Medicine, Imperial College London, London SW7 2AZ, UK

Oncology Safety, Drug Safety and Metabolism, IMED Biotech Unit, AstraZeneca, 1 Francis Crick Avenue, Cambridge CB2 0RE, UK

Kaiyuan Sun, Qian Zhang, Ana Pastore-Piontti, Matteo Chinazzi and Dina Mistry
Laboratory for the Modeling of Biological and Sociotechnical Systems, Northeastern University, Boston 02115, USA

Natalie E Dean, Diana Patricia Rojas and Ira M Longini Jr
Department of Biostatistics, College of Public Health and Health Professions, University of Florida, Gainesville 32611, USA

Stefano Merler and Piero Poletti
Bruno Kessler Foundation, 38123 Trento, Italy

Luca Rossi
Institute for Scientific Interchange Foundation, 10126 Turin, Italy

Alessandro Vespignani
Laboratory for the Modeling of Biological and Sociotechnical Systems, Northeastern University, Boston 02115, USA
Institute for Scientific Interchange Foundation, 10126 Turin, Italy

M Elizabeth Halloran
Vaccine and Infectious Disease Division, Fred Hutchinson Cancer Research Center, Seattle 98109, USA
Department of Biostatistics, University of Washington, Seattle 98195, USA

Index

A
Anthropometry, 136, 148, 211, 213, 215, 229, 231
Artemether-lumefantrine (AL), 146

B
Benzodiazepines, 69, 73, 77
Bhc Implementation, 82, 84
Bhc Package, 79-84, 86
Body Mass Index (BMI), 4, 126
Breast Cancer, 52, 54, 58, 66-67

C
Carboplatin, 54, 60-61, 63, 66
Cavitation, 40, 42, 45-46, 125-134
Chest Radiograph, 40, 42, 44-45, 134-135
Chronic Obstructive Pulmonary Disease, 26, 33, 35, 38-39
Coeliac Disease, 117-118, 123-124
Community Health Workers (CHWS), 79-80
Confocal Microscopy, 52, 54-55, 58, 60
Coronary Artery Disease, 26, 34, 37

D
Diabetes Prevention, 150-151, 154-155, 157, 161, 163-166
Disease Progression, 41, 49, 131
Drug Misuse, 167-169, 171-172, 174, 176-177
Drug Therapy, 34, 53

E
Enteropathy, 118, 209-210, 217
Epidemiology, 37, 41, 43, 48, 50-51, 68, 76, 89, 93, 97-99, 116, 124, 167-169, 178, 207, 219, 221, 233-234, 246-247
Exosomes, 52-53, 55-56, 58, 60-61, 63-67

F
Fisher's Exact Test, 42, 46
Functional Resonance Analysis Method, 179, 181, 183-185, 187-189, 191, 196-197

G
Generalized Linear Model (GLM), 68, 70

H
Health Deterioration, 1, 3-5, 7-13
Health Transitions, 1-4, 7, 13
Heart Failure, 26-27, 29, 32-39
Hemolysis, 53, 55, 66
Her2-positive, 52-54, 56-66
Hypoalbuminemia, 126

I
Infectious Diseases, 50, 89, 97, 99, 133, 203, 247
Intensive Statin Therapy, 26, 33

L
Latent Tuberculosis, 167-168
Logistic Regression Models, 1, 4, 57, 59-60, 169, 175-177

M
Malaria Transmission, 80, 84, 138, 143, 145, 147-148
Malaria-endemic, 101-102, 105, 146
Mechanistic Model, 89
Multi-disciplinary Rehabilitation, 18
Multi-morbidity, 31, 36

N
Neoadjuvant Therapy, 52-53, 61-63, 65
Newcastle-ottawa Scale, 136, 138, 147-148
Nmr Spectroscopy, 219, 221, 223, 228-229, 234
Non-communicable Diseases, 11

O
Opioid Abuse, 69, 74-75, 77-78
Opioid Disorders, 69-74
Oral Rehydration, 86, 88, 211

P
Pathological Complete Response, 52-54, 66
Pneumonia, 32, 35, 83, 86, 88, 99, 137
Primary Health Care, 117
Propensity Score Model, 70, 75

R
Randomised Controlled Trials, 25-27, 38, 207
Rapid Diagnostic Test (RDT), 79
Respiratory Diseases, 29
Risk Assessment, 157, 236

S
Schizophrenia, 26, 30, 33-35, 38-39, 203, 219, 233
Selective Reporting, 198-201, 203-207
Sepsis, 179-180, 182-188, 190-197
Serum Carnitine, 218, 228
Severe Acute Malnutrition (SAM), 137, 145
Socio-cultural Influences, 150-151, 156, 158, 161, 163-166
Stat Model, 19, 21-23
Student's T Test, 57-58

Stunting, 136-141, 143, 148-149, 209-210, 212, 214, 216-217

Sub-acute Ambulatory Care Services (SACS), 17

T

T Cell Responses, 101-102

Tamoxifen, 64, 67

Tb Transmission, 41, 48

Threonine Catabolism, 219, 232, 235

Tuberculin Skin Tests (TSTS), 42

Tuberculosis, 40-41, 45-48, 50-51, 80-81, 83, 87, 116, 125-126, 129, 132-135, 146, 167-168, 170-178

V

Vertical Integration, 79

W

Western Blot, 52, 54-55, 58, 60-61

Whole-genome Sequencing, 40, 50-51

CPSIA information can be obtained
at www.ICGtesting.com
Printed in the USA
BVHW010532240519
549125BV00017B/127/P